Y0-BSM-469

Cancer & the Environment

Cancer & the Environment

Edited by Lester A. Sobel

Contributing editors: Jeanne Burr, Joe Fickes, Lauren Sass **Indexer:** Grace M. Ferrara

Facts On File
119 West 57th Street, New York, N.Y. 10019

Cancer & the Environment

Published by Facts On File, Inc.,
119 West 57th Street, New York, N.Y. 10019.

Library of Congress Cataloging in Publication Data
Main entry under title:

Cancer & the environment.

Includes index.
1. Cancer   Environmentally induced diseases. 3. Cancer—United States. I. Sobel, Lester A. II. Fickes, Joseph. [DNLM: 1. Neoplasms—Drug therapy. QZ267 C638e]
RC263.C28   616.9'94'071   79-17369
ISBN 0-87196-283-7

9 8 7 6 5 4 3 2 1
PRINTED IN
THE UNITED STATES OF AMERICA

Contents

'DANGEROUS TO YOUR HEALTH' 1
DANGER AT WORK, DANGER FROM INDUSTRY 9
Cancer Deaths Increase, Jobs & Industry a Cause 9
PCB Under Attack 15
Asbestos 18
Hazardous Wastes 26
Other Industrial & Chemical Problems 30
Protection of Workers from Exposure to Carcinogens 38
DANGER IN THE AIR 43
War on Air-Borne Carcinogens 43
Stress on Auto Pollution 47
Widening Regulation 50
Energy Crisis Complicates Anti-Pollution Campaign 55
Cleanup Inadequate 60
Energy, Pollution & Health 64
SST, Other Ozone Threats & Skin Cancer 71
DANGER IN FOOD & DRINK & OTHER EVERY-DAY ITEMS 77
The Delancy Clause: All Food Carcinogens Banned 77
Danger in Sweeteners 82
Danger from Nitrite 91
Danger from Food Colors 93
Danger from DES in Livestock 94
PBB Case 97

Danger in Drinking Water ... 98
Cigarette Smoking ... 103
Other Cancer Hazards ... 112
MEDICAL RESEARCH, TREATMENT, PREVENTION & HAZARDS ... 115
War on Cancer ... 115
Treatment & Controversies ... 122
Danger in Medical Practice ... 127
Research on Virus & Cancer ... 136
RADIATION & CANCER ... 139
Energy, the Atom & Cancer ... 139
Nuclear Hazards to Health ... 146
Action Vs. Radiation Dangers ... 149
Cancer Dangers Stressed ... 153
The Three Mile Island Accident ... 159
Danger from Radioactive Wastes ... 171
A-Weapons & Tests ... 174
Other Radiation Problems ... 180
OTHER DANGERS ... 183
Danger in Pesticides ... 183
Environmental Developments ... 188
Diet & Nutrition ... 195
INDEX ... 199

'Dangerous to Your Health'

THIS FAMILIAR NOTICE APPEARS on every packet of cigarettes sold in the United States: "Warning. The Surgeon General has determined that cigarette smoking is dangerous to your health."

The warning is required by law because years of research and experience have implicated cigarette smoking as a cause of lung cancer. Evidence has been produced that smoking also is involved in cases of cardiovascular disease and other ills. But the cancer connection was the weapon that won the campaign to label cigarette smoking officially as a health hazard.

With similar justification, some observers say, the government could also require notices warning that:

- The air you breathe is dangerous to your health.
- The food you eat is dangerous to your health.
- The water you drink is dangerous to your health.
- The clothes you wear are dangerous to your health.
- Your home is dangerous to your health.
- Your job is dangerous to your health.
- Your school is dangerous to your health.
- Your doctor and dentist are dangerous to your health.
- Sunbathing is dangerous to your health.
- The area you live in is dangerous to your health.
- Industrial and government activities (foreign and domestic) are dangerous to your health.

In each case, as most of us are aware, the deliberately exaggerated health hazard referred to is the danger of cancer.

Carcinogens in minute quantities are reported in food, food additives, drinks, medicines, the air, the soil, the water. Radiation from industry, American and foreign weapons testing, medical and dental X-rays and natural ("background") sources are described as potential producers of cancer. Cancer-causing substances are said to have been found in the insulation in our homes and schools, in the pollution from factories that blankets many of our communities, in flame-retardants with which some clothing has been treated and in many materials that workers handle daily on the job.

In sum, the environment—or many things in it—may give you cancer.

This conclusion was expressed in the April 1977 issue of the *Journal of the National Cancer Institute* by Ernest L. Wynder of the Division of Epidemiology, American Health Foundation, and Gio B. Gori of the Division of Cancer Cause & Prevention, National Cancer Institute, National Institutes of Health. "Most cancers today appear to be induced by elements originating in man's environment rather than as a result of purely genetic or viral factors," the two scientists wrote. They specifically defined "environmental elements . . . as those originating wholly or largely outside the host's body." The authors noted that "with the increasing number of news reports regarding hazardous components [of the environment], the average citizen considers himself immersed in an uncontrollable sea of carcinogens."

Some concerned observers are beginning to question the accuracy of reports about the prevalence of so many claimed cancer-causing agents. "Almost daily," Rep. William C. Wampler (R, Va.) told the U.S. House of Representatives March 14, 1979, "the consuming public is being bombarded with news stories that hundreds of substances—in such items as bacon and hot dogs, saccharin, beer, asbestos, tobacco, spinach, pesticides used to control insects and weeds in food production, and cleaning fluids—that people breathe, touch, eat or drink or encounter in the workplace every day are suddenly suspected of causing cancer. These media announcements, generally unsupported by the scientific community, give the public a horrible fright. Of greater concern, however, many in the general public are beginning to wonder who and what to believe, because so many beneficial substances, long in use, are being linked to this ever-growing suspect list of substances that are alleged to cause cancer." Wampler continued:

Congress, which is a nonscientific body, has in the past been called upon to write legislation concerning carcinogens. . . . We have authorized various Federal agencies to regulate the use of chemicals that may pose a risk to cancer. We have not told them how to do it, but have entrusted them with the task of using their scientific expertise to formulate policies that would protect our population from harm while preserving the capability of our farmers and our industries to carry on their business, and the working people of this country to earn their bread and butter. Unfortunately, we were too optimistic in assuming that 'scientific validity' necessarily leads to 'workability.' We find that today no less than seven agencies operating from nine laws promulgated by several congressional committees are involved in assessing the cancer risk posed by various chemicals, and that they all have their own policies for doing so. The result—despite the recent efforts of a task force of the Interagency Regulatory Liaison Group to come up with a common Federal policy—has been haphazard application of controls on potential carcinogens that has left both the public and large segments of American agriculture and other industries in a state of confusion and uncertainty. . . .

. . . [T]his confusion is understandable, for there is no scientific consensus of opinion on risk assessment of chemical carcinogenesis. Implicit in cancer and toxic substances research is a large degree of uncertainty and a distressing scarcity of hard facts. The long-term effect of many chemicals is simply not known, nor is the validity of some of the tests currently used to measure the toxicity or carcinogenicity of a particular substance. Above all, there is little agreement on how the results of animal tests should be applied to humans. . . .

. . . [T]he universe of known chemicals is something on the order of 4.2 million, of which roughly 50,000 to 70,000 are in the inventory of Chemicals in Commerce being compiled under the Toxic Substance Control Act. In addition, there are probably between 1,000 and 2,000 new chemicals introduced every year. . . . [The Environmental Protection Agency] states that only 1,500 to 2,000 substances have undergone testing that is considered scientifically valid. Those chemicals were selected for testing on animals because they had, at one time or another, fallen under suspicion of being carcinogens. Results accumulated over recent years, according to EPA, indicate that between 700 and 1,000 substances, or roughly fifty per cent of those tested, show reasonable solid evidence of being animal carcinogens. Another measure of the approximate number of suspected carcinogens is the list maintained by the National Institute of Occupational Safety & Health (NIOSH). As of the 1977 edition, it named 2,091 compounds that were referred to as suspected carcinogens at least once in the scientific literature. . . . [T]he National Cancer Institute informs me that the U.S. Public Health Service Report No. 149 lists some 7,000 chemicals tested, including some tests which were fragmentary. Less than 1,000 of these chemicals tested show possibilities of carcinogenicity to animals. NCI states that only 600 to 800 of these animals tests were conducted using what they consider to be acceptable test methods. Finally, the National Cancer Institute cites findings in the reports of the International Agency for Research on Cancer. Volumes 1 through 16 identify only 247 of 368 chemicals that had positive animal tests, which might show some evidence of carcinogenicity to man.

Having established to some degree the extent of known chemical carcinogenesis in laboratory animals, the crucial question now becomes: How are these data to be extrapolated to humans so that the risk of cancer in man may be assessed? Here is where we find disagreement among scientists and divergence of policy among the regulatory agencies charged with controlling chemicals.

While it is generally agreed that the best method of documenting carcinogenicity in man is through epidemiological studies, it is also recognized that such studies have severe drawbacks. . . . The limitations on human studies are such that only thirty or so chemicals have definitely been identified as carcinogenic in man. For all practical purposes, then, the detection of carcinogenic activity of chemicals is necessarily based on animal experimentation. It is the process of interpreting the resulting data for application to humans that generates scientific and regulatory controversies. . . .

Yet, discussing data on cancer mortality rates in the United States, Dr. Samuel S. Epstein, professor of occupational and environmental medicine at the School of Public Health, University of Illinois Medical Center in Chicago, reported a growing consensus "in the scientific community that most human cancers are environmental. . . ." Epstein, in an article in the March 1977 issue of the *Bulletin of the Atomic Scientists*, noted a "marked geographical clustering of high cancer rates of various organs in white men and women in heavily industrialized areas." He asserted that "[s]uch data correlate cancer rates in the general community with living near certain industries." "[S]pecific exposures at specific occupations are an important cause of cancer deaths," he continued, "particularly among males." Epstein's article, which had appeared in part in the July/August 1976 issue of *Technology Review*, cited estimates indicating that five to fifteen per cent of "all current cancer deaths in males are occupational in origin."

The possibility of a direct connection between an occupation and a risk of a specific cancer has been known for more than 200 years. The English surgeon Percivall Pott reported in 1775 that most patients he examined with cancer of the scrotum were chimney sweeps. Even earlier, it had been noted that miners were fairly frequent victims of what is recognized as a lung cancer that was rare in the rest of the population. By the late nineteenth century, other occupationally linked cancers had been reported, and in recent decades, scores of carcinogens have been traced to the workplace.

Data on cancer mortality in the United States had been mapped on a county-by-county basis by researchers of the Epidemiology Branch, National Cancer Institute. Researchers Robert Hoover, Thomas J. Mason, Frank W. McKay and Joseph F. Fraumeni, Jr. reported in the September 1975 issue of *Science* that when they plotted the distribution for bladder cancer, "the tumor most strongly linked to occupational exposures," they found "clusters of elevated mortality [for white males] in heavily industrialized areas"; this pattern "was not duplicated in females." This obviously suggested "industrial hazards." The group cited Salem County, N.J., which "leads the nation in bladder cancer mortality among white men." The researchers attribute[d] this excess risk to occupational exposure since about 25% per cent of the employed persons in this county work in the chemical industry. . . ."

Environmental causes of cancer often involve an element of voluntary risk. This aspect of the situation was discussed by Admiral Hyman G. Rickover Aug. 1, 1979 in an address accepting the Winston Churchill Award of the International Platform Association. In his speech, entitled "The Need for Environmental Perspective," Rickover asserted that "the environmental risk having the greatest effect in the United States today is smoking. Smoking causes us about 325,000 deaths each year, . . . about one-quarter [of them] from lung cancer. Sixty years ago we had little lung cancer. Today more are dying from it than from automobile accidents."

Rickover, who headed the Navy's atomic program, suggested that the risks from radiation were misunderstood, even "widely distorted." He said:

> While accepting the many daily risks of living, many seem to be getting the idea that their demands for energy should be met on essentially a risk-free basis. Since this is impossible, attention should be focused on taking reasonable steps to safeguard the public, on developing realistic assessment of the risks, and on placing them in perspective. . . . At the start of the Navy's Nuclear Propulsion Program in 1946, I realized the need for careful attention to radiation. . . . [I]f nuclear ships were to be viable, there would have to be assurance that workers and crews not be subjected to excessive radiation. To emphasize this, I designed the shielding for our naval nuclear plants to be many times more stringent than required by the standards then in effect. As a result, the shielding built into the first nuclear submarine, the *Nautilus*, was so conservative that it continues to be far more than adequate to meet the considerably lower radiation levels permitted today.
>
> Insofar as the environment is concerned, naval plants have been so designed and operated that in each of the last eight years the total gamma radioactivity discharged to all harbors of the world has been less than two thousandths of a curie. This quantity is for the operation of over 100 ships and of all their support facilities. To give you an idea what this means, if one person were able to drink the entire amount of this radioactivity discharged into any harbor in all of 1978, he would not exceed the annual radiation exposure permitted by the Nuclear Regulatory Commission for an individual worker. . . .
>
> Scientists have stated for decades that radiation can cause harm. However, all of us have been subjected to radiation throughout our lives. . . . The en-

tire human race has been subjected to radiation, as has every living thing, throughout the entire evolution of our earth. The average person in the United States receives each year about one-tenth rem from natural radioactivity in the earth, in his body, and from cosmic radiation. The unit of radiation, rem, . . . is defined in terms of energy absorbed in body tissues. Receiving one rem of gamma radiation is equivalent to absorbing 100 ergs of radiation energy for each gram of body tissue. There are 454 grams in a pound. An erg is the amount of energy required to lift a mosquito weighing one thousandth of a gram about one centimeter. In terms of energy the rem is a small unit. A dose of one rem would raise body temperature only two millionths of a degree centigrade. We are not accustomed to fear background radiation; after all it is part of our natural environment. Yet in scientific terms it can be shown that its risk is not zero.

More is known about radiation than almost any substance that can affect humans. More money has been spent to learn the effects of radiation on humans than for any other hazard in our modern society. The main effect is cancer. . . . The combination of one-tenth rem per year background radiation, together with nearly the same average amount from medical diagnostic radiation, is estimated to cause almost one per cent of cancer deaths in the United States. In an average group of 10,000 people, 1,600 will die of cancer. Sixteen of these deaths will be from background and medical radiation. If the lifetime radiation exposure of 10,000 people is increased by an average of one rem per person—a total of 10,000 rem—it is estimated that one additional fatal cancer may occur.* . . .

Of all industrial and medical radiation workers in the United States, about 15,000 die each year from cancer. The total radiation exposure from their work adds an estimated 25 cancer deaths per year. Radiation from the nuclear accident at Three Mile Island may add one fatal cancer death to the public within fifty miles. Of the two million people living within this fifty-mile radius, 325,000 are expected to die of cancer from causes other than the radioactivity released from this accident.

The perspective on radiation can be improved by comparison. For example, I know an apparently healthy person who forty years ago received more radiation from medical chest X-rays than the total exposure all 15,000 radiation workers at nine shipyards received in 1978 from naval nuclear power plant work. . . . Another example: . . . rumors have persisted that radiation-induced cancer has killed the crew of the first nuclear-powered ship, the *Nautilus*. In 1978 the Navy traced each of the 96 officers and enlisted men of this first crew. . . . [A]ll the men associated with operating the nuclear propulsion plant were alive and well. . . .

The questions of risk and perspective had been taken up earlier by Richard J. Mahoney, executive vice president of the Monsanto Co. "We hear and read that a majority of human cancers—possibly as high as 70 per cent to 90 per cent—are due to

*This risk estimate was made in 1977 by the United Nations Scientific Committee on the Effects of Atomic Radiation and by the International Commission on Radiological Protection. It is within the range of estimates in the 1979 draft report of the U. S. National Academy of Sciences Committee on Biological Effects of Ionizing Radiations, and in the 1972 report of this committee.

environmental causes," Mahoney noted in a speech in St. Louis. "From this, many people leap to the conclusion that chemical food additives, pesticides and industrial chemicals are to blame. Yet, medical studies have shown repeatedly that the main human cancers do not stem from intentional or even inadvertant chemical contaminants in our environment. A . . . medical research paper noted that the overwhelming environmental causes of cancer are cigarette smoking and dietary considerations. . . . Control these two elements—cigarettes and diet—and you've controlled the cause of perhaps 95 per cent of environmentally caused cancers. . . ."

The work of Dr. John Higginson adds further complexity to the puzzle of the link between cancer and the environment. After studying South African black and U.S. cancer rates in the 1950s, as Daniel S. Greenberg notes in the *Washington Post* July 17, 1979, Higginson had theorized that perhaps two-thirds of non-skin cancers "are environmental in origin" and that men lived in a "carcinogenic soup" created by industrialization. Higginson later became founding director of the eleven-nation International Agency for Research on Cancer, established in Lyon, France in 1966. After a decade and a half of work at the Lyon agency, Greenberg reports, Higginson characterizes his early formulation as simplistic and misleading. Higginson is said to consider the environment only one of the culprits in the cancer problem. "Diet, stress, sexual and child-bearing patterns, and, especially, tobacco and alcohol consumption"—in two words, life style—appear to Higginson to be responsible for the variations in cancer rates. He hints that these may be more important factors than chemical pollution in causing cancer.

Despite some doubts raised by a minority of investigators as to exactly where to lay the blame for the scourge of cancer, most authorities seem to have no doubt that environmental causes bear an overwhelming share of the guilt.

There certainly is no doubt as to the fear cancer spreads or the damage it does. According to health officials, cancer is the second leading cause of death in the United States. (Heart disease is the first.) A million people in the country are under treatment for cancer, and it is expected that about 900,000 new cases of cancer will be diagnosed in the United States within a year after this book is published. Authorities predict that one out of every four Americans will ultimately develop cancer in some form and that more than half of us who do so will die of it. The dollar cost of cancer has been estimated at $30 billion a year—some $2 billion alone for hospitalization, additional billions for non-hospital treatment and about $12 billion lost to the economy and wage earners in time away from work.

This book is intended to serve as a record of the facts about cancer and the environment as they emerged during the 1970s. It is based largely on the accounts compiled by FACTS ON FILE in its weekly reports on current history. As in all FACTS ON FILE works, there was a sincere effort to keep this volume free of bias and to make it an accurate and useful reference tool.

LESTER A. SOBEL

New York, N.Y.
September, 1979

Danger at Work, Danger from Industry

Cancer Deaths Increase, Jobs & Industry a Cause

The incidence of cancer in the U.S. has increased to the point where it is authoritatively described as "a killing and disabling disease of epidemic proportions" (Dr. Samuel S. Epstein in Bulletin of the Atomic Scientists, March 1977). A major cause of the increase is said to be industry. The victims are reported to be workers in high-hazard industries, people who live near industrial plants that allegedly use cancer-causing materials, and consumers of carcinogenic products.

Cancer & the workplace. Sen. William Proxmire (D, Wis.) summarized in the Congressional Record Oct. 2, 1978 "the devastating effect [of job-related carcinogens] on workers in certain industries and how greatly the incidence of cancer exceeds that of the general population." Listing some of "the appalling statistics," he said:

A shoe worker is eight times more likely than the average American to develop cancer of the nasal cavity and sinuses and twice as likely to get leukemia.

A tire builder is twice as likely to get cancer of the brain or bladder.

A metal miner is three times as likely to develop lung cancer.

Printing pressmen on newspapers are more than twice as likely to get cancer of the mouth and pharynx.

Textile workers are nearly twice as likely to also develop cancer of the mouth and pharnyx.

Coal miners get stomach cancer at a rate 40 percent more than normal.

Furniture workers have an incidence of nasal cavity and sinus cancer 300 to 400 percent higher than normal.

Coke byproduct workers have a 181-percent excess incidence of cancer of the large intestine and a 312-percent excess incidence of cancer of the pancreas.

In short, a worker's occupation will determine his or her odds of contracting cancer and also the kind of cancer.

The data on estimates of cancer by occupation were prepared by the National Cancer Institute, the National Institute of Environmental Health Sciences, and the National Institute for Occupational Safety and Health.

The study became available a week after Health, Education, and Welfare Secretary Joseph Califano told the AFL-CIO's national conference on job health and safety that Government scientists estimated that 21 to 38 percent of all cancers are work-related. This buried the conventional wisdom propagated so long by industry that only 1 to 5 percent of cancers were job-related and, therefore, workers should just go ahead and whistle while they work.

Proxmire noted that these facts had appeared in the "Washington Window" column of the Sept. 30, 1978 issue of the AFL-CIO News. Among other statements in the column:

While scientists can pinpoint the excess incidence of cancer in certain occupational groups, they cannot always identify the specific cause.

The scientists say the excess incidence of cancer in these occupational groups is in addition to the risks involving exposure to known cancer agents.

These known agents include asbestos, arsenic, benzene, chromium, nickel, and petroleum products. There are an estimated 13,900 excess cancer deaths per year associated with exposure to asbestos. Exposure to other substances cause an additional 33,000 excess cancer deaths.

Some 1.5 million workers are exposed to arsenic and they run a threefold to eightfold risk of respiratory tract cancer.

Some 2 million workers are potentially exposed to benzene, with a fivefold risk of excess cancer deaths from leukemia.

Some 1.4 million workers exposed to nickel run a fivefold to tenfold risk of cancer of the respiratory tract.

Some 1.5 million workers exposed to chromium compounds run a ninefold excess risk of respiratory cancer. The 3.9 million workers exposed to petroleum products run a twofold to 33-fold excess risk based on studies of coke oven and gas workers.

Because cancer usually takes several decades to develop, and new substances are continually introduced, it is to be expected that the incidence of work-related cancer deaths will rise in the years ahead. Indeed, scientists say, job-related cancers now comprise a substantial and increasing fraction of cancer incidence.

Industrial chemical standards. The Labor Department announced Jan. 29, 1974 that it had approved permanent standards against 14 cancer-causing chemicals used mostly in the manufacturing of plastics, dyes and fire-resistant fabrics.

The new rules prescribed work practices, individual tolerance levels, plant contamination control plans, medical surveillance procedures, employe training programs and employer reporting standards.

Occupational cancer hazards reported. A conference on occupational carcinogenesis, held in New York March 24–27, 1975, included presentation of a study by David L. Bayliss, a researcher with the National Institute for Occupational Safety and Health (Niosh), which found that workers exposed to ultra-fine fiber particles might be in greater danger of getting respiratory cancer than those exposed to only large fibers. The major fiberglass companies were reported manufacturing ultra-fine fibers.

Richard A. Lemen, also of Niosh, reported to the conference that a recent study showed that two chemicals commonly used in industry, hydrochloric acid and formaldehyde, combined spontaneously to produce bischloromenthyl ether (BCME), one of the most powerful cancer-causing agents known. The study found that workers exposed to BCME ran a 2½ to three times greater risk of lung cancer than a control group not exposed. The findings could affect thousands of workers in such industries as textiles, particle board manufacture and biological laboratories.

Another study, presented by Dr. H. A. Anderson of the Mt. Sinai Medical School in New York, showed that asbestos workers carrying fibers home on their persons spread cases of fatal lung cancers to their wives and children.

Other studies disclosed by Niosh:

■ The discovery of a Soviet report linking chloroprene, a chemical used in the manufacture of the synthetic rubber Neoprene, to cancer had prompted E. I. du Pont de Nemours & Co., which made the rubber, to start a health study of the several thousands of its employes who had ever worked with the substance.

■ A study by a federal health agency in one U.S. gold mine disclosed an abnormally high rate of lung cancer among miners exposed to asbestos-bearing ore similar to that mined by the Reserve Mining Company in Silver Bay, Minn.

■ A study showed that people living near orchards sprayed with arsenic insecticide had 20% more cases of lung cancer than normal.

Worst industries for cancer?—A study performed by Research Triangle Institute for Niosh concluded in 1977 that the three most hazardous industries in terms of exposure of workers to presumed carcinogens were, in order of greatest hazard: (1) the manufacture of scientific and industrial instruments, (2) the fabrication of metal products and (3) the manufacture of electrical equipment and supplies.

In 12th place was the chemical industry, considered by many observers as the most likely to top the list.

Industry-cancer link suggested by new figures. A five-member federal research team from the National Cancer Institute said that a study of cancer death rates showed strong links between some types of cancer and certain types of industrial pollution. The report, first announced April 23, 1975, ended a four-year study of U.S. death certificates during 1950–69 covering 34 different types of cancer.

Results showed indications of high bladder cancer levels near heavy auto production, according to the researchers, as well as heavy bladder, lung and liver cancer levels around clusters of chemical industries. In New Jersey, which had heavy concentrations of chemical plants, it was pointed out that every county scored in the top 10% of the country for bladder cancer. High lung cancer rates were also reported near copper and lead smelters long associated with the disease.

The group said, however, that not all cancers could be related to industrial pollution. Many cancers were apparently linked to ancestry and eating habits, while melanoma, a skin cancer, was most prevalent in the southern states where sunlight, believed a cause of it, was strongest.

The cancer mortality rate (per 100,000) in the U.S. between 1950–69 was 174 for white males and 184 for nonwhite males. The highest mortality rates of the nation's 10 largest cities, for whites and nonwhites in the same period were: Baltimore, 233 and 257, Philadelphia, 221 and 244, New York City, 216 and 234, Cleveland, 212 and 229, and Detroit, 209 and 217.

The danger increases. Dr. Samuel S. Epstein reported in the March 1977 issue of the Bulletin of the Atomic Scientists that while fatalities from most other ailments are declining, the rate of increase in deaths from cancer (the U.S.' second greatest cause of death) "is more rapid than the rate of increases in population."

Epstein also found "general agreement" that the population and workforce is "continuously exposed to . . . chemical carcinogens in their air, water and food." New chemical agents that may pose cancer risks are also being "introduced into commerce and the workplace," he said.

Rep. George Miller (D, Calif.) called attention to questions that these new dangers raise. He said in a statement in the Congressional Record Oct. 4, 1977:

The dangers in the workplace in this generation are unlike those of the past. Safe working conditions have long been among the primary reasons for which workers agitated and organized, and similarly were among those first of workers' rights recognized by Government. In the past, those dangers, such as exposed machinery, crowded tenement conditions, fire perils, and the like, threatened workers' safety daily. One major accident could, and periodically did, result in the deaths of dozens of workers.

The dangers which affect workers today go far beyond those of the last, and early parts of this century. The dangers of the workplace to which contemporary workers are subjected are carried home to their families, and passed on to future generations. The hazards in some workplaces endanger not only the employees at that site, but can even jeopardize the well-being of an entire community.

There is an obvious question here, that being, should workers be subjected to these kinds of risks in order to earn an income and provide for their families? But there is another extremely important issue, and that is, who decides that workers are to be subjected to occupational hazards? . . . I find it extremely disturbing that someone is making decisions that there is an "acceptable level of risk" in some job, which in many cases really means that a decision has been made that some worker must risk his health and safety, and that of his family, in order that a particular business or industry operate under current design.

Who decides that a coal miner should work in a 30-inch seam? Who decides that an asbestos worker should be exposed to cancer-causing dust? And these questions can be asked repeatedly about many, many industries.

I really fear that a decision has been made that there must be some unhealthy industries in this countries, and that this decision presumes that there will be

Industry & Cancer

Among the human cancers that have been shown to be due to industrial exposure are the following: bladder cancer in aniline dye workers who handle **beta-napthylamine**; bone cancer due to swallowing radium; lung cancer caused by inhalation of chromium compounds, radioactive ores, asbestos, arsenic, and iron; cancer of the nasal sinuses and the lung in nickel mine workers, skin cancer due to handling some products of coal, oil shale, lignite, and petroleum.

Hazards to which industrial groups are exposed also have some implications for the general population. For example, air pollution from industrial wastes represents a potentially important source of carcinogens. When the air contains impurities, our lungs ordinarily are rid of them by coughing, or by more complicated processes within the lining of the bronchial tubes or lung tissue. But excessive or continuous exposure to inhaled impurities brings about changes in the bronchial linings and the lungs which may eventually result in disability and illness. If the impurities contain cancer-producing substances, prolonged exposure can lead to cancer.

—From *The Cancer Story* (U.S. Department of Health Education & Welfare)

workers subjected to the health hazards associated with these jobs. I have no doubt whatever that the people who make those decisions are not the ones who subsequently ruin their health by working at the job.

One hundred years ago, as the labor movement was first beginning to command the attention it now enjoys, decisions were made that we were not going to permit young children to climb among the whirring machines in the silk mills, and that we were not going to permit tailors to be crammed into tiny spaces despite safety hazards. Then, too, some complained that sacrifice was the price of industrial advancement. The problem which I am addressing today is only the modern variant of that dilemma between the maximization of profits and production versus the cost of human life.

Industrial cover-ups charged—Rep. Miller charged July 27, 1979 that there have been widespread cover-ups by corporate officials of cancer and other health hazards caused by industry. According to Miller:

> Today, we must face a fact which is both chilling and depressing: A number of products and industrial processes pose enormous health hazards to millions of people who work with them, purchase them, live near the sites where they are manufactured or disposed of.
>
> In recent months, we have become aware that corporate officials, in numerous cases, have known about these hazards, sometimes for decades, and yet have remained silent. As a result, hundreds of thousands, even millions, of people have been exposed to hazardous ma-

terials and processes which can cost them their health and even their lives.

There are many reasons why this situation has developed and why it has continued largely unchecked for so many years. One of the major reasons is that the responsible individuals who have consciously made these decisions to cover-up hazards have little to fear from the justice system. Too often, offending companies have been fined nominal amounts; in some cases, they have been awarded tax benefits allowing them to write off liability losses. This situation cannot continue.

When someone makes a decision to conceal information about a product or an industrial process, knowing full well that the product or processes jeopardizes someone's life, health or safety, I believe a criminal act has occurred.

ASBESTOS COVER-UPS

Over the course of the past year, I have personally led the investigation of health hazards in the asbestos industry. Relying on documents and statements of the companies themselves, we have pieced together a legacy of four decades of cover-up which has resulted in the exposure of millions of people to cancer-causing asbestos materials.

As long ago as the mid-1930s, the attorney for one of the major asbestos companies commented on medical studies on asbestos recently conducted at the Saranac Laboratory in New York:

> My own idea is that it would be a good thing to distribute the information among the medical community, *providing it is of the right type and would not injure our companies.* [Emphasis added]

The cover-up continued through the following decade. In the early 1950s, the medical director of one of the major companies recommended that a warning label be placed on asbestos; his advice was rejected by the corporate officials who had hired him for his medical expertise:

Later that decade, the Asbestos Textile Institute rejected a recommendation by Dr. Kenneth Smith of Johns-Manville that the institute fund a study of the correlation of asbestos exposure in non-primary workers and lung cancer. His recommendation was rejected, among other reasons, because ATI feared that it would "stir up a hornet's nest."

Although some in the asbestos industry claim that no certain correlation between asbestos and lung cancer was proven prior to Dr. Irving Selikoff's study of insulation workers in 1964, documents of the British Thermal Insulation Contractors Association illustrate that this information was being discussed in the trade in the mid-1940's.

Executives of the Johns-Manville Co. have testified that a formal corporate policy required that employees whose chest X-rays revealed abnormalities be told of the problem and relocated to less dusty areas of the factory. Yet documents, including the minutes of the Health Review Committee from the Manville, N.J. plant, and the testimony of the former manager of the Pittsburg, Calif., plant, indicate that these policies were not followed. In fact, many individuals were not told that their X-rays indicated possible lung damage attributable to asbestos exposure.

As late as last summer, there was a discussion among the members of the European Advisory Committee of the Asbestos International Association at which corporate representatives discussed ways to minimize hazard warning labels on asbestos products shipped to the European continent because—

> A label would put the continental industry in a difficult position . . . (There are) countries where it was felt it was still too early to start voluntary labelling, in fear of a possible negative influence on sales." (Emphasis added.)

. . .

KEPONE

Even before kepone was marketed, the Allied Chemical Co. subjected the substance to extensive laboratory tests which revealed its potential for causing cancer, liver damage and reproductive system failure. Despite tests which suggested numerous problems, Allied increased its production of kepone in the mid-1960s. Heavy amounts were dumped into the James River. In 1975, workers at the subcontracting factory, LSP Co. became ill, and in the resulting inspection, 75 cases of acute kepone poisoning were documented. Soil, air and water in the vicinity were contaminated.

alpha-Naphthylamine (CAS 134327) (29 CFR 1910.1004)

Synonyms: 1-NA, naphthalidam, naphthalidine, naphthylamine, 1-naphthylamine, 1-aminonaphthalene, Antioxidant - MB, C.I. Azoic Diazo Component 114, Fast Garnet Base B

Description: White, needle-shaped crystals, having an unpleasant odor.

Route of Entry: Inhalation, skin absorption, ingestion.

Use: Preparation of dyes and antioxidant for rubber, paint, plastics, and petroleum. Also used in manufacture of herbicides.

Health Hazard: Normally contaminated with 2-NA. Suspected to induce bladder tumors in humans; several metabolites have been shown to induce tumors in rats and mice.

Exposure Limits: Solid or liquid mixtures containing more than 1.0% by weight or volume.

—Identification for a container of a suspected carcinogen; from *Working With Carcinogens* (U.S. Department of Health, Education & Welfare)

BENZIDENE

In 1936, Dr. Wilhelm Hueper told officials of the DuPont Co. that benzidene was carcinogenic. At the time, Hueper was an employee of DuPont.

In 1948, the chief medical officer of the DuPont Co. presented a paper at an international medical conference in London at which he argued that benzidene was not a carcinogen. Three years later, according to Dr. Michael Williams, the medical officer to the Imperial Chemical Industries Dyestuffs Division, was told by the same company official that.

> We here know very well that benzidene is causing bladder cancer, but it is company policy to incriminate only the [other] . . . substance, Beta-naphthylamine.

There are numerous reasons why these hazards were not fully disclosed. As Dr. Hueper wrote in 1943,

> It is, therefore, not an uncommon practice by the parties financially interested in such matters to keep information on the occurrence of industrial cancer well under cover.

In several situations, corporate officials cited fears of possible litigation or compensation claims by affected workers; in other cases, the costs of cleaning up or fixing a product was a factor. But in each case, certain corporate officers made a conscious decision to subject unsuspecting and innocent people to hazards which could imperil their safety and even their lives. . . .

PCB Under Attack

PCB dangers. The attack on polychlorinated biphenyls (PCBs) had begun in the mid-1960s.

PCBs were considered a toxic environmental pollutant. They had caused liver cancer and reproductive failures in laboratory animals and some workers using the chemicals had reported various ailments, such as allergic dermatitis, nausea, dizziness, eye and nasal irritation, asthamatic bronchitis and fungus infections.

Prevalence of the PCBs in the environment was not discovered until 1966, although industrial use began in the 1930s, because the PCB chemical structure was similar to that of DDT. Like DDT, the PCB was not readily biodegradable in the environment. Its industrial use in the U.S. was confined to manufacture of electrical capacitors and transformers. They were utilized abroad in die casting, fireproof sealants and coatings of various kinds.

The commissioner of the Food & Drug Administration, Dr. Charles C. Edwards, said Sept. 29, 1971 that PCB use constituted a "potential but not immediate health hazard." His statement was issued while opponents pressed efforts to ban the chemical and incidents of PCB contamination were reported involving turkeys, fish and packaged dried foods.

Edwards reported that the Monsanto Co., the only U.S. producer of the chemical, would restrict sales to "essential closed-system uses, with no use in food or feed plants." A complete ban, he said, was "not feasible." FDA officials Sept. 30 disputed reports of a PCB ban in Britain, but the British embassy in Washington said that day that a "voluntary ban" had been in effect since March.

Rep. William F. Ryan (D, N.Y.), a leading critic of the chemical's use, conceded Sept. 29 that there was no acute PCB hazard at present, but pointed to the long-term environmental effects. He pledged to continue his efforts to legislate a total ban.

A conference of Nobel Laureates in Goteborg, Sweden asked for restrictions on PCB use, according to the Sept. 22 New York Times. They said of PCB marine pollution that "concentrations may reach levels sufficient to damage ecosystems irreversibly on a worldwide scale before the damage is recognized."

■ The Senate Environment Subcommittee heard a report Aug. 4 that 5 Japanese died and 1,000 suffered a severe skin disease in 1968 due to PCB concentrations of 200 parts per million in cooking oil. Robert Riseborough, University of California professor, reported that some women afflicted subsequently bore stillborn or defective children.

In testimony the same day, the Alabama Game and Fish Division told the committee that spotted bass caught in a creek near a Monsanto plant in Anniston in 1970 had PCB concentrations as high as 360 parts per million. Bass and catfish caught in a nearby lake were found to contain from 10 to 127 parts per million.

■ Swift and Co. informed the FDA Aug. 6 that 50,000 turkeys ready for processing at its Detroit Lakes, Minn. plant had residues of PCB of up to 35 parts per million. (FDA guides allowed 5 parts per million for poultry.) The turkeys were removed from processing.

■ Some 60,000 eggs contaminated by a PCB leak at a Wilmington, N.C. feed plant were believed to have reached Washington-area consumers, FDA officials said Aug. 18. The eggs were among 400,000 containing more than 0.5 parts per million of the chemical, the maximum allowed under FDA guides. An agency spokesman said there was no danger from "the short term exposure."

■ The FDA reported Sept. 27 that a variety of dried packaged foods had been found to contain PCB, in unacceptable levels in the case of shredded wheat and noodle dinners. The contamination was traced to cardboard packing made from recycled paper, which in turn contained carbon paper and printing ink treated with PCB. Such PCB treatments ceased in June, according to the agency, and the food processing companies had stopped using the cardboard involved.

4,4′-Methylenebis(2-chloroaniline) (CAS 101144)
(Note: 29 CFR 1910.1005 revoked 20 August 1976)

Synonyms: MOCA
DACPM
di-(4-amino-3-chlorophenyl)methane
methylene-4,4′-bis(o-chloroaniline)
p,p′-methylenebis(alpha-chloroaniline)
p,p′-methylenebis(o-chloroaniline)
3,3′-dichloro-4,4′-diaminodiphenylmethane
4,4′-diamino-3,3′-dichlorodiphenylmethane
4,4′-methylene(bis)chloroaniline
4,4′-methylenebis(o-chloroaniline)
Curalin M
Curene 442
Cyanaset

Description: Yellow or light tan solid usually in pellets or small clumps or powder form.

Route of Entry: Inhalation and skin absorption.

Use: Used widely as curing agent for urethane liquid-castable elastomers and foams; also as curing agent for epoxy and epoxy-urethane resins.

Health Hazard: Induces cancer in mice and rats though not conclusively proven carcinogenic for humans.

Exposure Limits: Solid or liquid mixtures containing more than 1.0% by weight or volume.

—Identification for a container of a suspected carcinogen; from *Working With Carcinogens* (U.S. Department of Health, Education & Welfare)

The PCBs were being lost into the environment through vaporization, leaks and spills, at least 10 million pounds of them each year, EPA chemist Thomas E. Kopp told the conference Nov. 19. Kopp said at least 10 plants in the U.S. were dumping PCBs directly into waterways and two others into municipal sewage systems.

Curb on PCB use recommended. A curb on the industrial use of polychlorinated biphenals (PCBs) was advocated by Interior Assistant Secretary Nathaniel P. Reed Nov. 21, 1975. The proposal was made on the third and final day of a conference in Chicago on PCBs called by the Environmental Protection Agency.

EPA Administrator Russell E. Train, who opened the conference, told of the discovery of PCBs in the drinking water of Winnebago, Ill. and Sellersburg, Ind. and of suspicion of PCB content in drinking water of Bridgeport, Conn., Escondido, Calif. and New Bedford, Mass.

The conference heard Nov. 20 from Dr. Frederick W. Kutz of the EPA's national human monitoring program that possibly 41% to 45% of all Americans had some PCBs in their tissues. Charles R. Walker, senior environmental scientist with the U.S. Fish and Wildlife Service, said PCBs had been found in fish and wildlife in widely scattered parts of the country.

Interior Assistant Secretary Reed told the conference Nov. 21 the rivers and lakes of the country were "in mortal danger" from the PCBs. In recommending a federal curb on their use, he said they should be restricted solely to transformers and capacitors.

Train called on industry Dec. 22 to find substitutes for PCBs voluntarily because of their "serious threat" to human health and the environment.

The chemicals were a "suspected carcinogen," he said, and the agency planned to seek an eventual halt to all PCB production and use in the U.S.

Toxic substances bill. Congress Sept. 28, 1976 gave final approval to a bill requiring pre-release testing of potentially dangerous chemicals. President Ford signed the bill Oct. 12. The legislation, long sought by environmentalists, passed the House, 360-35, and the Senate, 73-6, both on Sept. 28.

The bill instructed the Environmental Protection Agency to require chemical manufacturers to test products that might be hazardous to human health or to the environment. Manufacturers were required to notify the EPA 90 days in advance of the manufacture of a new product (or the preparation of an existing product for a "significant new use), giving the EPA the opportunity to require additional testing of the product or ban it.

The bill, in its sole reference to a specific chemical, banned the manufacture, sale or distribution of polychlorinated biphenyls (PCBs), unless the EPA ruled that their continued use did not present a hazard to human health or the environment. The ban was to take effect, for PCBs not in enclosed systems, one year after the bill's enactment; the ban would extend to the manufacture of all PCBs two years after enactment, and to the sale and distribution of all PCBs two-and-a half years after enactment.

EPA Administrator Russell E. Train had called Feb. 26 for "effective toxic substances legislation."

Train's appeal came in the wake of recent disclosure of Kepone poisoning of workers in a Hopewell, Va. plant and the closing of the Hudson River to fishing because of PCB contamination.

The PCB situation in the Hudson derived from General Electric Co. plants in Fort Edward and Hudson Falls in Washington County, N.Y., where the chemicals were used in making capacitors and other electronic equipment. New York State accused GE Feb. 9 of having violated state water quality standards by its PCB discharges into the Hudson. "PCBs are toxic substances which pose grave risks to public health and have severely damaged fish resources," state environmental commissioner Ogden R. Reid said. "The Hudson River's water, sediments, organisms and fish are highly contaminated with PCBs."

The state agency acted Feb. 25 to close part of the Hudson to most commercial fishing. All fishing was banned in one 40-mile section.

Acting under the bill, the EPA Jan. 19, 1977 issued rules barring the industrial discharge of polychlorinated biphenyls directly into American waterways. Train said the PCBs "have been shown to be highly toxic, persistent and nonbiodegradable." They "may cause cancer in humans," he said, and they were known to cause skin disease and liver problems in humans and reproductive anomalies in test animals.

Congress had set a deadline of Jan. 1, 1979 for an end to the manufacture of PCBs; the deadline to end processing and distribution was June 1, 1979. The EPA regulations called for compliance with the discharge ban within a year.

One of the chemicals' users, General Electrical Co., reported Feb. 7 that it had found two new compounds to replace

PCBs. GE and New York State Sept. 8, 1976 had signed an agreement for a co-operative $7 million program to end PCB pollution of the Hudson River.

PCB contamination developments. An Environmental Protection Agency suit filed in federal district court in Chicago March 17, 1978 accused Outboard Marine Corp. of having discharged two million pounds of PCB into Waukegan Harbor in Lake Michigan over an 18-year period. The suit charged that the discharges came from the company's Johnson Outboards facility, which made outboard motors.

The EPA requested that the firm be ordered to remove the PCB from the sediment in the harbor. The government sought a penalty of up to $10,000 a day for each day the PCB was discharged, up to a maximum penalty of $20 million.

The company, which said it no longer used PCB at the facility, had filed suit March 1 requesting financial assistance for removal of the PCB from the harbor and instructions on how to do it. The suit was filed against the federal and Illinois environmental agencies.

Animal feed contaminated by PCB in a warehouse fire in Puerto Rico in April 1977 was the subject of a massive recall by the FDA April 12. Ralston Purina Co. said it had voluntarily notified the FDA "as soon as" it became aware of the contamination. More than 800,000 pounds of feed were recalled and disposed of in special hazardous-waste areas. Hundreds of thousands of chickens that had eaten the feed and millions of eggs in the U.S. had to be destroyed.

Final PCB Rules Issued. The Environmental Protection Agency issued final regulations April 19, 1979 banning the manufacture of PCBs and phasing out most uses of the chemicals.

Manufacture of the toxic chemicals, used primarily as insulating fluids and coolants in electrical equipment, already had been stopped.

The ban was required under the Toxic Substances Control Act.

Limited use of PCBs would be allowed for up to five more years in some existing equipment. Replacement of the substances thereafter would be prohibited.

The Food & Drug Administration June 28 sharply reduced the levels of PCBs that it would allow in food.

The new FDA limits would affect fish, poultry and dairy products shipped in interstate commerce after Aug. 28, an agency spokesman said. The FDA had originally set PCB tolerance levels for such foods in 1973. However, recent studies linking PCBs to liver tumors and reproductive problems in test animals had shown, the spokesman said, that "these chemicals are more toxic than previously thought."

The FDA lowered the permissible levels of PCBs in fish and shellfish to two parts per million from five parts per million. The impact of these restrictions on commercial fishing was estimated by the FDA as a loss of about $6 million worth of fish per year.

Other new FDA reductions on PCB levels were: 1.5 parts per million for milk and other dairy products, down from 2.5 parts per million; and three parts per million for poultry products, down from five parts per million.

According to the FDA, a certain amount of food contamination by PCBs was unavoidable, because the chemicals were already present in the soil and water. Since PCBs were highly stable chemicals, the agency said, their initial absorption into food could not be eliminated by later processing.

Asbestos

The Johns-Manville Corp. is the free world's biggest producer of asbestos fiber. Henry Ward Johns, founder of the company, died in 1898. It is assumed that the chronic lung condition that killed him was asbestosis, an ailment caused by inhaling asbestos fibers. He was not the last victim. By 1979, Johns-Manville was fighting more than 1,500 lawsuits from people with cancer or other diseases that they blamed on asbestos. Owens-Corning and other past or current asbestos producers were co-defendants. The U.S. Health, Education & Welfare (HEW) Department esti-

Medical detective 614.4 R75
or
Medical detective 340.6 Im 7m
C78m

G C 977.102
C 49A Medical directory

mated that perhaps 11 million Americans had received hazardous asbestos exposure since 1940, the greatest proportion of them in World War II shipyards. HEW predicts that 67,000 of them will die annually for 30 years of asbestos-caused cancer or other asbestos-caused ailments.

Asbestos controls urged. The National Research Council, in a report prepared for the Environmental Protection Agency, asked Oct. 7, 1971 for tight controls to keep asbestos dust out of the atmosphere. The report said since it was unknown how much asbestos dust could be inhaled without health damage, it would be "highly imprudent to permit additional contamination of the public environment."

Inhalation of the dust by asbestos workers had been linked to lung disease and cancer. The council cited among sources of atmospheric asbestos pollution spray fire-proofing of buildings and dust from demolition of buildings with asbestos used for insulation and wallboard.

The Environmental Protection Agency Dec. 3 proposed new curbs on industrial atmospheric emission of asbestos, mercury and beryllium.

No specific standard was set for the emission of asbestos into the air, but the rules would require the use of filters to clean gases during mining and manufacturing of asbestos products such as floor tiles, brake linings, paper and textiles. Spraying of buildings with asbestos for fireproofing and insultation would be banned, except for indoor spraying, where air treatment would then be required.

Curbs tightened. The Labor Department's Occupational Health & Safety Administration Dec. 7, 1971 ordered a reduction in the maximum asbestos exposure levels for manufacturing and construction workers from 12 to 5 fibers per milliliter. It was the department's first use of emergency powers under the Occupational Safety and Health Act.

The decision came five days after publication in the New England Journal of Medicine of a report that 38% of a group of pipe coverers exposed to "safe" levels of asbestos over long periods showed evidence of lung scarring.

Six months later the agency June 6, 1972 set new standards for asbestos exposure levels in plants but delayed their implementation for four years.

The standard of an average of five fibers per cubic centimeter (c.c.) of air over an eight-hour period set in December 1971 would remain. But beginning July 7, 1972 no concentrations of 10 fibers per c.c. would be permitted at any one time. Starting July 1, 1976 the average standard would be reduced to 2 fibers per c.c.

The new regulations were criticized June 12 by Dr. Irving Selikoff of Mount Sinai Hospital in New York, who predicted that thousands of workers would continue to die of asbestos-related diseases, including bronchial cancer, under the new rules.

New EPA curbs. The EPA March 30, 1973 issued new rules limiting industrial emissions of asbestos, mercury and beryllium.

The rules would bar visible emissions of asbestos in asbestos mills and in plants using the substance, including textile and construction materials factories, unless air cleaning devices were used, and would bar the use of asbestos mine tailings for road surfacing.

The EPA estimated that the asbestos regulations would add $45 million annually, or 8%, to building demolition costs.

Workers' hazards detailed—Dangers faced by asbestos workers were detailed by Paul Brodeur in the Nov. 19, 1973 issue of the New Yorker magazine. Citing Brodeur's article, Walter F. Mondale, then a senator, told the U.S. Senate April 2, 1974:

> In the article, Mr. Brodeur reviews the history of health standards pertaining to industrial exposure to toxic materials such as asbestos. It was not until 1970, when Congress passed the Occupational Safety and Health Act, that any significant legislative action was taken to

Asbestos (CAS 1332214) (29 CFR 1910.1001)

Synonyms: Actinolite, Amianthus, Amosite, Amphibole, Anthrophyllite, Ascarite, Chrysotile, Crocidolite, Tremolite

Description: Fibrous minerals having heat and chemical resistance.

Route of Entry: Inhalation.

Use: Long fibers: Fireproof garments, curtains, shields, clutch facings, and brake linings; filter media.

Short fibers: Insulating boards, shingles, pipe coverings, molded products, reinforcement of plastics, and cements.

Health Hazard: Causes asbestosis, lung and intestinal cancer, and mesothelioma.

Exposure Limits: 2 fibers (longer than 5 micrometers) per cubic centimeter of air.

—Identification for a container of a suspected carcinogen; from *Working With Carcinogens* (U.S. Department of Health, Education & Welfare)

protect our Nation's workers from workplace hazards. And it was not until June 6, 1972, that, over strong industry protest, a safety standard was created for asbestos fibers. To say the least, in view of the fact that investigations have revealed that cancer accounts for approximately 75 percent of the excess deaths among asbestos-industrial workers and that even slight exposure has been proven to cause asbestosis, mesothelioma, and other malignant tumors, the 1972 ruling was long overdue.

Mondale inserted the article in the Congressional Record. In the article, Brodeur was quoted as reporting:

. . . Of all the industrial hazards, none was considered to be more serious than occupational exposure to asbestos. Indeed, mortality studies conducted by Dr. Irving J. Selikoff, the director of the Mount Sinai School of Medicine's Environmental Sciences Laboratory, and by Dr. E. Cuyler Hammond, vice-president for epidemiology and statistics of the American Cancer Society, indicated that one out of every five deaths among asbestos-insulation workers in the United States was due to lung cancer; that almost one out of every ten deaths among these men was due to mesothelioma, an invariably fatal tumor of the linings of the chest or abdomen which rarely occurs without some, even if slight, exposure to asbestos; that another one out of ten deaths among them was due to asbestosis, which is scarring of the lungs resulting from inhalation of asbestos fibres; and that almost half of the men were dying of some form of asbestos disease. . . .

The San Jose Mercury commented editorially May 9, 1979:

For decades, American industry seems to have kept hoping that the problem of asbestos-related lung disease would just go away.

The problem not only refused to go away but obstinately got bigger. At this point, it's grown into a $2 billion problem. That's the amount at stake in more than 1,500 lawsuits filed by people who claim exposure to asbestos gave them cancer or other lung disorders.

There is evidence the industry knew more than 40 years ago that asbestos produced a non-malignant but disabling lung disorder called asbestosis. In 1956, Johns-Manville's own medical director urged the industry to investigate the possible connection between asbestosis and lung cancer. The industry shelved the idea.

In 1964 a definitive study proved beyond all reasonable doubt the link between asbestos and cancer. Yet as late as 1973 we hear the director of environmental affairs for Raybestos lamenting that the board of directors had not responded to his warnings.

Rulings against Reserve Mining plant. U.S. District Court Judge Miles W. Lord in Minneapolis April 20, 1974 ordered Reserve Mining Co. to halt discharges of industrial wastes from its Silver Bay iron ore processing plant into Lake Superior and the air. After a trial lasting almost nine months, Lord ruled that asbestos and other fibers in the wastes posed substantial cancer hazards to five communities in Minnesota and Wisconsin using Lake Superior as a drinking water source.

The immediate effect of the order was the closing of both the plant, which processed taconite, a low-grade iron ore, and the company's taconite mine inland from the lake. But a three-judge appeals panel, acting on an appeal by the company, issued a temporary stay of Lord's order April 22 and allowed the plant to resume operations pending a hearing.

In his ruling, Lord noted evidence that prolonged exposure to minute fibers found in the discharges had been associated with asbestosis—a lung disorder—and cancer of the lungs, gastrointestinal tract and larynx. Lord said the exact scope of the hazards was impossible to gauge immediately, since asbestos-related diseases did not develop until 15–20 years after initial exposure. According to reports during the trial, Reserve had been dumping 67,000 tons of taconite wastes into the lake daily for 17 years.

Lord rejected company objections that closing the plant would cause severe economic hardship in the area, ruling that people in Duluth, Minn. (with over 100,000 residents, the largest community affected by the pollutants) should not be "continuously and indefinitely exposed to a known human carcinogen in order that the people in Silver Bay can keep working." (The plant processed about 15% of the iron ore produced in the U.S. and, with the mine, had a work force of 3,100.)

Lord also noted that he had repeatedly encouraged the company to devise an alternative method of disposing of the wastes on land. The company had failed to do so, Lord said, and had engaged in delaying tactics while continuing the taconite dumping. Contending that Reserve's two parent companies, Armco Steel Corp. and Republic Steel Corp., were among the wealthiest in the nation, Lord rejected as "absurd" a company proposal for federal and state assistance in paying for an on-land disposal system.

The "intransigence" exemplified by the proposal, and the company's request for a ruling that no health hazards existed, forced him to order an immediate halt to the discharges, Lord said.

The suit against Reserve had been brought by the federal government, the States of Minnesota, Wisconsin and Michigan, and a coalition of environmentalist groups.

Across the border in Canada, a New Democratic Party member of the Ontario provincial legislature said Dec. 16 that an unpublished report prepared for the international Joint Commission in September showed that potentially cancer-causing asbestos fibers were contaminating the water of Great Lakes cities, including Toronto and Niagara Falls. The report identified the Reserve Mining Co. of Silver Falls, Minn. as "a major Lake Superior source" of asbestos fibers.

Dr. Morton Shulman, the legislator who divulged the report, said filtration systems in Ontario did not properly remove the asbestos fibers from the water.

The U.S. Court of Appeals in St. Louis March 14, 1975 ordered Reserve Mining to take immediate steps to reduce air pollution at its plant in Silver Bay, Minn. and to plan to end water pollution within a "reasonable" time.

The Court of Appeals, noting the plant was a major employer in the area, criticized the order to close the plant "in the absence of proof of a reasonable risk of imminent or actual harm."

But it said the plant's discharges "give rise to a potential threat to the public health," and were a threat "of sufficient gravity to be legally cognizable." It found the air problem "more significant" than the water discharge because of the asbestos contaminant in the discharges. When inhaled, asbestos was linked with increased cancer incidence.

As for the water contamination, the court said the taconite disposal operation must be moved to an on-land site that must be approved by the state of Minnesota. It did not set the precise limit for "reasonable" time, but it said if the site could not be set up, the plant at Silver Bay would have to be closed.

The court noted that the health factor imparted "a degree of urgency to this case that would otherwise be absent from an environmental suit in which ecological pollution alone were proved."

U.S. District Judge Edward J. Devitt in St. Paul May 4, 1976 fined Reserve Mining and its parent firms more than $1 million for polluting Lake Superior.

Devitt ordered that $837,500 be paid to the state of Minnesota because of violation of water discharge permits pertaining to the dumping of taconite wastes into Lake Superior.

Another $200,000 was to be paid to state and environmental organizations that brought suit against Reserve Mining. This fine was assessed to cover legal costs and as punishment for "misconduct" in failure to furnish requested data.

Another $22,920 was ordered by the court to be paid the city of Duluth for "furnishing interim clean water facilities and supplies" to residents in the area involved.

Reserve wins dump site—A Minnesota court Jan. 31, 1977 upset a decision by two state environmental agencies declining permits for Reserve Mining Co. to dump waste containing asbestos fibers on a land site preferred by the company.

The agencies, the State Pollution Control Agency and the Department of Natural Resources, had rejected the permits because of concern that the asbestos fibers—a possible carcinogenic agent—would be blown from the site into the nearby Silver Bay community.

The state agencies preferred a dump site farther inland. The company opposed this alternative as too costly an operation.

The mining and processing firm was under federal court order to halt by midnight July 7 its current discharge of the waste into Lake Superior.

Reserve's owners said July 7, 1978 that the firm would remain in business in Minnesota and proceed with a $370-million pollution-control project.

The owners said that the company expected to meet a federal court deadline of April 15, 1980 for ending the dumping of wastes into Lake Superior.

Construction of the disposal site, a six-square-mile basin, had been initiated June 1, 1977. (A previous deadline of July 7, 1977 to end the dumping in the lake was deferred.)

The latest court ruling in the case, on April 14 by the Minnesota Supreme Court, favored the state agencies. It required the company to comply with their air and water pollution standards.

The company had argued that limits set by the agencies on the quantity of harmful fibers emitted into the air or water should be related to a "medically significant" amount.

In rejecting the argument, the court said the agencies could bar any release of the harmful fibers into public waters. As for an air standard, the court upheld the agencies' rule requiring no more fiber content in the air around the site than in the air of a control area, such as a neighboring city.

Several times during the long litigation, Reserve Mining's owners held out the prospect of having to abandon the plant because it would become uncompetitive with the additional burden of pollution-control costs.

The decision to continue operation of the company was announced at a news conference by Armco Chairman William Verity and Republic Chairman William De Lancey.

Another participant was Minnesota Gov. Rudy Perpich, who said the resolution of the dispute satisfied environmental needs and preserved more than 3,000 jobs.

Asbestos found in 5 water supplies. The Environmental Protection Agency said April 30, 1976 that asbestos fibers had been detected in drinking water supplies for Boston, Philadelphia. Atlanta, San Francisco and Seattle.

The samplings were "inconclusive," the EPA cautioned, because later samplings held no asbestos content.

The asbestos was found as part of a two-year study of water supplies for 10 cities. No asbestos was found in samples taken from the water supplies of the test group's other five cities—Chicago, Dallas, Denver, Kansas City and New York.

Workers get $20 million award. A $20-million settlement was awarded Feb. 8, 1978 to 445 Tyler, Tex. asbestos-plant workers who had sued the U.S. government and several private companies in 1974 for negligence in having allowed them to work, unaware of the danger, with the harmful substance.

The settlement, on a consolidation of lawsuits, had been reached in the fall of 1977 but sealed until Feb. 8, when the Justice Department informed the court—U.S. District Judge William Steger in Beaumont, Tex.—that the federal government had agreed to pay $5.75 million as its share of the settlement.

The Tyler plant, which manufactured asbestos pipe insulation, was closed in 1972.

In their suits, the workers had argued that under the Occupational Health and Safety Act of 1970, it had been HEW's and the Labor Department's responsibility to alert workers to job-related health risks.

Asbestos Workers Get Health Warning. The Health, Education and Welfare Department said April 26, 1978 that it was warning current and former asbestos workers about the health risk associated with working with the substance.

The nation's physicians also were to be given information from the government on detection of asbestos poisoning in their patients.

The department estimated that between 8.5 million and 11.5 million persons, still living, had worked on jobs with the lethal material since the beginning of World War II. That included 1.5 million to 2.5 million workers currently exposed to asbestos on the job.

The largest group of workers exposed to asbestos was thought to be the approximately 4.5 million who worked in shipyards during World War II. Asbestos, a fireproofing and insulation material, was used extensively in ships to insulate boilers, steam pipes, hot water pipes and nuclear reactors.

The advisory prepared for physicians warned that asbestos exposure as short as a month could result in disease many years later because of the inhaled dust.

The advisory cited studies of heavily exposed workers that found lung cancer had caused approximately 20 to 25 of each 100 deaths 20 or more years after initial exposure.

Another 11% to 14% died from other cancers, such as of the esophagus, stomach or abdominal cavity, the study found. In some groups, as many as 7% of the workers died of asbestosis, a disabling respiratory disease also known as "white lung disease."

The warning to workers advised them to stop smoking. Asbestos workers who smoked, according to studies, were up to 30 times more likely to develop lung cancer than nonsmoking workers, and up to 90 times more likely to develop lung cancer than nonsmokers who had not been exposed to asbestos.

A statement issued by HEW Secretary Joseph A. Califano Jr. said in part:

> Asbestos is the term used for a group of fibrous materials that do not burn and are excellent thermal insulators In the past four decades asbestos has been used for a great number of purposes—more than 3,000 uses have been identified—with two-thirds of all asbestos used in the construction industry. Ship construction has been an activity with especially high use of asbestos, since the substance is effective in insulating boilers

steampipes, hot water pipes and nuclear reactors.

Unfortunately, numerous studies have indicated that exposure to asbestos in settings, like the workplace, where it is concentrated, significantly increases the risk of incurring four serious diseases: lung cancer, asbestosis (a progressively debilitating lung disease that impairs breathing and increases risk of serious illness or death from respiratory infections like pneumonia), mesothelioma (a cancer of the chest and abdominal cavities) and certain gastro-intestinal cancers.

Both the Surgeon General's advisory and public information campaign will suggest certain actions that individuals exposed to asbestos can take to reduce or mitigate the health threat to the greatest extent possible. They will stress that no single step has a more important effect in reducing risks from two of the most common diseases associated with asbestos—lung cancer and asbestosis—than stopping cigarette smoking.

Our best estimates of the increased risks associated with asbestos exposure are based on HEW supported studies of workers heavily exposed to asbestos before the government began to regulate asbestos in the workplace in the late 1960's and early 1970's. As a result of recent government regulation, current workers, without previous exposure, can be expected to face smaller risks than those exposed in the past.

The risks for past workers regularly exposed to asbestos are estimated to be as follows:

Lung Cancer. A non-smoker who has been exposed to asbestos is three to four times more likely to develop lung cancer than a non-smoker who has not been exposed. However, a smoker who has been exposed to asbestos is up to 90 times more likely to incur lung cancer than a non-smoker who has not been exposed, and up to 30 times as likely to incur lung cancer than a non-smoker who has been exposed.

At present, it is estimated that 20-25 percent of workers, both smokers and non-smokers, exposed to asbestos before the era of government regulation die of lung cancer.

Asbestosis. Only individuals exposed to asbestos contract asbestosis which afflicts approximately 7 percent of the number of workers exposed in the past. Asbestosis is an irreversible and progressively disabling lung disease that impairs breathing, and individuals with the disease are much more likely to die of respiratory ailments, like pneumonia, than individuals who do not have asbestosis. The Surgeon General advises me that clinical experience indicates a person who smokes and has been exposed to asbestos faces a greater risk of developing asbestosis and of dying from a respiratory ailment than an asbestos exposed individual who does not smoke.

Mesothelioma. As with asbestosis, only those individuals exposed to asbestos appear to contract this disease. Approximately 7–10 percent of those exposed to asbestos in the past die of this cancer.

Gastro-intestinal cancer. Individuals exposed to asbestos in the past are estimated to be about twice as likely to die of gastro-intestinal cancers—including cancers of the esophagus, stomach and colon—as nonasbestos exposed individuals. Approximately 8 to 9 percent of asbestos-exposed individuals die of these types of cancer.

In addition to the 4.5 million persons who worked in shipyards during World War II, it is estimated that 500,000 to 1.4 million persons have been employed in shipyards since the War. Other occupations in which there has been significant exposure to asbestos include asbestos mining and processing; construction work involving insulation; building demolition; roofing; and automotive work in brake and clutch lining installation and repair.

EPA enforcement limited. The Supreme Court Jan. 10, 1978 ruled, 5–4, that the Environmental Protection Agency was limited in its authority to enforce prohibitions on asbestos pollution in the air. Specifically, the high court upheld the dismissal of an indictment against Adamo Wrecking Co. of Michigan, which had been prosecuted for violating an EPA regulation based on the 1970 Clean Air Act. The regulation had required Adamo, and all other wrecking firms, to wet down and remove asbestos materials from a building before it was demolished.

Adamo contended that the EPA was not legally empowered to issue "work practice" orders, which were a list of procedures under which companies could meet pollution standards. The EPA argued that the procedures were necessary because of the difficulty of measuring the amount of asbestos in the air.

Justice William H. Rehnquist, writing for the majority, agreed with a lower court judge that Congress, in enacting the Clean Air Act, had intended that the EPA set "a quantitative limit on [pollution] emissions," rather than issue work procedures.

Justice Potter Stewart, joined by Justices William J. Brennan Jr. and Harry A. Blackmun, dissented, saying that the majority ruling frustrated "the intent of Congress to establish a speedy and unified system of judicial review under the Act."

Justice John Paul Stevens, dissenting separately, criticized the majority for making "the asbestos standard, and any other work practice rule . . . unenforceable."

The case was *Adamo Wrecking Co. v. U.S.*

EPA revises rules—The Environmental Protection Agency June 15, 1978 amended its 1973 asbestos regulations to limit the amount of asbestos that could be released into the atmosphere in the renovating or demolishing of buildings.

The revision extended coverage of careful handling to asbestos-containing materials that could be crushed by hand. Such materials were to be wetted and removed before wrecking began or otherwise handled in such a way, such as in containers, to prevent release of the asbestos.

Asbestos was described by EPA Deputy Administrator Barbara Blum as "a dangerous pollutant which has been directly linked to cancers of the membranes lining the chest and abdomen in humans."

Asbestos Danger in Schools Cited. The Environmental Defense Fund announced Dec. 21, 1978 that it had asked the government to require that public schools be inspected for asbestos dangers.

The petition, filed with the Environmental Protection Agency, was supported by the National Education Association, the AFL-CIO American Federation of Teachers and the National Parent-Teachers Association.

Asbestos, sprayed on ceilings and walls, had been used extensively in the past for insulation, fireproofing and soundproofing. Such uses had been banned in school construction by the EPA in 1973.

The EPA was operating a program for inspection of schools by local authorities for asbestos dangers. But, according to the Defense Fund, only 6,333 of the nation's 87,000 public schools had been inspected thus far.

The Defense Fund said 15% of the schools inspected had been found to contain potentially dangerous asbestos.

In New York City, where asbestos was being found in a third of the schools inspected, two schools had been closed because of the problem.

In the few states that had inspected 20% or more of their schools, the percentages of schools deemed to have dangerous levels of asbestos ranged from 5% in Rhode Island and Massachusetts to 48% in Indiana.

Rep. George Miller (D, Calif.) held hearings of two House Labor & Education subcommittee in 1978 on the problem of asbestos' dangers to health. He told the House in a statement Jan. 31, 1979:

One of the most serious problems which was brought to the attention of the subcommittee earlier this month was that asbestosis materials were widely used in the construction of schools during the period 1946–72. One recent survey found asbestos materials in one-sixth of all schools surveyed. In some, the asbestos level in the air was 100 times the normal ambient level. Asbestos was used for fireproofing, insulation, and soundproofing, and was mixed in cement and tiles, used as pipe insulation, and sprayed on walls and ceilings.

Over time, some of this asbestos material has deteriorated and found its way into the air, where it can be inhaled by students and school employees. Especially when the asbestos materials have become friable, or are within easy reach of students, the likelihood of the release of asbestos fibers is very great. Additional problems are caused by broken insulation around pipes and water and air damage.

The problem in our schools is particularly severe because children, according to leading medical experts, may be especially susceptible to environmentally caused cancers. Asbestos related cancers also take as long as 30 years or more to develop. If a young child is exposed, therefore, his or her likelihood of surviving well into the post-latency period, when the cancer becomes manifest, is far greater than in the case of an older worker.

There are very inadequate controls governing asbestos in the school environment. There is currently no safety standard applicable to schools. Although the use of sprayed asbestos was banned by the Environmental Protection Agency in 1973, there is no program to survey schools and remove hazardous asbestos, except on a voluntary basis. Local school boards do not have the technical expertise to test their schools, nor the financial resources to pay for the containment or removal of hazardous substances. Although administrative relief is being sought under the Toxic Substances Control Act, resolution of the current petition may require years, and we cannot afford to wait. Doctors told our committee that there is no safe level of exposure to asbestos; cancers have appeared in people who were exposed for only a few weeks several decades in the past.

Voluntary Hair Dryer Recall Sought. The staff of the Consumer Product Safety Commission April 19, 1979 asked makers of some hand-held electric hair dryers to voluntarily recall their products from the market. Such a recall could involve 12 million dryers.

The CPSC action was the result of reports that more than 100 models of portable hair dryers manufactured by nine major companies contained asbestos heat shields or linings. Asbestos was a known cancer-causing agent, thus posing the threat that particles of the substance might be blown in the faces of, and inhaled by, hair-dryer users.

The hair-dryer problem was brought to light in an investigative report by WRC-TV, a Washington, D.C. station, in collaboration with the Environmental Defense Fund. The CPSC had not determined to what extent the hair dryers were health hazards.

Some manufacturers and retailers of the hair dryers had suspended their sale, but there was no industrywide plan for dealing with the product.

Hazardous Wastes

One aspect of the problem of cancer and the environment is the matter of disposing of industrial wastes that might prove carcinogenic. It was realized quite early that radioactive wastes posed such a problem. By 1978, however, it became widely known that some discarded non-radioactive chemicals also threatened nearby populations.

Niagara Site a Disaster Area. The Love Canal of Niagara Falls, N.Y. was declared a disaster area by President Carter Aug. 7, 1978 because of dangers from long-buried waste chemicals.

A warning that "a great and imminent peril to the health of the general public" existed in the area had been issued Aug. 2 by New York State Health Commissioner Robert P. Whalen.

Whalen recommended that pregnant women and children under two leave the area immediately. He cited a "significant excess" of miscarriages and birth defects in the area. The rate of miscarriages was 50% more than average. Of 24 children in the area, four were mentally retarded.

Hooker Chemicals and Plastics Corp., a unit of Occidental Petroleum Corp., had used the Love Canal area as a dump site for its toxic wastes from 1947 to 1952. In 1953, the company sold the site to the Niagara Falls board of education for $1.

After several years of heavy rains, the waste chemicals began to surface in 1976 on the school playground and yards and basements of homes.

Tests of the material revealed more than 80 different chemical compounds, at least seven of them suspected carcinogens.

Evacuation of families from the area began Aug. 4. Money for rent and moving expenses came from New York State and the Niagara Gazette, which had received a $6,000 grant from the foundation of its parent company, the Gannett chain.

Federal funds became available after President Carter declared the site a disaster area.

Hooker Corp. Aug. 7 offered to help pay for a ditch to drain the dump. The company, which had made no secret that the site was a toxic waste dump, disclaimed any liability for damages.

New York Gov. Hugh L. Carey said Aug. 7 the state would join with the federal government "on a 50-50 basis" to pay for cleaning up the area. The state also purchased the houses of residents wanting to move. By April 12, 1979, some 235 of 239 families in the area had moved.

Hooker Corp. had known as early as 1958 of the seepage of the toxic chemicals, according to data released April 10, 1979 by the House Commerce Subcommittee on Oversight & Investigations.

A former official of the chemical company told the House panel that Hooker had informally warned the board of education. But he said residents of the area had not been warned for fear of causing legal problems for the school board.

The congressional panel had obtained the company documents from the Securities and Exchange Commission, which had received them during an unrelated investigation of a merger fight between Hooker's parent company, Occidental Petroleum Corp., and Mead Corp.

A Senate panel also was looking into the Love Canal situation and the problem of the dumping of toxic wastes.

At a hearing April 11, Assistant Attorney General James W. Moorman told the Senate Judiciary Committee that more than 40 million tons of toxic substances were being generated every year in the U.S. and "we don't know where all this poison is going."

"We now have one attorney spending full time on toxic-waste dangers," he said. "But neither my department nor the EPA have any legally trained investigators to work on other Hooker-type cases."

Moorman said the Justice Department had been working with the EPA, the Environmental Protection Agency, on the Hooker case for more than a year.

EPA Report on Hazardous Dump Sites. The Environmental Protection Agency said Nov. 21, 1978 that faulty disposal of hazardous waste posed "an extremely serious environmental problem."

The warning accompanied the agency's first nationwide inventory of hazardous waste sites.

The survey found more than 32,000 sites that "may contain hazardous waste in any quantity which now or potentially could cause adverse impact on public health or the environment."

At least 103 of the sites were described as "current threats."

One of the agency's findings was that disposal of dangerous waste continued to be a problem because up to 90% of hazardous waste continued to be improperly discarded.

The EPA Dec. 14 proposed regulations to control such disposals.

The regulations would cover generation, or production, of the wastes, transportation, treatment and disposal.

Companies that generated 100 kilograms (about 220 pounds) or more of hazardous wastes would be required to provide full information about the nature of the material and to keep track of their disposal on a permanent basis.

Permits would be required for disposal sites. One of the requirements was that the facilities carry $5 million in liability insurance. The sites themselves would have to be secure by federal standards.

The EPA and the states would police the waste-management sites.

The cost of the new rules for 17 major industries affected, according to EPA estimates, would be about $750 million a year, compared with $155 million these industries already spent annually for management of hazardous wastes.

EPA Administrator Douglas Costle admitted that the cost was high but he estimated it to be 0.5% of the annual production value. If groundwater supplies could be safeguarded at that price, he said, "it is a bargain."

The proposed regulations did not extend to past dumping of hazardous wastes or the cost of clean-up of wastes already dumped.

Nor did they apply to disposal of nuclear wastes, an area covered by separate laws and regulations.

Curbs set on five toxic chemicals—The EPA Jan. 3, 1977 had set rules to curb water pollution caused by five highly toxic chemicals. The rules barred any discharge of the pesticides aldrin-dieldrin and DDT into waterways. "Stringent restrictions" were imposed on discharges of benzidine, endrin and toxaphene.

Carter Proposes Cleanup Plan. President Carter asked Congress June 13, 1979 for legislation that would establish funding and authority for cleaning up hazardous oil and chemical spills and dump sites.

In letters to the House and Senate, the President cited in particular the old chemical dump at the Love Canal.

"This case clearly demonstrates the unacceptable costs of improper hazardous waste disposal," Carter said in his letters to congressional leaders.

Benzidine (CAS 92875) (29 CFR 1910.1010)

Synonyms: 2-amino diphenyl
4,4'-diaminobiphenyl
4,4'-diaminodiphenyl
4,4'-diphenylenediamine
p-diaminodiphenyl
C.I. Azoic Diazo Component 112
Fast Corinth Base B
4,4'-biphenyldiamine

Description: White or reddish-gray solid occuring as crystals, flakes, or powder.

Route of Entry: Skin absorption.

Use: Intermediate in production of sulfur, azo, and aniline dyes; clinical detection of blood; security printing; and quantitative analysis.

Health Hazard: Induces bladder tumors in humans primarily by absorption through the skin. Also carcinogenic to rats and mice.

Exposure Limits: Solid or liquid mixtures containing more than 0.1% by weight or volume.

—Identification for a container of a suspected carcinogen; from *Working With Carcinogens* (U.S. Department of Health, Education & Welfare)

The President proposed establishment of a $1.63-billion fund over the next four years to handle the cleanup costs. The fund would come largely from taxes on businesses producing the hazardous materials: 80% of it would be raised through fees on the oil and chemical industries.

The 20% remainder of the fund would be provided by federal, state and local governments.

At a White House news conference, Administrator Douglas Costle of the Environmental Protection Agency said that a substantial part of the cost of cleanup probably would be passed on to the consumer.

"Both industry and consumers have financially benefited from cheap and unsafe disposal practices in the past, and therefore both should share in the remedies we must now pursue," he said.

Several environmental groups issued a joint statement strongly endorsing the President's initiative. But they objected to what they considered an inadequate provision to reimburse victims of spills or waste sites for medical expenses or loss of property or jobs.

Robert Roland, president of the Chemical Manufacturers Association, protested the proposal. "The bill unfairly singles out the chemical and related industries to bear a disproportionate burden of cleanup costs," he said. "In so doing it fails to adequately reflect society's responsibility for resolving a problem which everyone has helped create and for whose solution everyone should help pay."

The President's plan did not cover nuclear waste materials.

Threat in Michigan. Rep. Guy Vander Jagt (R, Mich.) said in a June 22, 1979 statement in the Congressional Record that potentially cancer-causing industrial wastes had also been dumped in Dalton Township, Muskegon County, Mich. He said:

> . . . This community of several hundred has suffered from the dumping of highly toxic wastes on their land. In 1971 over 300 barrels of poisonous chemicals, some suspected carcinogens and others proven to be cancer-causing, were scattered throughout Dalton Township. The liquid, toxic contents of these barrels found their way into the groundwater eventually thoroughly contaminating the only source of drinking water for some 90 families.
>
> Since the discovery of the contaminated wells over 2 years ago, Dalton Township residents have had to ship bottled water into their homes so that further contamination would not take place. Needless to say, the expense and inconvenience of this distressing and troublesome episode greatly taxes the resources of these people.
>
> Engineering studies show that the best solution is to link the township with a neighboring city's existing water system. The solution exists, but the cost, estimated $3 million has proven prohibitive leaving the residents of Dalton Township with no recourse but to continue expending money for a supply of water that does not even temporarily meet their needs.

Culver on Dangers & Costs. In a statement in the Congressional Record June 20, 1979, Sen. John C. Culver (D, Iowa) discussed the dangers of improperly dumped industrial wastes, some of which had been found to be cancer-causing. He said:

> These dangers are significant. Over 50,000 chemicals are in commercial production in this country, and the environmental and health effects of many of them have not been sufficiently studied. There are an estimated 35,000 hazardous waste disposal sites in this country, and recently the Environmental Protection Agency stated that as many as 2,000 of them are leaking hazardous, toxic, or mutagenic wastes into soils, streams, or groundwaters. The costs of cleaning up these unsafe sites range as high as $40 billion. The implication of these figures, in terms of public health and safety, degradation of the environment, and containment and cleanupcosts, is staggering.
>
> In Charles City, Iowa, 24 pollutants proven to be carcinogenic, toxic or mutagenic, including benzine and arsenic have leached from one waste disposal site into the Cedar River. The cost of containing or removing the wastes may reach several million dollars. However, if the waste seeps through the limestone bedrock into the underlying Cedar Valley Aquifer, the principal water supply for most of northeastern Iowa would be contaminated. Who would pay the clean up costs if that took place? Who could pay for it—or for 2,000 more sites like "Love Canal" or the "Valley of the Drums"?
>
> Congress must take the lead in enacting laws which give adequate protection to health and environmental values. Reasonable and effective regulation is required before the damage to human life and the environment becomes irreversible.
>
> Correcting the errors of the past with respect to inactive and abandoned waste sites will be a formidable challenge. The cost will be substantial and require a concerted effort on the part of both government and industry to find the resources needed to mitigate the worst effects of these "chemical time bombs." The Resource Protection Subcommittee, which I chair, is currently holding a number of hearings in Washington, D.C., and around the country on legislation to establish a hazardous waste reserve fund to contain and clean up sites that pose unacceptable risks to human health and the environment.

Other Industrial & Chemical Problems

GAO study scores OSHA. The General Accounting Office, Congress' auditing agency, March 23, 1977 released a report critical of the Occupational Safety and Health Administration and the National Institute of Occupational Safety and Health, a research organization in the Department of Health, Education and Welfare.

The study said millions of workers were exposed daily to substances known to cause cancer and other diseases. Yet final protective procedures had been imposed by the government for only 15 such poisons in the previous five years. The report estimated that the two agencies together had spent $727 million during the period. The GAO warned that unless the agencies speeded up their issuance of health regulations, it would "take more than a century to establish needed standards for substances already identified as hazards."

U.S. access to medical data upheld. U.S. District Judge Dennis R. Knapp in Charleston, W. Va. Dec. 22, 1977 upheld the right of federal probers to inspect a company's medical records and work histories of past and present employes.

The National Institute for Occupational and Safety and Health (NIOSH) had sought access to the data, under the 1970 Occupational Safety and Health Act, at Du Pont Co.'s Belle, W. Va. plant. The inquiry stemmed from a worker's request for an evaluation of hazards at the plant because of concern over an apparently large number of cancer cases.

Du Pont asked the consent of current and former Belle employes to disclose their personal medical records, but it refused to grant NIOSH access to the records of the employes who declined consent. The company's caution was based on possible violation of the constitutional right of privacy.

In Knapp's opinion, the issue "isn't whether a right of privacy exists respecting the information sought, but rather whether the record indicates that such a right will be abridged. We think not."

Knapp stressed, however, that the data was protected and he set restrictions in NIOSH's handling of it. It must not be disclosed to any other sources, he said, and must be returned intact to Du Pont within a year.

List of Chemicals Set. The Environmental Protection Agency Dec. 22, 1977 ordered companies to report to it the names of all chemicals they produced or imported.

The action was taken as the first major step toward implementation of the 1976 Toxic Substances Control Act.

The agency planned to compile and publish an inventory of the chemicals. An estimated 70,000 chemicals were produced by the country's 5,400 chemical makers and petroleum refiners.

Large producers, those with more than $5 million in chemical sales in 1977, were required to report the quantities of chemicals they made and the manufacturing sites.

EPA Administrator Douglas Costle said the inventory would be "the first road map of the chemical problem" in the U.S.

CPSC Adopts Rules on Cancer Agents. The Consumer Product Safety Commission June 1, 1978 voted unanimously to adopt regulations making it easier for the agency to identify and ban cancer-causing agents from consumer products.

The new rules established formal procedures for screening, classifying, evaluating and regulating potential carcinogens. For example, the regulations permitted the commission to take "precautionary action" without establishing proof of a chemical's harm.

Under the rules, suspected cancer-causing substances would be placed into one of four categories, based on the evidence of their danger. Chemicals in the first category would be banned outright. Substances in the remaining categories would be subject to continuing investigation and regulation by the CPSC.

Anesthetic gases linked to ills. A survey involving 29,000 operating room personnel indicated that they had abnormally high rates of disease and birth defects among their children, it was reported Oct. 14, 1974. Long-term exposure to waste anesthetic gases, the National Institute of Occupational Health and Safety-sponsored study said, was apparently linked to increased cancer rates among women, unusually high incidence of liver and kidney disease among both men and women, abnormal numbers of spontaneous abortions and birth defects among children of women working in operating rooms, and a 25% greater than normal rate of birth defects among children fathered by anesthetists.

Action against vinyl chloride. The Labor Department Oct. 1, 1974 issued rules designed to curb workers' exposure to vinyl chloride, a basic material in manufacture of plastic products. The substance, a gas processed from solid polyvinyl chloride, had been shown to induce angiosarcoma, a rare and incurable form of liver cancer.

Under the new standards, vinyl chloride in the air in plastics plants would be limited to one part per million (ppm) parts of air, averaged over eight hours, beginning Jan. 1, 1975. Until that time, the limit would be 50 ppm, the same as had been set in temporary emergency standards issued April 5. Beginning Jan. 1, 1976, workers would be required to wear respirators if concentrations exceeded the 1 ppm limit. During 1975, respirator use would be optional up to 25 ppm. The old limit in effect before the April emergency action had been 500 ppm.

Earlier actions had been taken to limit exposure outside the plastics plants. In a report released Sept. 16, the EPA estimated that 200 million pounds of vinyl chloride a year escaped into the air around the plants. EPA Administrator Russell E. Train said there was no evidence of an "imminent hazard" to people near the plants, but there was sufficient potential danger to warrant EPA emission rules, which he said would take several months to formulate. The EPA study estimated that emissions could be reduced by 90% with available control technology.

The U.S. Court of Appeals in New York Jan. 31, 1975 upheld the Labor Department regulations.

The Supreme Court March 31 refused to delay implementation of U.S. Occupational Safety and Health Administration standards designed to reduce workers' exposure to vinyl chloride gas. The Firestone Plastics Co. and the Society of the Plastics Industry Inc., a trade association, had petitioned the court, asking it to stay the new standards while it considered whether to hear a challenge to the standards themselves. The new standards, whose effective date was April 1, set vinyl chloride exposure levels at one-fiftieth of the previous standards.

The Consumer Product Safety Commission (CPSC) Aug. 16 announced a ban on the use of vinyl chloride as a propellant in household aerosol sprays. The CPSC said the gas was not currently being used in newly-manufactured aerosols, but that some produced several months earlier might contain it. The CPSC ban primarily affected paints and paint removers, adhesives and solvents.

In a series of actions April 3-24 involving other aerosol products containing vinyl chloride, the EPA and the Food & Drug Administration (FDA) ordered recalls and banned further sales of some brands of cosmetics, medicinal products and deodorants (FDA), and 29 brands of indoor pesticides (EPA). The EPA added five more pesticides to the banned list, it was reported May 29.

The EPA Dec. 16, 1975 issued a proposed standard requiring a 90% reduction in air emissions of vinyl chloride gas from plastics factories.

Mark Green suggested in the Washington Post Jan. 21, 1979 that industry frequently overestimates the cost of protecting workers against carcinogens. Citing vinyl chloride, he wrote:

> In the early 1970s, for example, chemical manufacturers announced that a proposed federal standard on vinyl chloride, a proven cause of cancer, could cost 2 million jobs and $65 billion to $90 billion. "The standard is simply beyond the compliance capability of the industry," their trade association declared. The standard was adopted and the industry has flourished—without any job losses and at a cost that is one-twentieth of the original industry estimate.
>
> Similarly, in one of a growing number of regulatory battles within the Carter administration, Energy Secretary James Schlesinger recently suggested that Labor Secretary Ray

bis-Chloromethyl ether (CAS 542881) (29 CFR 1910.1008)

Synonyms: BCME | dimethyl-1,1-dichloroether
bis-CME | sym-dichloro-dimethyl ether
chloro(cholromethoxy)methane
sym-dichloromethyl ether
chloromethyl ether

Description: Colorless liquid with a suffocating odor.

Route of Entry: Inhalation

Use: Alkylating agent. May form spontaneously from reaction of hydrochloric acid and formaldehyde; therefore, traces may be found in cotton finishing operations, and in manufacture of flameproofing agents, insecticides, bactericides, antibiotics, dispersing agents, water repellants, and rubber. NOTE: Normally present as a contaminant in methyl chloromethyl ether.

Health Hazard: Induces lung cancer in humans, rats, and mice.

Exposure Limits: Solid or liquid mixtures containing more than 0.1% by weight or volume.

—Identification for a container of a suspected carcinogen; from *Working With Carcinogens* (U.S. Department of Health, Education & Welfare)

Marshall block a proposed worker exposure standard for beryllium, another known carcinogen, because of its supposed $150 million cost. Energy officials later conceded that their estimate was derived from "a gross estimate based on rule of thumb"—provided by other than beryllium manufacturers.

Allied chemical also seen as hazard—A chemical widely used in the metal and dry cleaning industry was found in preliminary tests to cause cancers of the liver and other organs in mice. The chemical, trichloroethylene, was a close relative of vinyl chloride. An April 26, 1975 report said an internal government "memorandum of alert" had been issued by the National Cancer Institute to prompt consideration of further studies and the protection of exposed workers. Trichloroethylene was used mainly as a degreasing agent in the metal industry and by auto mechanics, and as a solvent in the dry cleaning and clothing industries. It was also used as an anaesthetic in minor operations and in the processing of certain foods such as decaffeinated coffee.

Du Pont Co. said in a letter in Science magazine that recent tests had shown that rats inhaling small amounts of a commonly used solvent had developed malignant tumors in their nasal cavities. The company warned the nation's laboratory workers to handle the solvent, hexamethylphosphoramide or HMPA, with the same precautions they would take with a cancer-causing agent, it was reported Oct. 28. The government's National Institute for Occupational Safety and Health (Niosh) estimated that 5,000 workers were currently exposed to HMPA, about 90% of them in research laboratories.

Niosh said, in a letter to occupational health experts, that ethylene dibromide (EDB), an industrial chemical, had proved to be a "strong" carcinogen in rats and mice. The agency said the EDB was used as a grain fumigant and as an additive in 88% of the automobile gasolines sold in the U.S. According to the July 14 report, 650,000 persons employed in service stations were exposed to the leaded gasoline as well as 8,900 persons who did fumigating. It was reported that the major manufacturers of EDB were starting to investigate the health records of workers to determine if precautions should be instituted regarding the handling of the chemical.

Arsenic curb proposed. Tighter controls for industrial use of inorganic arsenic were proposed by the Labor Department Jan. 19, 1975 with a warning that it was "strongly implicated" as a cause of cancer. The department had received evidence in 1974 from several chemical firms of an abnormally high rate of lung and lymph cancer among workers exposed to the chemical, which was used in a variety of products, such as pesticides, herbicides, glassware and wood preservatives. The department proposed that the exposure limit of .005 milligram per cubic meter of air on an eight-hour basis be tightened to .004 milligrams. Above .002 milligrams, protective equipment and regular medical examinations would be mandatory. For any 15-minute period, a maximum of .01 milligrams was proposed.

A study released Jan. 16, 1977 charged the Canadian government with misleading Yellowknife residents about arsenic contamination. It said the city's 12,000 residents were being exposed to "horrendously high" levels of arsenic.

A study prepared by the National Indian Brotherhood, the United Steelworkers of America and the University of Toronto disputed 1975 federal studies that found no evidence of exposure to dangerous amounts of the poison. The study said union workers in the goldmining industry at Yellowknife had been found to have as much as 278 parts per million in their hair, and traces of more than five parts per million had been discovered in Yellowknife soil and snow. (The World Health Organization's maximum acceptable level was five parts per million.)

Prolonged exposure to arsenic had been linked to various cancers, brain disorders, paralysis, gastrointestinal disorders and other serious illnesses. Government statistics had indicated a cancer death rate for Yellowknife, the capital of the Northwest Territories, that was twice as high as the national average. Arsenic was found in Yellowknife's gold-bearing ore and was released into the air by the smelting process.

Coke oven emissions guide set. The Labor Department issued regulations Oct. 20, 1976 to protect workers from harmful emissions from coke ovens.

The regulations included specific engineering and work-rule controls. The emission of benzene-soluble particulates, considered a relevant measure of the risk of lung cancer to the worker, was to be limited to .15 milligrams per cubic meter of air averaged over an eight-hour period. The informal industry limit was .2 milligram of "coal-pitch-tar volatiles," said to be a comparable grouping to the benzene-soluble particulates. The government found emissions ranging up to 1.5 milligrams in some plants.

The new standards called for attainment of the .15 level by Jan. 20, 1980. Steps to achieve that standard were to begin when the new regulations took effect on Jan. 20, 1977.

Coke, used in steel-making, was produced by about 65 plants employing 22,000 workers. Protection for the coke-oven workers had been sought by the AFL-CIO United Steelworkers union. The cost of compliance was a major in-

4-Aminodiphenyl (CAS 92671) (29 CFR 1910.1011)

Synonyms: 4-ADP, biphenylamine, biphenyline, p-aminobiphenyl, p-aminodiphenyl, p-biphenylamine, p-phenylaniline, xenylamine, (1,1'-biphenyl)-4-amine, 4-aminobiphenyl, PAB

Description: Colorless crystals darken to yellowish-brown when exposed to air.

Route of Entry: Ingestion, inhalation, and skin absorption.

Use: Not in production or use since 1955.

Health Hazard: Induces bladder tumors in humans. Also causes cancer in rats, mice, and dogs. Traces are found as contaminant in diphenylamine.

Exposure Limits: Solid or liquid mixtures containing more than 0.1% by weight or volume.

—Identification for a container of a suspected carcinogen; from *Working With Carcinogens* (U.S. Department of Health, Education & Welfare)

dustry objection to the standards. When controls were first proposed in 1975, the industry contended that the cost would be about $500 million in capital investment and $295 million in annual operating costs. The government estimate of the cost of compliance with the final version of the rules was $200 million a year.

A petition for review of the Labor Department action was filed later Oct. 20 in the U.S. Circuit Court of Appeals in Philadelphia by the American Iron and Steel Institute, the industry trade association, and six steel companies.

Exposure to benzene curbed. The Labor Department April 29, 1977 issued an emergency order to reduce a worker's exposure to benzene. The chemical had been identified as a cause of leukemia.

The order, effective May 21, was expected to cover 150,000 workers in 1,200 plants.

The permissible level of exposure for a worker was reduced to one part from 10 parts of benzene per million parts of air over an eight-hour average.

The emergency order was issued pending development of permanent standards. Labor Secretary Ray Marshall stressed that the need to act was urgent. "The sad fact is," he said, "that because of exposure to benzene, many workers have died and many are now suffering from leukemia, an irreversible form of cancer."

But the temporary benzene standard never went into effect because of court challenges by the oil industry, a major employer of the workers involved.

The Labor Department issued new rules Feb. 2, 1978 to limit worker exposure to benzene.

Because "the available scientific evidence establishes that employee exposure to benzene presents a cancer danger," Dr. Eula Bingham said in announcing the new rules, "this standard limits employee exposure to benzene to the lowest feasible level." Bingham was director of the Labor Department's Occupational Safety and Health Administration (OSHA).

The rules would require employers to limit worker exposure to the chemical to a maximum of one part per million parts of air over an eight-hour period or five parts per million for any 15-minute period.

The new standard would be a 90% reduction from the department's current permanent standard for an eight-hour period.

Benzene was used in the production of other chemicals that were used in the manufacture of rubber, plastics, resins, disinfectants and pharmaceuticals. It also was used as a component of motor fuels and in the production of detergents, pesticides, and solvents and paint removers.

About 11 billion pounds of benzene were produced in the U.S. annually. The new rules would affect up to 600,000 workers, the department estimated.

The American Petroleum Institute took immediate exception to the new standard in a statement issued later Feb. 2. "OSHA has ignored the fact that there is no evidence that the former exposure standard for benzene is unsafe," it said. "No one disputes that exposure to large amounts of benzene can be harmful, but the new standard is far too rigid and unnecessary."

The statement cautioned that the new standard "may make compliance economically unfeasible."

OSHA Issues Rule for Acrylonitrile. The Occupational Safety and Health Administration issued an "emergency" standard Jan. 16, 1978 to cut worker exposure to acrylonitrile, a chemical widely used in making synthetic fibers and other plastics. The chemical had been linked to cancer in laboratory tests and employee studies.

The new standard would require worker exposure to air-borne acrylonitrile to be limited to no more than two parts per million parts of air, averaged over an eight-hour period. The old standard was 20 parts per million.

A ceiling of 10 parts per million was set for any 15-minute exposure period (no such provision had been in the previous standard).

The requirement was issued on an "emergency temporary" basis.

OSHA Sept. 29 issued a final regulation to limit worker exposure to acrylonitrile.

The new standard would limit worker exposure to acrylonitrile to two parts per million parts of air over an eight-hour period.

The effective date of the rule was Nov. 2 but companies would be given two years from that time to install "engineering controls" to attain the standard.

An OSHA spokesman said the "principal focus" of the new standard was on 5,000 workers at 43 plants operated by 19 producers and major users of acrylonitrile.

The estimated costs of meeting the standard were $110 million in capital outlays and $12 million in annual operating costs (agency estimates).

New Jersey Cancer Rate Studied. The federal government's National Institutes of Health would analyze the factors that made New Jersey's cancer mortality rate the highest in the nation, state environment officials said Jan. 12, 1978. A computerized data bank system would monitor how New Jersey's industry—which used, processed and disposed of many of the 188 known or suspected carcinogenic chemicals—contributed to the state's cancer death rate, which was 14% higher than the national average.

Sleepwear flame-retardant banned. The Consumer Product Safety Commission April 7, 1977 banned production and sale of children's sleepwear treated with a flame-retardant chemical known as Tris because

Coke oven emissions (No CAS number) (29 CFR 1910.1029)

Synonym: Coal tar, aerosol.

Description: Usually black heavy smoke emitted by coke ovens.

Route of Entry: Inhalation and skin absorption.

Use: Byproduct of process to produce coke from coal. Used as raw material for various chemicals and as a source of fuel.

Health Hazard: Causes skin, lung, kidney, and bladder cancer.

Exposure Limits: 150 micrograms per cubic meter (ug/M^3) benzene solubles averaged over any-8-hour period.

—Identification for a container of a suspected carcinogen; from *Working With Carcinogens* (U.S. Department of Health, Education & Welfare)

it was believed able to cause kidney cancer. The commission ordered the recall of 20 million Tris-treated garments from stores and directed them to give refunds to customers who returned treated garments unwashed. However, it did not issue a recall of Tris-treated garments currently in use, as it had been urged to do.

Tris (2, 3 dibromopropyl phosphate) had been used heavily in polyester and acrylic-polyester sleepwear for children in order to meet federal fire safety regulations. Animal tests performed by the National Cancer Institute had indicated a link between Tris and cancer.

The ban had been sought by the Environmental Defense Fund.

U.S. District Court Judge George Hart April 28 ordered the CPSC to extend its ban on Tris to all uses of the chemical. This order had had the effect of a ruling that all branches of the industry—the chemical makers, yarn producers, textile mills, garment manufacturers and retailers—should share the financial burden of the recall and of refunds to consumers. Hart ruled in a suit brought by the American Apparel Manufacturers Association, which had sought to protect the children's garment manufacturers from having to pay the entire cost.

(Hart May 3 essentially repeated the order in ruling against a separate suit brought by Velsicol Chemical Co. that sought to limit liability for the recall and refunds to the garment industry.)

Hart's ruling was upheld by a federal court of appeals May 19. The appeal had been filed by the American Textile Manufacturers Institute.

■ F.W. Woolworth Co. May 18 signed a consent order settling a Justice Department suit, filed May 17, charging the company with noncompliance with the CPSC ban. Woolworth admitted no violation and agreed to recall all Tris-treated garments from its stores.

Judge reverses ban—U.S. District Court Judge Robert F. Chapman in Columbia, S.C. June 23 ruled that Spring Mills, Inc., a South Carolina textile mill, did not have to comply with the Tris ban and did not have to repurchase $2 million worth of Tris-treated material, as ordered by the CPSC Chapman based his order on a finding that the CPSC "had violated its own rule-making procedures" in banning Tris. He said the commission had failed to give Springs Mills an opportunity for a hearing on the ban.

Chapman June 23, acting on Spring Mills' request, upset the CPSC's April ban on the production and sale of children's sleepwear treated with Tris.

Chapman chided the CPSC for violating "procedural safeguards enacted by Congress" in not holding public hearings before imposing the ban.

The judge June 26 enjoined the federal government from ordering the recall of Tris-treated children's wear from the market.

The 4th U.S. Circuit Court of Appeals in Richmond, Va. Aug. 12 refused to reinstate the ban.

The CPSC then filed suit against two chain stores Aug. 19 and Aug. 22 to prevent the sale of children's sleepwear treated with Tris. The first suit was brought against R.H. Macy & Co. in New York City, the second against Zayre Corp., in Boston. U.S. District Court Judge Richard Owen, acting on the CPSC complaint, Aug. 20 ordered Macy's to stop selling the garments in question.

The Environmental Defense Fund Sept. 29 said it had urged three major retailers to stop selling children's sleepware treated with the chemical Fyrol FR-2. The chemical was used by some manufacturers as a flame retardant. The fund believed that Fyrol FR-2, like Tris, could cause cancer if absorbed through the skin. According the fund, the retailers contacted were J. C. Penney Co. Inc., Federated Department Stores Inc. and K-Mart Apparel Corp., a subsidiary of S. S. Kresge Co. (Federated and the CPSC Aug. 31 had agreed on a consent order settling a CPSC complaint on the sale of Tris-treated clothing.)

Reimbursement vetoed—President Carter Nov. 8, 1978 pocket vetoed a bill that required the government to reimburse clothing manufacturers who suffered losses because of the ban on the use of the chemical Tris in children's sleepwear.

The reimbursement bill, which obtained final passage in the House Oct. 12 and the Senate Oct. 13, would have provided an estimated $51 million to manufacturers. Proponents had argued that the businesses should be aided by the government since federal regulations had caused them to lose money. The bill was opposed by consumer groups.

In his veto message, Carter said that the legislation would have "established an unprecedented and unwise use of the taxpayers' funds to indemnify private companies for losses incurred as a result of compliance with a federal standard." He called the ban on Tris "fully justified."

The President, in an accompanying message, asked the Small Business Administration to seek out small cutting and sewing firms that might suffer serious harm because of the veto, "and assist them as much as possible under existing loan programs."

The Consumer Product Safety Commission May 5 had voted to ban the export of children's clothing treated with Tris.

The CPSC's latest action reversed a vote it had taken in October 1977 to allow the exports. At that time, the commission had decided it lacked the legal authority to interfere with the overseas sales of the clothing.

The May 5 vote was prompted by reports that U.S. clothing manufacturers were unloading millions of dollars worth of Tris-treated garments on foreign markets at "distress" prices, usually one-sixth the value of the merchandise.

Protection of Workers from Exposure to Carcinogens

Working With Carcinogens' (a Department of Health, Education & Welfare publication) describes some methods of protecting workers against exposure to carcinogens:

There are four basic methods of limiting employee exposure, and none of these is a simple management decision.

The ***use of an alternative noncarcinogenic material*** is the best method. Changes in product performance, processing, availability of materials, economics, by-products, etc. must be considered. However, more critical, unless the toxic effects of the alternative have been thoroughly evaluated, a seemingly safe replacement, after many years of use, may be found to induce other serious health effects.

Containment or ***isolation of the process*** is the second method preferred. Here, noncarcinogenic chemicals are charged to processing equipment, reacted to form a carcinogen, which is further reacted with other materials to form noncarcinogenic end products, all within the closed system of the process equipment. Local ventilation (hoods or suction lines) should be used to ensure that possible leaks, such as from packing glands or seals of stirrers and pumps, do not allow the carcinogen to enter the environment. Another method is to maintain the process equipment at a slight vacuum so that any leakage is that of external air into the equipment. A variation of this is to enclose (isolate) the process equipment in an enclosure or room which is at a lower pressure than the outside atmosphere.

A third alternative is the ***isolation of employees.*** It frequently involves the use of automated equipment operated by personnel observing from a closed control booth or room. The control room is maintained at a greater air pressure than that surrounding the process equipment so that air flow is out of, rather than into, the room.

The least preferred method is the use of ***personal protective equipment.*** This equipment—respirators, goggles, gloves, barrier creams, air-supplied suits, etc.—should not be used as the only means to prevent exposure during routine operations. The use of personal protective equipment is **required:**

where a leak develops
when a spill occurs
while control mechanisms are being tested, installed, repaired, or are not yet available
where local exhaust at a process equipment opening is insufficient to completely control the escaping substance
while charging carcinogens into otherwise closed systems and where splashing or release of dusts or vapors is likely to occur
when portions of a closed system are impossible to decontaminate prior to opening for maintenance operations
where a breakdown of local controls could result in a serious health hazard
where engineering contro . are impossible or inadequate, such as demolition work involving asbestos products

. . .

Routine surveys should be made by competent industrial hygiene and engineering personnel to ensure that controls are effective. Routine air sampling and swipe samples of work surfaces in and near regulated areas should be used to monitor the effectiveness of controls and work practices in preventing dispersion of the carcinogens. For some substances, analysis of the blood, sputum, urine, or specific body tissues may show when workers have been exposed to conditions which allowed carcinogens to enter the body.

. . .

REGULATED AREAS

A "Regulated Area" must be established by an employer wherever carcinogens are manufactured, processed, used, repackaged, released, handled, or stored. Regulated areas are defined as ***areas where entry and exit is restricted and controlled.*** Only **authorized employees** are allowed in such areas. A daily roster of employees entering regulated areas must be maintained. The rosters, or a summary of the rosters, must be kept for 20 years.

Entrances to regulated areas must be posted with signs stating:

CANCER-SUSPECT AGENT
AUTHORIZED PERSONNEL ONLY

Signs and instructions informing employees of the procedures that must be followed in entering and leaving a regulated area must be posted at the entrance to, and exit from, regulated areas.

The standards **prohibit** the following in regulated areas:

drinking beverages or storage of beverage containers
eating or storage of food
use or storage of cosmetics
smoking or storage of smoking materials
chewing of tobacco or other products for chewing or storage of such products.

Where employees are required to wear protective clothing and wash or shower, the employer must provide clean change rooms and washing and shower facilities. It is especially important that employees use these facilities before leaving at the end of the work shift. Toilets in regulated areas must be in a separate room.

Except for outdoor systems, regulated areas must be maintained at a lower atmospheric pressure than the surrounding nonregulated areas. In other words, ventilation must be such that air cannot move from the regulated area into nonregulated areas. Equipment, materials, or other items taken into, or removed from, a regulated area must be moved in such a manner that the nonregulated areas do not become contaminated by the carcinogens. Procedures for decontamination of materials, equipment, and the decontamination accessories must be developed and used.

. . .

Emergency deluge showers and eyewash fountains supplied with potable water must be located near, within sight of, and on the same level as locations where a direct exposure to carcinogens having corrosive or highly irritating properties (BPL and EI) would most likely occur as a result of equipment failure or from improper work practices.

. . .

MAINTENANCE AND DECONTAMINATION

In areas where direct contact with carcinogens may occur, such as where leaks or spills are cleaned up, or where contaminated systems or equipment are repaired or maintained, employees must wear clean, impervious garments, including gloves, boots, and continuous air-supplied hoods.

Entrances to areas where such work is performed must be posted with signs stating:

CANCER-SUSPECT AGENT EXPOSED IN THIS AREA

IMPERVIOUS SUIT INCLUDING GLOVES, BOOTS, AND AIR-SUPPLIED HOOD REQUIRED AT ALL TIMES

AUTHORIZED PERSONNEL ONLY

The protective garments and hoods must be decontaminated **before** they are removed, and employees must shower after removing them.

Danger in the Air

War on Air-Borne Carcinogens

Despite dispute about the extent of the danger, there are generally accepted indications that some substances that produce cancer come to the victims in the air they breathe. Cancer and other ailments are said to be caused often by fibers, dust and fumes breathed by workers in industrial plants, by factory exhausts breathed by residents of industrial areas, by emanations from autos and trucks and by such other air-borne sources as cigarette smoke and radioactive fallout.

It was reported 20 years ago that U.S. motor vehicles annually spewed into the air some 21.2 billion pounds of "cancer-bearing" hydrocarbons. Cancer-causing asbestos in brake linings may be sprayed into the air wherever motor vehicles are driven. Cigarette smoking is implicated as a cause of lung cancer—affecting non-smokers who breathe the smoke as well as smokers—and air pollution is said to increase susceptibility to smoking-caused lung cancer.

Industry seems to be a great offender. The industry-polluted air of the District of Columbia, it is assumed, has helped give the district the U.S.' highest rate of cancer deaths—168.2 per 100,000 persons. Industrial Maryland is second with a rate of 143.7. New Jersey, with many chemical plants in the state and on its borders, is third at 142.8. Rhode Island is fourth with 142.4. Utah, actively seeking industry, has the lowest rate, 94.6, but a factor may be the Mormon population's avoidance of cancer-implicated cigarettes and alcohol.

The growth of air-borne causes of cancer and other ills has led to an outcry for a cleanup of the air.

Federal guidelines. Guidelines for controlling air pollution were made public Feb. 10, 1969 by Health, Education & Welfare Secretary Robert H. Finch. The guidelines, levels at which sulphur oxides and particulate matter were considered harmful to health: Sulphur oxides averaging .1 parts per million in 24 hours; particulate matter averaging 80 micrograms per cubic meter annually.

Low-pollution auto sought. A federal program to spur competition to develop a low-pollution vehicle for the 1970s was announced Aug. 26, 1969 by Dr. Lee DuBridge, President Nixon's science adviser. The Transportation Department would provide $2.2 million in 1969—and possibly double or triple that amount the following year or two—for research on gasoline and other internal combustion engines and on unconventional steam and electric gas turbine engines that would propel vehicles with a minimum of pollution expulsion. The funds would be shared by the auto makers and other companies developing unconventional engines.

DuBridge made the announcement after President Nixon met at the Western White House in San Clemente, Calif. with his Environmental Quality Council.

The Administration announced July 16, 1970 a research program to develop two alternatives to the internal combustion engine by 1975. John J. Brogan—who was to head the new program within the Health, Education and Welfare Department—said that with the help of the federal project, private industry should be able to produce low-pollution cars by 1980, when strict auto emission standards were scheduled to go into effect.

Trust suit settled. The Justice Department Sept. 11, 1969 announced the settling of an antitrust suit charging the nation's largest auto manufacturers with conspiracy to retard the development and use of air-pollution control devices. Under a consent agreement filed in U.S. District Court in Los Angeles, the department dropped its charges against General Motors Corp., Ford Motor Co. and Chrysler Corp. The auto companies, while admitting no guilt, agreed not to conspire to obstruct anti-smog devices and said they would give royalty-free patent licenses on air pollution inventions and technical information to any company seeking to install such devices.

The consent decree also barred the companies from: (1) restricting publicity about research and development on anti-pollution devices; (2) jointly assessing patents submitted by inventors; or (3) jointly responding to information requests by government regulatory agencies. Company spokesmen denied the charges made in the suit but said they preferred the consent arrangement to a lengthy trial.

Four years later, in a decision made public Nov. 26, 1973, U.S. District Court Judge Manuel L. Real of Los Angeles dismissed 34 consolidated antitrust suits which had accused auto manufacturers of conspiring to delay development of pollution control devices. The suits had been filed by a number of states and localities.

Real said there was a "temptation" to depart from traditional application of antitrust law because of the seriousness of auto pollution. He decided, however, that antitrust laws were meant to preserve "free and unfettered competition" and were not intended as a "panacea" for all social damage caused by industry.

However, Real criticized the auto makers, charging them with conduct "that occasionally bordered on the legerdemain" in their response to public pressure to reduce air pollution. He said the industry's "cross-licensing agreement" on control technology might have hampered development.

Nixon curbs leaded gas. President Nixon Oct. 26, 1970 ordered that all federal vehicles must use low-lead or unleaded gasoline whenever possible. The President also urged the nation's governors to impose similar regulations on state vehicles.

In announcing the action, Russell Train, chairman of the Council on Environmental Quality, said its purpose was "to reduce air pollution and to increase the market for low-lead and unleaded gasoline."

In a letter to the governors, Nixon said joint federal and state action "would offer the gasoline and refinery marketing industries a sizable incentive to produce and distribute low-lead and lead-free gasoline" and "the motorist will be able to buy them and thus make a major contribution to the cleaning up of our air."

Robert L. Kunzig, administrator of the General Services Administration, said the order would apply to gasoline bought as soon as existing stocks were depleted. He said 54% of the present government fleet could be operated on low-lead fuel and that all new vehicles bought by the government would be able to use such fuel. However, officials said Oct. 31 that the order did not apply to existing contracts for bulk purchases of gasoline and that for the next year, most of the fuel bought by the government would be leaded gasoline.

1970 air pollution damage. The EPA estimated Oct. 21, 1974 that air pollution had caused $12.3 billion in damage to human health and property in 1970. The agency said its 1970 estimate, the latest available, was lower than a 1968 estimate because of more complete data and reductions in air pollution..

'72 rules eased. The Department of Health, Education & Welfare Nov. 10, 1970 published final 1972 auto pollution standards, which were slightly less stringent than exhaust limits that had been proposed in July. The rules said new cars produced in the fall of 1972 must emit 25% less hydrocarbons and 17% less carbon monoxide than 1971 models. In July the government had proposed a 35% hydrocarbon reduction and a 20% carbon monoxide reduction, but the auto industry had claimed that there was not enough time to meet these requirements.

Nader probers vs. Muskie. A group of student investigators, sponsored by Ralph Nader's Center for the Study of Responsive Law, said May 12, 1970 that Sen. Edmund S. Muskie (D, Me.) should be "stripped of his title as 'Mr. Pollution Control'" because he had "failed the nation in the field of air pollution control." The charge, contained in a 523-page report released at a Washington, D.C. press conference, centered on the 1967 Air Quality Act, which Muskie had sponsored with Sen. Jennings Randolph (D, W. Va.).

At the press conference, John C. Esposito, chairman of the law, science and medical student group that prepared the air pollution report, said Muskie and Randolph had "worked hand in hand" to create the 1967 act, which so far had been a "'business as usual' license to polluters." The task force report charged that Muskie's insistence on "a cooperative approach with industry" killed a tougher bill proposed by former President Lyndon Johnson that would have set uniform national emission standards for every industry. The group said "not one particle of air pollution from smokestacks has been reduced as a result of the so-called regional approach which is the heart of the [Muskie] act."

In response to the report, Muskie said May 13, "We intend to strengthen the [air pollution] law this year." He said he welcomed "constructive suggestions from any source, including the Nader report." He said the 1967 law was geared towards regional air quality standards tied to national criteria, "not for the dark, secret, conspiratiorial reasons suggested by the Nader report," but because "national emissions standards were described as minimal standards, which we feared might tend to find acceptance as maximum controls." He said national standards "would apply only to industries which could be regarded as 'national' polluters" and not to "other sources which contribute to degradation of the air in our real problem areas."

Clean air bill passed. Both houses of Congress Dec. 18, 1970 approved by voice votes a strong clean air bill requiring development of an automobile engine within six years that would be cleansed of 90% of the pollutants currently emitted by engines. President Richard Nixon signed the bill Dec. 21, 1970.

The deadlines for the cleaner car engine were 1975 for elimination of the hydrocarbon and carbon monoxide pollutants and 1976 for elimination of nitrogen oxide pollutants.

In other areas, the bill called for establishment of national air quality standards, to be put into effect within 5½ years for 10 major polluting substances. An additional two years for compliance could be granted upon the request of a governor in special cases involving a polluting plant.

An order against a polluter could be issued by the administrator of the Environmental Protection Agency (EPA), who would have further recourse to the Justice Department and, if the Justice Department did not act, could file suit himself. Fines of $25,000 a day and jail sentences of a year were applicable against first offenders; second offenses were liable to double penalties.

Other provisions authorized the federal government to require a new plant to have the latest pollution control equipment and the EPA administrator to set zero emission levels for substances deemed hazardous.

The original version of the measure, passed by 73–0 Senate vote Sept. 22, had been worked out in Sen. Edmund S. Muskie's pollution subcommittee.

Although the bill, as it emerged from the Senate Public Works Committee Sept. 11, provided a possible one-year extension of the 1975 auto pollution deadline, the auto industry claimed the requirement was technically impossible to meet.

Sen. Robert P. Griffin (R, Mich.) supported the industry position in the only lengthy floor debate against the bill. To Griffin's protest that the exhaust emission requirement would raise the price of cars, Muskie replied that the principal issue was public health.

Jet plane pollution accord. The major U.S. airlines agreed Jan. 20, 1970 to meet a 1972 deadline proposed by the Nixon Administration to end smoke pollution from jet airliners. Health, Education and Welfare (HEW) Secretary Robert H. Finch and Transportation Secretary John A. Volpe, after meeting with officials of 31 carriers, said the airlines had agreed to begin installation within 90 days of antipollution devices on JT8D jet engines.

The engines, produced by the Pratt & Whitney division of United Aircraft Corp. and used to power the Boeing Co.'s 727 and 737 jets and the McDonnell Douglas Corp.'s DC9, allegedly caused 70% of all pollution from jets. Industry spokesmen claimed that jet smoke accounted for only 1% of air pollution in the nation, but officials of the HEW National Air Pollution Control Administration argued that the problem around major airports was considerably more severe.

The airlines earlier had told federal officials that installation of antipollution devices could be completed by 1974, but the Nixon Administration had threatened to support restrictive legislation if the industry refused to speed up the program.

EPA sets clean air standards. The Environmental Protection Agency April 30, 1971 announced "tough" national pollution standards that would limit permissible amounts of six major air pollutants by 1975. The standards, described by EPA Administrator William D. Ruckelshaus, were issued under provisions of the 1970 Clean Air Act.

To satisfy the standards, Ruckelshaus said, there would have to be "drastic" changes in industrial and electric power practices and in "commuting habits" of persons living near large metropolitan areas. He said many electric generating plants would have to switch from high-sulphur coal to "clean" fuel and warned that the consumer's electric bills might go up.

Ruckelshaus June 29 issued final rules for reducing auto exhaust pollutants as required by the Clean Air Act of 1970. Ruckelshaus said the standards were "stringent" and would "challenge the ingenuity of American industry." He also predicted that the cost of meeting the standards by the 1975 and 1976 deadlines would be "substantial, both to the industry and the consumer."

The 1970 act required a 90% reduction in carbon monoxide and hydrocarbon emissions on 1975 models and a 90% reduction in nitrogen oxide emissions on 1976 models. The new EPA rules said this would limit emissions in grams per mile to the following levels: carbon monoxide, 3.4; hydrocarbons, .41; nitrogen oxides, 3 (1973 models), .4 (1976 models).

Air quality improved. The EPA reported May 7, 1973 an improvement in air quality in many urban areas in the 1960–1971 period. The agency noted, however, that the assessment dealt only with sulfur oxides and particulate matter, not with carbon monoxide and other pollution caused by motor vehicles.

About half of the 200 regions surveyed showed a general decrease in pollutants, but 27 areas showed an increase from 1968 to 1971. In the latter category were eight of the 28 rural areas checked, including such scenic regions as Glacier National Park, Mont. and Black Hills National Monument, S.D.

Stress on Auto Pollution

N.J. orders annual tests. New Jersey environmental officials Jan. 6, 1972 ordered into effect a program of annual vehicle inspections, to enforce strict new limits on automobile exhaust pollution.

All gasoline-fueled vehicles weighing 3 tons or less would be given a 30-second exhaust test each year; those exceeding legal emission limits or having visible exhausts would be marked with a red sticker, banning them from the road within two weeks if not brought up to standards.

The program was to begin on a voluntary basis July 1, become mandatory after a year and become annually more stringent until 1975. Standards would vary depending on model year.

Hawaii to limit autos. Hawaii Gov. John A. Burns (D) signed a bill setting up a Transportation Control Commission, that would make annual recommendations to the legislature on the maximum number of automobiles and other transportation vehicles to be permitted on each island, it was reported May 25, 1972.

California used car rule. A California regulation effective in September 1972 required that all cars in model years 1955–65 be fitted with exhaust controls when the vehicles changed ownership or were brought into the state, at an individual cost of as much as $85.

The state's Air Resources Board ruled Oct. 25 that 1966–70 model cars would have to install a new emission control device, costing up to $35 a car, by early 1975. Cars in the South Coast Air Basin, stretching from northern San Diego County to Santa Barbara, would have to be equipped by February 1974.

EPA eases rules. The EPA proposed Nov. 6, 1972 that catalytic converters in automobile exhaust controls be required to last for only 25,000 miles, rather than 50,000 as originally proposed. It was a concession to automobile manufacturers who claimed they might not otherwise be able to meet the 1975 model year deadline for a 90% reduction of pollutants.

EPA asks LA gas rationing. Environmental Protection Agency (EPA) Administrator William D. Ruckelshaus Jan. 15, 1973 announced an air pollution-control proposal for the Los Angeles Basin. The plan included a gasoline rationing system designed to reduce automobile use by up to 82% during summer months by 1977. But Ruckelshaus said he had "grave doubts" that such a plan was feasible, and said it had been issued only to meet a court order and to stimulate further debate on how to meet federal pollution guidelines or on whether to adjust the standards to the special social and meteorological conditions of the area.

The EPA had been ordered by a U.S. district court in November 1972 to come up with a plan for the region, the only area in the country for which a state had not submitted a plan for reaching the national standard of .08 parts per million (ppm) of photochemical oxidants.

Under the plan, rationing would be undertaken beginning in 1975, with rations changing each month and enforced either by consumer coupons or limited distribution to retailers. The plan included other measures, but without rationing, Ruckelshaus said, pollution would still exceed the limit by one-half.

Ruckelshaus said the proposal would have severe effects on the region, which he said was uniquely dependent on automobiles for transportation and for its "lifestyle," with nearly 6 million motor vehicles for its 10 million population. He denied that the proposal had been aired to pressure Congress to modify the 1970 Clean Air Act, which he called "a great success" nationally.

Court bars enforcement delay. The U.S. Court of Appeals for the District of Columbia ordered EPA Jan. 31 to rescind its approval of a two-year delay in enforcement of some primary air pollution control standards for 17 states, pending further study to determine whether the control technology was available.

Under the 1970 Clean Air Act, states had been required to submit plans by Jan. 31, 1972 for meeting primary ambient standards for six pollutants, and the maximum quantity of the substances in the air consistent with public health, by May 1975. EPA Administrator William D. Ruckelshaus had ruled in 1971 that states could delay submission until Feb. 15, 1973 of those parts of the plans relating to transportation controls, which would limit carbon monoxide and photochemical oxidants, because the technology of emission control and the experience of transportation alternatives were not sufficiently developed. Ruckelshaus had further announced May 31, 1972, that he had accepted the request of 17 states for a two-year delay in the 1975 deadline for enforcing those parts of the plans.

The Clean Air Act had allowed for two-year extensions, but the court ruled that EPA could not grant the delays until after the plans were filed and analyzed. The court ordered the agency to require the 17 states to submit plans by April 15 for full compliance by 1975, and barred the agency from approving a delay unless it determined that compliance was impossible.

The suit had been brought by the Natural Resources Defense Council.

EPA delays auto curb. The Environmental Protection Agency April 11, 1973 granted the automobile industry a one-year delay in 1975 emission control standards but set relatively strict interim standards for that year.

Following the recommendation made at EPA hearings by General Motors Corp. March 12 and Ford Motor Co. March 13, EPA agreed to two sets of 1975 standards, one for California, which was particularly plagued by air pollution, that would reduce hydrocarbon and carbon monoxide emissions about two-thirds of the way toward the original 1975 goal, and one for the rest of the country, which would go about half way toward the original goal.

The California limits would be .9 grams of hydrocarbons and 9 grams of carbon monoxide per mile, while the national standard would be 1.5 grams of hydrocarbon and 15 grams of carbon monoxide.

Cars built for the California market, about 10% of national production, would be equipped with catalytic converters, the device that all the Detroit automakers had chosen to meet the 1975 goals, but which they said presented still unresolved operational problems.

The 1970 Clean Air Act had provided for a one-year delay, if the EPA administrator found that automakers had tried to meet the goals in "all good faith." Ruckelshaus said the good faith issue had been "particularly troublesome" with regard to Chrysler Corp., and said he might have ruled against Chrysler "if Congress had provided me with some sanctions short of the nuclear deterrent—in effect—closing down that major corporation."

Ford fined $7 million. The Ford Motor Co. was assessed $7 million in civil and criminal penalties in U.S. court in Detroit Feb. 13, 1973 for violating the Clean Air Act by improperly servicing 1973 model cars undergoing emission control tests during 1971 and 1972.

Ford was fined $3.5 million, the maximum penalty under the law, for 350 counts of criminal violation, and entered into a consent decree for $3.5 million more in civil penalties. The company was also ordered to keep better records of its test procedures, and to warn all employes that violations could make them liable to punishment by the courts or by the company.

U.S. Attorney Ralph B. Guy Jr. said the settlement "helps demonstrate that the government means business in enforcing the provisions of the Clean Air Act."

Curbs for urban areas. The EPA June 15, 1973 announced transportation curbs for 17 urban areas in an effort to curb air pollution generated by motor vehicles. The agency also approved a traffic control plan submitted for New York City. The goal, said EPA Acting Administrator Robert W. Fri, was to force a change in the public's "long-standing and intimate relation to private automobiles," and to bring urban areas into substantial compliance with the Clean Air Act of 1970 by July 1, 1975.

The EPA proposed its own compliance schedules after most jurisdictions failed to submit pollution control plans or submitted deficient plans.

The EPA Oct. 15 issued final rules for the 17 urban areas. The rules generally followed those announced in June.

The major departure from the earlier proposals was an easing of planned gasoline sales limitations for Los Angeles and several other areas. Under the new rules, such areas as Los Angeles, San Francisco and Houston-Galveston, Tex. would face "contingency" restrictions on fuel sales by 1977 if they were otherwise unable to meet pollution standards. Even the eased fuel restrictions could be further postponed, EPA Administrator Russell E. Train said, if Congress acceded to EPA's proposals to soften some of the provisions of the 1970 Clean Air Act.

Most of the areas involved were ordered to institute restrictions on inner-city parking, encourage car-pooling and promote the use of mass transit.

The Houston-Galveston area was also required to curb stationary pollution sources by prohibiting construction or modification of industrial installations which might add to hydrocarbon concentrations.

The EPA Nov. 20 announced transportation control plans for the Washington metropolitan area and Chicago designed to curb downtown auto traffic and increase reliance on mass transit.

Under the Washington plan (which included parts of Maryland and Virginia), a commuter parking surcharge would be imposed in mid-1975 beginning at 50¢ a day rising to $2 a day by 1977. The revenues would finance mass transit improvements.

The Chicago proposal called for restrictions on downtown stopping and standing, parking surcharges to finance mass transit, a program of annual vehicle emission inspection for all of Cook County similar to one already in effect in Chicago and installation of catalytic converters on taxis.

EPA bars catalyst delay. EPA Administrator Russell Train Nov. 6, 1973 rejected any delay in imposition of emission control standards for 1975 model autos, despite evidence that catalytic exhaust converters planned for use by manufacturers could create new hazards possibly more dangerous than the hydrocarbons and carbon monoxide they were designed to control.

Train told the Senate Public Works Committee that sulfur-related pollutants produced by the catalysts would not reach potentially dangerous levels until well into the second year of use of the converters. By that time, Train said, the EPA would have had time to determine whether fears of health hazards were justified. If so, the problem could be met by requiring installation of additional equipment on cars and removal of sulfur from gasoline.

A dispute had developed within the EPA over the issue of sulfur pollution, it was reported Oct. 15. EPA researchers had reported that catalysts, while oxidizing carbon monoxide and hydrocarbons, would convert small amounts of sulfur in gasoline into sulfates and sulfuric acid mists, which would be harmful to persons suffering from bronchitis or asthma, and—in high concentrations—could be related to lung cancer and heart disease. It was also found that the converters emitted small particles of platinum, a potential source of respiratory ailments.

While researchers urged a delay in installing converters to allow further study, regulatory officials in the agency contended that a delay of the 1975 standards was unjustified, since concentrations could not reach problem levels until a large proportion of all autos were equipped with converters. Although he rejected a postponement of controls, Train told the committee the EPA would step up research on sulfate emissions and consider proposing rules limiting sulfur in fuel.

A spokesman for Mobil Oil Corp. told the committee Nov. 5 that removal of sulfur from gasoline was an unrealistic goal which would require major refinery investments and aggravate the fuel shortage by adding to the burden of an "already overloaded" industry.

Widening Regulation

EPA delays state plans. The Environmental Protection Agency (EPA) May 31, 1972 announced its rulings on clean air plans submitted by the states. Eleven states and three other jurisdictions received complete approval, while 27 cities in 18 states were granted two-year extensions beyond the 1975 deadline for meeting primary health emission standards for six classes of pollutants.

For the most part, EPA Administrator William Ruckelshaus said, the agency was granting the additional time because it was still "having difficulty relating transportation controls to air pollution."

Ruckelshaus reported that large parts of some state plans had been disapproved, and warned that the EPA had legal authority to write its own rules in such cases if revised plans were not approved by July 31.

Ruckelshaus said that the number of Americans living in areas exceeding primary pollution standards would drop by 1975 to 80 million from the 1972 figure of 170 million, while by 1977 "essentially every urban area should have air that meets the primary standards."

The jurisdictions receiving complete approval were Alabama, American Samoa, Colorado, Connecticut, Florida, Guam, Mississippi, New Hampshire, North Carolina, North Dakota, Oregon, Puerto Rico, South Dakota and West Virginia.

The EPA proposed changes in the air plans of 24 states and the Virgin Islands June 14, including tougher controls in 10 states to meet federal emission standards for nitrogen oxides and hydrocarbons.

The 10 states facing tougher emission controls were Georgia, Louisiana, Maryland, Massachusetts, Michigan, Missouri, New Jersey, Tennessee, Texas and Washington. The other 15 jurisdictions faced changes in measurement techniques, record-keeping or public access to data. The EPA also announced June 14 that the effective date for the nitrogen oxide emission limit of 100 micrograms per cubc meter would be delayed 11 months to July 1, 1973, because of evidence that previous measurement methods had been unreliable.

The states had been required to devise practical measures in each air quality region that would reduce the concentration per cubic meter of air of six classes of pollutants below maximum levels set by the EPA in 1971. The plans were to include, besides conventional controls of existing plant emissions and waste incineration, methods to reduce automobile use through traffic control, parking limits and better mass transit systems.

No deterioration permitted—A three judge panel of the U.S. Court of Appeals for the District of Columbia upheld without comment Nov. 2 a lower court decision barring EPA Administrator William D. Ruckelshaus from accepting any state air pollution control plan that would tolerate a significant deterioration of air quality even in regions whose air met the strictest federal standards.

In appealing the lower court ruling, Ruckelshaus had said the decision would effectively prevent nearly all industrial or residential development in rural areas. But the four environmental groups whose suit resulted in the new rule had proposed that EPA interpret "significant" deterioration as a rise by 10% or five micrograms per cubic meter, whichever was greater, in any of five categories of pollutants in a region's air.

EPA orders Delaware curb. The Environmental Protection Agency (EPA), in the first regular legal action under the 1970 Clean Air Act, March 8, 1972 ordered Delmarva Power & Light Co. of Delaware City, Del. to cut back on sulphur dioxide emissions that violated the EPA-approved state pollution control plan.

The power company had obtained a court order enjoining the state Water and Air Resources Commission from enforcing the state plan, which had called for a 40% sulphur dioxide emission cut for New Castle County by Jan. 1. The EPA gave the company 30 days to comply, by purchasing low-sulphur fuel, or face penalties of up to $25,000 a day.

The Supreme Court Jan. 15, 1973 refused to review the EPA order. It thereby upheld the order, which required Delmarva to stop burning high-sulphur fuel. The Getty Oil Co., Delmarva's fuel supplier, had challenged the order. Getty had since agreed to supply lower-sulphur fuel immediately, and switch to 1% sulphur content fuel by Jan. 1, 1974, it was reported Jan. 16.

Aircraft curbs. The EPA Dec. 4, 1972 announced a series of curbs on aircraft pollution emissions to go into effect between 1974 and 1979, including a ban on the venting of unburned fuel during and after takeoff. The agency attributed much of the delay from Sept. 27, 1971, when the proposals were legally due, to the need for testing and data collection; discussions with the Federal Aviation Administration on safety factors in the new rules had also contributed to the delay.

But the EPA then announced July 6, 1973 that the proposals for aircraft engines would be relaxed and that the effective dates would be delayed. Most rules which had been scheduled to become effective between 1974 and 1979 would be postponed to the 1979–1981 period.

The EPA dropped a proposed rule to impose maximum emission levels on engines manufactured after 1975, and standards set for a second deadline of Jan. 1, 1979 were relaxed to a "more technically feasible level." For large airliners, the new rules specified a 60% reduction from current levels of carbon monoxide emissions and reductions of 50% for nitrogen oxides and 70% for hydrocarbons.

A rule requiring installation of smoke suppressors on Boeing 707s and Douglas DC-8s was postponed from 1976 to 1978.

The rules affected all civilian aircraft except helicopters and supersonic transports.

The EPA also announced an agreement with the Federal Aviation Administration for a trial program to cut emissions while planes were on the ground. Under the plan, airliners at airports in Los Angeles and Washington would taxi with one engine shut down.

New industrial rules. The EPA June 5, 1973 issued rules limiting emission of particulates and hydrocarbons in seven categories of industry. The rules, which would affect new plants and modifications of existing plants that would increase their emissions, called for reductions ranging from 80%–99.7% of uncontrolled levels.

The industries affected were: asphalt concrete plants, petroleum refineries, petroleum storage tanks, secondary lead smelters, secondary brass and bronze ingot production plants, iron and steel plants using basic oxygen furnaces and sewage treatment plant incenerators. The agency allowed 45 days for comment before putting the rules into effect.

Federal contract curbs proposed. Under rules proposed June 21 by the EPA, industrial recipients of federal contracts, loans or grants would lose federal funds if convicted of criminal violations of the 1970 Clean Air Act. Non-criminal violations would nullify contracts larger than $100,000. The rules would also affect subcontractors indirectly benefiting from government business.

Power plant & smelter rules relaxed. The EPA Sept. 6, 1973 issued new rules for electric utilities and nonferrous-metal smelters which would retain the agency's "primary" emission standards (protection of human health) but allow an alternative to the previously required installation of expensive "scrubbing" equipment on plant smokestacks to meet the standards.

According to old rules, companies had to decide under state deadlines whether to install the scrubbing mechanism to curb pollution or to burn costly low-sulfur fuels. The new alternative would allow many plants to continue emitting pollutants at current levels until company-operated monitors determined that maximum allowable concentrations might be reached. Plants would then be required to cut back operations or close temporarily.

Critics of the rules had predicted blackouts in urban areas if power plants were allowed to emit pollutants until the stagnant air conditions common in summer months forced cutbacks in operations when power demand was highest. Acting EPA Administrator John R. Quarles Jr. said Sept. 6, however, that utilities in large urban areas would not be allowed to take advantage of the alternative.

Some critics said the rules would stifle the incentive to develop better plant equipment to clean emissions. Laurence I. Moss, president of the conservationist Sierra Club, also noted that the rules would put antipollution enforcement "in the hands of industry." The rules were to take effect in 30 days.

U.S. Steel pollution cases. The State of Pennsylvania and Allegheny County filed a civil suit in the County Court of Common Pleas Feb. 11, 1972 against U.S. Steel Corp., to obtain compliance at the company's Clairton steel works with county air pollution limits. The suit was settled Sept. 25 when U.S. Steel signed a consent decree to begin a massive program of air pollution abatement at the plant.

Allegheny officials said the plant, the world's largest private steel mill, poured 225 tons of pollutants a day into the atmosphere, creating a public nuisance, endangering health, and violating the state's constitutional guarantee of clean air. United Steelworkers local president Daniel Hannan supported the suit, citing high rates of lung cancer and other ailments among employes.

The corporation's vice president for environmental control, Harold Mallik, said Feb. 11 "there is no way to bring the works into compliance," although $15 million had already been spent on controls and another $25 million was pledged. The company claimed that its practice of quenching hot coke with polluted water from other plant processes, creating polluted steam, was necessitated by laws against dumping the tainted water into local sewer systems. County officials said other area steel plants successfully treated such polluted water.

Over $17,000 in fines had been levied against U.S. Steel since November 1971, when the County Air Pollution Appeals Board denied the plant's request for a waiver.

U.S. Steel signed the consent decree after it had obtained assurances that the Environmental Protection Agency would approve a compromise under which the state promised to extend the company's compliance deadline from 1975 to 1977.

A federal spokesman said the settlement was the most expensive commitment by any company to combat pollution. The Wall Street Journal said Nov. 30 steel industry sources estimated total costs at $70 million.

The EPA and U.S. Steel reached agreement, reported Sept. 11, 1974, for air pollution control measures at the firm's steel and cement facilities in Gary, Ind. The consent decree settled a suit filed by the government and a countersuit by the company.

According to an EPA spokesman, the Gary facilities were "the largest industrial air pollution source to date to be put on an enforcement clean-up schedule." The EPA said the shutdown of older facilities and installation of pollution abatement equipment required in the agreement would eliminate 70,000 tons of particulate emissions a year. The control program would be undertaken in steps through Nov. 30, 1976.

Faced with a federal court order to either shut its No. 4 hearth in Gary or pay a fine of $2,300 a day for as long as 90 days to keep the facility open, the U.S. Steel Corp. closed down the 10 open-hearth furnaces that comprised the plant, effective Jan. 1, 1975. A federal judge had issued the ruling setting the options Dec. 26, 1974, after hearing arguments on the firm's request for a six-month extension of a consent decree ordering the shutdown of the Gary works because of failure to implement anti-pollution measures. Federal and local agencies had charged that emissions violated air quality regulations.

In remarks reported Jan. 3, Russell Quarles, EPA deputy administrator, said the EPA had allowed U.S. Steel reasonable time to install clean furnaces and he accused the corporation of "an unacceptable degree of delay." The American Iron and Steel Institute reported Jan. 2 that U.S. Steel's permanent closing of the Gary furnace was the industry's first such action taken under an environmental order.

According to the Wall Street Journal Jan. 10, most of the facility's 549 workers had been laid off when the operation closed. U.S. Steel had forecast total layoffs of 2,500, including temporary furloughs in related industries.

U.S. Steel agreed May 31 to pay Alabama $35,000 in air-pollution fines for a gradual phase-out over the next 13 months of five open-hearth steelmaking furnaces near Birmingham. The deadline for compliance with local, state and federal clean-air laws was midnight May 31, and Alabama clean-air authorities had refused to grant the company extra time to clean up its Birmingham operation, which emitted 7,500 tons of reddish iron dust into the environment every year.

The state authorities directed the company to work out a "reasonable settlement" with the state Attorney General, Bill Baxley, who insisted that a token fine must be a condition of any agreement to operate in violation past the deadline. Without any agreement, the company faced possible state and federal prosecution.

The federal Environmental Protection Agency, entering the dispute with the company and state and local officials at impasse, refused to grant the company another year to clean up the Birmingham operation and ordered it to begin phasing out the violating facilities within five weeks.

The company reached a compromise with the federal officials May 30, but Baxley declined to accept it without the principle of the fine. "They have this intolerable, bully-boy attitude that the law does not apply to them," he commented. The company had threatened to close its hearths rather than pay a fine, and it had contended that construction difficulties had delayed replacing the violating facilities with more modern ones.

Under the final compromise, the company, in addition to paying the $35,000 fine, would close two of the open-hearth furnaces by June 30, the remaining three by June 30, 1976.

Baxley's comment: "Even giants must obey the law."

In a June 16, 1977 consent decree, U.S. Steel again agreed to end clean-air violations at the Gary plant and at its Universal Atlas Cement division, also in Gary. A $250,000 fine was part of this settlement for failing to meet the EPA's 1976 deadline. The company simultaneously agreed to install $70 million worth of water-pollution-control equipment and to pay a $4 million fine for not meeting the EPA's clean-water deadline.

The EPA's order setting a July 1 deadline had been upheld by a three-judge panel of the U.S. Circuit Court of Appeals in Chicago May 13.

In the consent decree entered in U.S. District Court in Hammond, Ind. June 16, a new deadline of Aug. 1, 1980 was set for having the pollution-control equipment in place.

The equipment was expected to reduce the discharge of pollutants into Lake Michigan and the Grand Calumet River, which flowed into the lake.

Curbs on Anaconda plant upheld. The U.S. Court of Appeals for the 10th Circuit held in Denver Aug. 8, 1973 that the EPA could enforce its order that the

Anaconda Co. remove 89% of sulfur oxide emissions from a smelter in Montana. The ruling overturned a lower court decision delaying enforcement of the EPA action against the company by requiring the EPA to prepare an environmental impact statement on the emission curbs.

The ruling said the lower court had improperly interfered before completion of the EPA's administrative proceedings, an action which, the appeals court said, would "frustrate" the EPA's "sole mission to improve the quality of the human environment."

The EPA had acted after Montana Gov. Forrest H. Anderson had refused to submit to the EPA a plan drawn up in December 1971 by the Montana Board of Health, which had called for a 90% reduction. Anderson said the plan might drive the smelting industry out of the state.

Anaconda claimed it could meet federal ambient air standards for the region surrounding the plant by reducing emissions by only 40%, at a cost of $30.7 million. The company said it would have to spend an additional $60 million to meet the higher standards.

Federal Judge Fred M. Winner ruled in Denver Dec. 6 that the EPA had to prepare an environmental impact statement before setting sulphur oxide emission limits for the Anaconda plant.

Pennsylvania air plans upheld. Judge Francis L. Van Dusen of the U.S. Court of Appeals for the 3rd Circuit upheld most parts of automobile pollution control plans imposed by the EPA for the Philadelphia and Pittsburgh areas, it was reported July 5, 1974.

The plans called for installation of emission control devices on all autos in the two metropolitan areas by 1977, and required the state to arrange car pools and other commuter services.

Rejecting arguments by the state, Van Dusen upheld the constitutionality of provisions of the Clean Air Act of 1970—the authority for imposition of the plans—which required states to enact laws and regulations implementing federal laws.

Auto standards backed. The National Academy of Sciences said in a report released Sept. 6, 1974 that it had found no "substantial basis" for changing the automobile emission standards set by the Environmental Protection Agency (EPA). The study had been commissioned by the Senate Public Works Committee after auto manufacturers had petitioned for relaxed rules in hearings held in late 1973.

While totally supporting the rules curbing two of the three types of auto emissions—hydrocarbons and carbon monoxide—the report said some minor changes might be considered for regulations applying to the third type, nitrogen oxides.

The study concluded that economic benefits that could be expected from implementation of the standards would be "commensurate with the expected costs." The report also estimated that as many as 4,000 deaths and four million illness-related work days missed each year could be currently attributed to auto pollution in urban areas.

The academy complained that while the available evidence provided sufficient support for the standards, the "data base" found in previous studies was unsatisfactory. The report urged that federal expenditures for auto pollution studies be substantially increased.

Scientists back timetable—The National Research Council June 4, 1975 released a report by a special panel of scientists that said the current timetable for reducing exhaust pollution from automobiles was feasible and its goals attainable without impairing the drive for fuel economy. The council was a unit of the National Academy of Sciences and the National Academy of Engineering.

The report said the schedule mandated by legislation should be kept for reduction of the two major car pollutants, hydrocarbons and carbon monoxide. It said the timetable, through the 1978-model year, could be met by use of catalytic converters, and further, that the potential danger from emissions produced by the converters of sulphuric acid and acid sulphates had been exaggerated by the Environmental Protection Agency.

The panel recommended establishment of a sulphuric-acid emission standard beginning with the 1978-model year, and it suggested that the problem could be eased substantially by dropping the sulphur content of gasoline, at a cost of one cent to two cents a gallon.

On another exhaust pollutant from cars, nitrogen oxide, the panel favored retention of the statutory standard of .4 grams a mile for 1978 models. It said if the standard were relaxed at all, it should not be in heavy pollution areas.

Energy Crisis Complicates Anti-Pollution Campaign

The growing energy dilemma added to the difficulty of efforts to keep hazardous pollution out of the air. Few sources of energy could be used without increasing pollution and the danger of causing cancer or other ailments.

Oil firms seek waiver. Oil distributors said Jan. 26, 1973 that they had asked Pennsylvania, New Jersey, New York, Connecticut, Massachusetts and Rhode Island to reduce air pollution standards in order to permit the burning of home heating oil with a sulfur content higher than currently allowable.

New York City acted Jan. 24 to permit Texaco, Inc. to sell fuel oil with a sulfur level eight to ten times higher than the law allowed. The variance was effective for 45 days but it included a pollution tax on every barrel of high sulfur oil sold.

Texaco lost its waiver bid in New Jersey, where it supplied 12% of the home fuel, according to the Washington Post Jan. 26.

W.Va. grants delay. The West Virginia Air Pollution Control Commission bowed to a demand by Gov. Arch A. Moore Jr. and granted a two-year delay Feb. 1 on 1975 fly ash and sulfur dioxide emission limits for the American Electric Power System.

The utility had claimed that it could not obtain enough low-sulfur coal, and threatened to import coal from Western states in competition with the local product. Environmentalists replied that the state had enough reserves of adequate coal, and said high-moisture Western coal would produce excessive fly ash in power plants built for dryer coal.

Nixon asks relaxation of clean air rules. President Nixon held a two-hour conference with 15 Administration officials Sept. 8, 1973 on the problems of energy supplies, development of alternative sources of fuel and increased production from U.S. oil reserves. Following the meeting, the President made an appearance at a White House press conference on the energy situation conducted by John A. Love, director of the Office of Energy Policy.

Nixon urged that the states relax antipollution laws in an effort to overcome the expected shortage of fuel oil during the winter. Although the federal government had no power to limit state laws, Nixon said Love would meet with governors and local officials from the Northeast and Midwest during the next two weeks to lobby for modifications in environmental standards. States would be asked to permit the burning of higher sulfur grade oil by utilities and other large users which had been diverting short supplies of low sulfur content heating oil from residential consumers. The Administration also planned to allow increased imports of higher sulfur fuel oil.

Nixon also said he was determined to give "new impetus" to development of nuclear power and licensing of new plants.

Nixon also noted that the U.S. possessed an estimated half of the known world reserves of coal, but lacked the technology to convert the fuel into a clean energy supply.

Train differs with White House—Russell E. Train, who was confirmed by an 85–0 Senate vote Sept. 10 as administrator of the Environmental Protection Agency, said Sept. 11 that he would oppose relaxation of clean air standards unless the Administration implemented a mandatory allocation program for fuel oil at the same time that antipollution rules were eased.

A mandatory program, Train said, would insure that low sulfur oil was allocated for areas where air pollution levels were high.

Another EPA official, Assistant Administrator Robert L. Sansom, had objected to Administration efforts to link environmental restrictions to the worsening energy shortage. "The heating oil problem is going to be blamed on the environmentalists instead of on the restrictions on oil imports," Sansom said Aug. 20.

New York relaxes anti-pollution laws—New York City and state officials, reacting to a critical shortage of low sulphur content fuel oil, authorized the city's Consolidated Edison Co. to burn oil containing more than the .3% sulphur limit allowed under anti-pollution laws.

The city's Environmental Protection Administration acted Nov. 19 to temporarily ease the sulphur restrictions, but officials warned that burning of the dirtier fuel oil would result in an increase of at least 10% in the amount of sulphur dioxide in the air. An estimated 50% of the city would have unhealthy levels of the gas, in contrast to the current level of 20%, spokesmen said.

Consolidated Edison's request that the burning of coal be allowed was denied on grounds that an intolerable level of filth would be added to the city's air; however, state officials ruled Nov. 27 that the power company could burn coal in two generating stations within the city.

Parking curbs dropped. The Environmental Protection Agency Jan. 10, 1974 announced that it was withdrawing the portions of its urban auto control plans which would have imposed parking surcharges and commuter taxes in nine metropolitan areas.

EPA Administrator Russell E. Train said the decision was based on "firm Congressional guidance" in the form of proposed legislation prohibiting federal imposition of the surcharges. However, Train noted that the EPA action would not prevent states and localities from imposing similar plans.

The urban areas involved were Washington, Boston, Newark, N.J., Chicago, and, in California, Los Angeles, San Francisco, San Diego, Sacramento, and the San Joaquin Valley.

The EPA, however, served notice Aug. 12 that it intended to enforce fully the other portions of the federally devised restrictions on traffic and auto-related air pollution in major metropolitan areas.

Technically, the latest action involved only Boston, but an EPA spokesman said it should be viewed as an example of the agency's intentions.

Under the Boston plan, employers of 50 or more persons were required to submit mass transit and car pool incentive programs designed to reduce employe parking by 25%. About half of the affected companies had complied by the July 31 deadline, and the EPA warned that failure to comply by an extended deadline of Aug. 19 could result in legal action.

The plan for the Boston area also included restrictions on downtown nonresidential parking, a freeze on commercial garage construction and a requirement for installation of emission control devices on older cars.

Clean air rules eased. By voice votes in the House June 11, 1974 and in the Senate June 12, Congress approved a compromise measure setting rules for conversion to coal by oil- and gas-burning plants and extending to the 1977 model year the EPA's strict standards for auto exhaust emissions. President Nixon signed this Energy Supply & Environmental Coordination Act of 1974 June 22.

The principal differences between House and Senate versions had been in the coal-conversion standards. The conference committee measure, which leaned towards the original Senate bill, provided that the administrator of the Federal Energy Administration (FEA) could order immediate conversion to coal if a plant could comply with the emission standards of the Clean Air Act. If the plant could not comply immediately, conversion could be ordered after acquisition of control equipment or low-sulfur coal.

Plants which converted to coal voluntarily between Sept. 15, 1973 and March 15, 1974, or converted afterwards under FEA order, would be exempt from strict compliance with state emission rules, if emissions did not exceed EPA standards set for the affected air quality region.

Two other provisions in the Senate bill—EPA exemption from environmental impact statement requirements, and extension of funding for enforcement of the Clean Air Act—were included in the compromise measure.

The Nixon Administration requests, designed to meet the demands of the energy crisis, had gone to Congress March 22.

The proposed amendments to the Clean Air Act of 1970 represented a compromise between the White House Office of Management and Budget (OMB), which had backed sweeping revisions, and Environmental Protection Agency (EPA) Administrator Russell E. Train, who had opposed too drastic a weakening of air quality standards.

EPA retreats on air rules. The Environmental Protection Agency Aug. 16, 1974 published revised regulations under which states would have the primary role in setting air pollution standards for areas where the air was cleaner than required by current federal regulations. Courts had ruled in 1972 and 1973 that states could not allow "significant deterioration" of existing clean air. (The new rules were issued by the EPA Nov. 27.)

The thrust of the proposed regulations would be to give states the option in setting priorities between industrial growth and the preservation of clean air.

States would be allowed to designate their clean-air areas according to three classifications: Class I, with very strict limitations on pollution increases and allowing almost no change in existing air quality patterns; Class II, with slightly easier pollution limits and an allowance for "moderate" air quality deterioration; Class III, for areas where major industrial or other growth was desired and where pollution increases up to current federal standards would be allowed. In all cases, major new industrial installations would be required to use the best available technology to control emissions.

Deputy EPA Administrator John R. Quarles Jr. said the agency would initially place all clean-air regions in Class II, but after adoption of final rules, states would be free to make reclassifications. State designations would be subject to EPA approval, but only to the extent of determining whether states had followed proper procedures in setting the designations. State designations of federally-owned lands would have to be cleared by the federal agency involved.

The proposal dealt only with land use and industrial development; other pollutants such as auto emissions were not covered.

The relaxed regulations were upheld by a three-judge panel of the U.S. Court of Appeals for the District of Columbia Aug. 2, 1976.

The appeals court, in a unanimous decision, held that the regulations balanced the need for clean air with the need for continued community development.

The challenge against the regulations had been brought by the Sierra Club, utilities and the American Petroleum Institute. The utilities, for example wanted the EPA's authority restricted to areas failing to meet the Clean Air Act's standards. The Sierra Club argued against permitting any deterioration of air quality.

EPA delays some standards—The EPA Dec. 24, 1974 postponed for six months, until July 1, 1975, the enforcement of clean air standards that would require a review of plans for shopping centers, highways, stadiums and airports. The restrictions would have limited auto pollution that tended to concentrate in such facilities.

The decision to suspend the rules followed Congressional intervention in the form of a prohibition against EPA expenditure of any funds on "indirect source" enforcement in the current fiscal year, ending June 30, the Wall Street Journal reported Dec. 26.

The suspension was made indefinite by the EPA June 30, 1975 in the face of continued resistance from Congress and industrial sources.

Quality standards eased. The Supreme Court ruled April 17, 1975 that federal law allowed states to exempt some violators from compliance with air pollution clean-up regulations without federal approval so long as the state as a whole met U.S. air quality standards. The case had arisen when the Environmental Protection Agency approved an air clean-up plan for Georgia imposing immediate pollution limits but giving the state power to grant exceptions to polluters not immediately able to comply.

Administration backs scrubbers. The Ford Administration, reversing the recommendation of the Nixon Administration, announced its support of an EPA finding that required utilities to use "stack-gas scrubbers" to remove sulfur oxides and particulate matter from smokestack gases, the Wall Street Journal reported Nov. 29, 1974.

The EPA had reported Sept. 25 that the scrubber technique for cleaning up dirty emissions from power plants had been found to be efficient and reliable. The EPA said its findings could clear the way for burning plentiful high-sulfur coal while maintaining the standards of the Clean Air Act.

(Scrubbing involved passing smokestack gases through a liquid spray to remove most sulfur oxides and particulate matter.)

Some power industry spokesmen had contended that scrubber devices were unreliable and too costly, and that the leftover sulfur sludge would create disposal problems. The EPA report said the sludge could be valuable for landfill and road building.

The EPA said that during the past 11 months the number of planned or operating scrubber units had grown from 44 to 93 (at 51 power plants). Overall, the report said, 110 coal-fired power plants needed such controls to meet federal standards, at an estimated eventual cost of $5.4 billion.

The EPA report coincided with an announcement that Philadelphia Electric Co. had agreed to install scrubber units on three generators, at a total cost of $68 million. A company spokesman said customers would pay $50 million–$75 million less a year than if the company were forced to switch to low-sulfur fuels.

Utah power project dropped. A consortium of utility companies announced April 14, 1976 the cancellation of a coal-fired electric power plant project on the Kaiparowits Plateau in southern Utah. The project, according to William R. Gould, executive vice president of Southern California Edison Co., "was beaten to death by the environmental interests."

Southern California Edison was the principal partner in the project with 40% ownership. The other partners were San Diego Gas and Electric Co. 23.4% ownership and Arizona Public Service Co. with 18%.

The $3.5 billion plant would have been on federal land at Four-Mile Bench, 30 miles north of the Glen Canyon on the Colorado River. The site was within 200 miles of eight national parks and three national recreation areas. The plant would have burned more than 1,000 tons of coal an hour; this was expected to produce about 300 tons of air pollutants per day.

Environmental interests fighting the project included the Environmental Defense Fund and the Sierra Club. The project, which would have been the largest coal-fired plant in the country, was planned to supply electricity for Arizona and Southern California.

Gould attributed the cancellation to "a series of uncertainties" relating to costs, regulatory approvals and anticipated environmental lawsuits.

A letter signed by 31 members of Congress had been sent to Interior Secretary Thomas S. Kleppe April 9 seeking a delay in a U.S. decision to permit the Kaiparowits project. The petitioners wanted an independent evaluation "of the need for the project" and an opportunity for Congress to establish new national air quality standards.

Ford backs standards delay. In his State-of-the-Union message Jan. 15, 1975, President Ford had proposed a revision and deferment (for five years) of the automotive pollution standards. He said his proposals "will enable us to improve new-automobile gasoline mileage by 40% by 1980."

Nader contests carmakers' stand—Consumer advocate Ralph Nader released to the press Jan. 21 his letter to President Ford contesting the carmakers' contention they could not attain the 40% improvement in gasoline mileage requested by the President and still meet the 1977 emission standards. Accompanying the release of the letter was a previously undisclosed study by the Federal Energy Administration that the Big Three could attain the 40% fuel economy without any easing of pollution standards.

After the President proposed in the State of the Union message the five-year moratorium on standards to gain the 40% fuel improvement, Nader said Jan. 15 the President "appears to have been deceived by the auto industry. General Motors has already improved its fuel efficiency by 28% from its 1974 to 1975 model year."

Standards delayed. EPA Administrator Russell Train announced March 5, 1975 that he was granting automobile makers a one-year delay in meeting antipollution standards set for 1977-model cars. The one-year delay was the maximum allowed under current legislation, and Train recommended that Congress extend the current emission standards through 1979 models and impose new interim standards.

Train said the action was not based on industry objections. Industry had maintained that the new standards would result in higher prices and more fuel consumption because of the installation on cars of catalytic converters—the antipollution devices to control two major pollutants, hydrocarbons and carbon monoxide. The delay, Train said, was based solely on the agency's recent discovery that catalytic converters produced sulphuric acid emissions that could accumulate, from mass use of the converters, to unacceptably high levels and be a serious health risk for asthmatic persons.

He said the agency was formulating a standard for sulphuric-acid emissions. Such converters already were installed on about 85% of 1975 U.S. automobiles.

The current standards, which Train proposed to delay through 1979, limited hydrocarbon emissions to 1.5 grams per mile and carbon monoxide to 15 grams per mile. For further interim emission standards, he proposed .9 gram of hydrocarbons per mile and nine grams of carbon monoxide per mile for 1980 and 1981 models.

Train also proposed to tighten the nitrogen-oxide emission standard from the 3.1 grams previously recommended by President Ford to two grams per mile.

At the opening of hearings on the Big Three carmakers' request for a freeze on emission standards through 1977—the industry had received a one-year deferment in meeting 1976-model emissions standards and wanted to extend the deferment through the 1977-model year—Train told the industry representatives Jan. 21 that "the economic vitality of the auto industry is closely related to the economic health of our nation, but at the same time the continued reduction of pollution from autos is vital to the physical health of the American people and public health must be our highest priority."

Environmentalists denounce decision—EPA's decision to delay the car exhaust standards was denounced by spokesmen for the Clean Air Coalition at a press conference March 6. They made these points: With the delay, carbon monoxide pollution would double by 1985 from the level set by Congress in the 1970 Clean Air Act; the small fraction—5%—of cars currently on the road equipped with catalytic converters could be provided, at a cost to the consumer of only a penny or two per gallon, with low-sulphur gasoline producing little sulphate emission; "cars in 1977 using low-sulphur gasoline could meet the statutory standards of Congress for carbon monoxide and hydrocarbons and still have lower sulphate emissions than today's cars."

Further standards delay urged. President Ford asked Congress June 27, 1975 for another delay in imposing final standards on pollution emissions from automobiles. He asked for a four-year delay, which had been sought by the industry. The final standards for emission content—no more than .41 grams of hydrocarbons per mile, 3.4 grams of carbon monoxide and .4 grams of nitrogen oxides—would not be required until the 1982 model cars. The interim standards—1.5 grams for hydrocarbons, 15 grams for carbon monoxide and 3.1 grams for nitrogen oxides—would apply in the meantime.

The President based his recommendation on the recent discovery that catalytic converters used to curb the major car exhaust pollutants produced another emission problem, the formation of noxious sulphates in the atmosphere. The President also said the stricter standards would cut gasoline mileage and raise car prices.

Cleanup Inadequate

Progress report. EPA Administrator Russell E. Train said May 30, 1975 that there had been "significant progress" in cleaning up the nation's air but there was "still a long way to go." The assessment was made on the eve of the deadline, May 31, under the 1970 Clean Air Act for regional compliance with air-quality standards.

According to the EPA, 156 of 247 regions of the country were not meeting the standards for at least one pollutant, and some did not meet the standards for several pollutants. In the breakdown, 60 regions failed to meet the statutory standards for particulates (dust, smoke and soot), 42 for sulphur oxides, 74 for oxidants, 54 for carbon monoxide and 13 for nitrogen dioxide.

Southern California continued to lead the list for the worst auto pollution. The highest levels for sulphur dioxides, emitted by factories and utilities, and for total particulates, were in the Northeast from New England to Ohio. Los Angeles, Chicago and Philadelphia were among the cities failing to meet the standards for each of the five measured pollutants. The New York area, including northern New Jersey and southern Connecticut, was not within the standards for carbon monoxide, oxidants and nitrogen dioxide.

On an industry basis, the steel industry was "at the top or close to the top of the list" for noncompliance, Train said. "There isn't one steel facility in the U.S. that is in compliance with clean-air regulations at this time." A major problem was old equipment that was difficult to improve, although there had been some progress, Train noted. The steel industry had reduced its particulate emission by four million tons a year since 1970, but a reduction of another 1.5 million tons a year would be necessary to meet the standards.

Train cited the electric-power industry as another major source of pollution and noted that the EPA had had "enforcement problems" with the industry throughout the country.

On the progress side, the EPA reported that sulphur dioxide concentrations nationally had been reduced about 25% since 1970, mainly in metropolitan areas; the national level of particulate pollution had decreased 14% from 1970 to 1973; the number of measurements exceeding carbon-monoxide standards had fallen 50% since 1970, nationwide; 78% of 20,000 major stationary polluters—power plants, factories and municipal incinerators, etc.—were in compliance with emission rules or on schedule toward clean-up.

The delay in compliance with the air standards was attributed to a variety of reasons, aside from the complexity of the entire situation: court challenges of enforcement, weakness of some state regulations, lack of compliance by companies plus unsuccessful enforcement by the EPA or states, unforeseen problems such as the recession and energy shortage. Train said he thought it was possible to meet energy needs without sacrificing clean air "if we are careful," but he warned that "if we are not, energy demands could unravel much of our progress to date."

Train also noted that some of the regions and individual plants standing in noncompliance with the standards had been granted extensions of the deadline by the agency.

Continued improvement—The EPA Dec. 8, 1976 reported a general improvement of the nation's air quality over a five-year period ending in 1975.

The agency's survey found that air pollution still constituted a health hazard for 30% of the nation's population, but a spokesman said, this was a one-third reduction since 1970. The number of persons exposed to harmful smoke and dust particulate levels fell from 73 million in 1970 to 49 million in 1974, the EPA said.

The greatest improvement was said to have taken place in the Northeast and Great Lakes areas and in urban California. Carbon monoxide pollution in those areas lessened about 5% a year in most areas, "due mostly to federal emission standards on autos," the report stated.

In California, where state standards on auto emissions were stricter than the federal ones, considerable progress was reported. In the smog-infested Los Angeles area, where air pollution levels exceeded health standards an average of 176 days per year in the 1960s, the figure was reduced to 105 days per year by 1975.

A mixed report was found on sulfur dioxide levels. In urban areas, the agency reported a 30% decrease in the five-year period but only a slight decline on a nationwide basis. The discrepancy was attributed to industrial dispersal from cities to rural areas. The agency warned that rural sources of sulfur dioxide, "such as smelters, pose the greatest threat to the maintenance of sulfur dioxide standards."

The general reduction in air pollution during the five-year period was credited largely to antipollution equipment in factories, the decrease in industrial activity because of the 1974–75 economic recession, a reduction in trash-burning and the stricter emission controls on cars.

AMC fined $4.2 million by California. The California Air Resources Board fined American Motors Corp. $4.2 million Jan. 5, 1975 for violating the state anti-pollution law. It also banned the sale of the three AMC models involved, the Matador, Hornet or Gremlin models equipped with eight-cylinder engines.

The fine was the largest ever assessed by the state against a carmaker, but the board offered to accept 25% of it, or $1.1 million, as payment if the company agreed to spend the remainder on emission-control and fuel economy of its cars. The offer was made, the board said, so as not to jeopardize the firm's financial base or competitive position in the industry.

Thomas Quinn, chairman of the state agency, said AMC executives had denied any intentional wrongdoing and had attributed the problem "to lack of attention, poor maintenance of test facilities and neglect." An AMC statement from Detroit Jan. 5 called the California action "unjustified" and the size of the fine "unreasonable."

A two-fold violation of the state law was charged—that the company had submitted "totally false" test reports to the state and that cars exceeding the state's pollution standards had been sold in the state. The state required test reports on 2% of all cars built for California sale. The state board found the data submitted inconsistent with its own inspections, which revealed that 85% of the models involved emitted too much carbon monoxide or oxides of nitrogen. The California standards limited carbon monoxide emissions to nine grams a mile and oxides of nitrogen to two grams a mile. These were stricter than the federal standards of 15 grams and 3.1 grams, respectively.

California bars Chrysler engine. The California Air Resources Board levied a $328,200 air-pollution fine against Chrysler Aug. 16, 1975 and barred the sale of cars with its biggest engine, which displaced 440 cubic inches. The agency acted after what it termed "completely inadequate response" to two recalls it had ordered.

The fine, equivalent to $50 for each of 6,564 offending cars shipped into

California during the year, was paid by Chrysler under protest. The money was held in escrow pending litigation. A Chrysler spokesman said the board had threatened to bar sale of 1976 models unless the matter was cleared up. The stop-sale order on the 1975 models was rescinded Aug. 18 after the company reached agreement with the board to test the unsold models involved, about 1,000, and certify they met the antipollution rules.

New York gets clean-air orders. The Environmental Protection Agency issued orders to the state and city of New York Sept. 29, 1975 to establish tolls by mid-1977 on the 11 bridges over the East and Harlem Rivers. The bridges currently were toll-free.

A second order issued at the same time required the city to put into effect by mid-1977 a plan to reduce the volume of automobile traffic entering Manhattan each morning by 10%.

The orders were part of a series of formal notices issued by the EPA requiring the state and city to implement traffic control and air-pollution clean-up under the 1970 Clean Air Act. The agency contended that the imposition of tolls would cut traffic and, thus, car pollution.

Other orders dealt with such things as curbs on parking, taxi cruising and truck deliveries.

The initial response from the state indicated an effort would be made to devise an alternate plan for tolls and to have the order revised.

The EPA had issued a timetable April 15 for city and state action on various segments of the clean-air program for the city. It said the city had failed to "effectuate and enforce specific increments" of a transportation control plan approved in 1973.

The orders were upheld April 26, 1976 by the U.S. Court of Appeals for the Second Circuit.

The court directed the U.S. District Court, which had held hearings on the case, to issue orders immediately to enforce four provisions of the plan and to "conduct an expeditious hearing" to enforce any of the other 28 provisions that were being violated.

The four provisions to be effected immediately were imposition of tolls on the East River and Harlem River bridges, a ban on cruising by taxis on certain key midtown streets, reduction of parking space in the central business district and a restriction against truck deliveries during peak congestion periods.

In a unanimous opinion, written by Judge Walter R. Mansfield, the three-man appeals court found the 1973 plan binding and enforceable against both the city and state under the 1970 Federal Clean Air Act. Mansfield said that carbon monoxide pollution in the city, 95% of which was attributable to motor vehicles, had actually increased "since pre-plan days by some 25%." Thus, he said, violations of the plan "were significantly harmful to public health."

Mansfield also upheld the right of citizen groups to bring suit in antipollution cases. Congress had made it clear that such groups were "not to be treated as nuisances or troublemakers," he said, "but rather as welcomed participants in the vindication of environmental interests."

The suit was brought by the Natural Resources Defense Council, a nonprofit law firm of environmentalists, on behalf of Friends of the Earth and other environmental groups. The appeals court rejected the environmentalists' bid to roll back the city's 50¢ transit fare.

Policy permits new plants. The EPA Nov. 10, 1976 announced a new policy to permit increased air pollution from new plants if offsetting reductions in pollution were made elsewhere so that there was no net increase in a region's pollution.

Most of the nation's air-quality-control regions were in violation of the clean-air standards set under the 1970 Clean Air Act so that strict enforcement of that law would allow new plants only if they were non-polluting.

The new policy was announced in a speech in Anaheim, Calif. by John R. Quarles Jr., EPA deputy administrator.

He described the action as "a trade-off policy" under which more pollution in one area could be traded off for cleaner air elsewhere. He also called it a "compromise" between the strictures of the environmental law and the demands for industrial growth.

Environmentalists immediately deplored the action. The National Clean Air Coalition said later Nov. 10 it was "a legally questionable undercutting and distortion" of the Clean Air Act.

Delay on auto emission rules. The Carter Administration April 18, 1977 urged that imposition of automobile emission standards be delayed for some time, but not for as long as the automobile industry wanted.

The Administration's views were presented by Environmental Protection Agency (EPA) Administrator Douglas M. Costle to a House Commerce Committee subcommittee. The panel was considering amendments to the 1970 Clean Air Act.

Under existing legislation, 1978 model cars were supposed to comply with the following emission standards: no more than .41 grams per mile of hydrocarbons, 3.4 grams per mile of carbon monoxide and .4 grams per mile of nitrogen oxide. (Currently, permissible levels of those emissions were: hydrocarbons, 1.5 grams per mile; carbon monoxide, 15 grams per mile, and nitrogen oxide, 2 grams per mile.)

The Carter Administration proposal would delay imposition of the standard for hydrocarbons for one year (making it effective for 1979 and later model cars); would require reductions in carbon monoxide levels to 9 grams per mile for 1979 models and 3.4 grams for 1981 and later models, and would require reduction of nitrogen oxide emissions to 1 gram per mile for 1981 and later model cars.

The EPA, under the Administration proposal, would decide in 1980 whether to require the lower standard of .4 grams per mile for nitrogen oxide emissions. If the lower standard were adopted, it would apply to 1983 model cars.

Administration views on other pollution issues—The Carter Administration also:

- Supported amendments requiring coal-burning power plants to use "the best available technology," including scrubbers, to clean their emissions.

- Favored amendments barring deterioration of air quality in areas with air cleaner than was required by national standards.

- Endorsed extensions of up to five years in the time that stationary sources of pollution would be given to comply with federal standards, and proposed strong economic sanctions for non-compliance. Companies not complying with standards, the Administration urged, should be fined the amount they had saved by not complying. The Administration said that a limit, proposed in the House, of $5,000 a day on noncompliance fines should be dropped.

The Carter Administration also asked Congress to let the EPA continue for a year its policy of restricting new sources of pollution in areas already violating clean air standards unless offsetting reductions of pollution were made elsewhere in the area. Businessmen and city officials from the older industrial cities of the Northeast and Midwest had complained that the policy stifled growth.

Air cleaner, but smog worse. The Environmental Protection Agency reported Dec. 21, 1977 that the U.S. was making "significant progress" in cleaning up its dirty air although the smog problem had intensified.

While the level of other major pollutants had decreased since the Clean Air Act was enacted in 1970, the levels of smog, composed of photochemical oxidants, had increased slightly in some parts of the country.

"We're still a long way from having healthy air throughout the country," EPA Administrator Douglas Costle commented.

Sulfur dioxide pollution decreased 27% from 1970 to 1976, the agency reported, carbon monoxide levels dropped 20% during the period and smoke and dust levels declined 12%.

Energy, Pollution & Health

Coal linked to pollution deaths. Scientists at the Brookhaven National Laboratory in New York issued a warning that increased reliance on coal for energy, a key element of President Carter's energy program, could increase substantially the number of persons dying prematurely as a result of air pollution. The New York Times July 17, 1977 said the scientists estimated that air pollution from oil and coal burning power plants currently caused 21,000 premature deaths annually east of the Mississippi River. By 2010, the number would grow to 35,000 a year, assuming coal replaced oil generally.

The Brookhaven researchers said their results assumed coal burning plants used 'scrubbers' that cut sulfur emissions by 80%. If the plants used scrubbers that were 90% effective, the number of premature deaths would be fewer, the scientists said.

In its July 16, 1979 issue, Newsweek discussed the situation editorially:

> The good news about coal is that we have huge domestic quantities of it—enough to last more than 600 years at current consumption rates. The bad news is that we have to use it. The health, safety and environmental threats posed by mining and burning coal are severe; its emissions cause respiratory ailments, contain carcinogens and release more carbon dioxide into the atmosphere than any other fossil fuel, raising the possibility of a "greenhouse effect"—a warming of the atmosphere that could cause catastrophic climatic changes.
>
> Mining it in the arid West, where it lies near the earth's surface, degrades hard-to-reclaim land. Mining it in the East, where it is trapped deep within the Appalachian hills, means a nightmare of labor and safety problems. Transporting it is awkward and expensive. Burning it is dirty. Coal is hardly the energy savior many proponents have claimed, and it should not be burned where the resulting pollution exceeds the health-related air-quality standards. . . .

Sulphur-dioxide monitoring asked. An agreement to monitor air pollution was reached by 14 European nations, led by Norway, in Geneva Jan. 19, 1977. They called for each government to set up ground stations by Sept. 1, 1977 to monitor flows of sulphur dioxide across their borders. The stations were intended to be the first step in a program to reduce the emission-flow levels by pinpointing the flows that contributed directly to pollution.

Norway in particular had been the target of sulphur-dioxide flows for years and had continually attempted to get other nations to reduce the amount of sulphur used in power stations and other industries. Emissions from sources in England and other North European countries drifted over Norway and combined with rain and snow to form acid rains that contaminated Norway's rivers and forests.

The Norwegian Institute for Air Research released statistics, reported Jan. 17, that showed a record rate of sulphuric rainfall in southeastern Norway. It reported that in one recent heavy period of rain and snow, almost one-third of the annual total of sulfuric rainfall had fallen and left a ton of sulfuric acid on each .38 square miles of territory. The acid rain had sometimes been heavy enough to form a film on the water and to kill fish and some vegetation.

In addition to Norway, the nations that signed the agreement were: Austria, Belgium, Denmark, Finland, East Germany, West Germany, Hungary, Ireland, Italy, the Netherlands, Poland, Portugal and Sweden. France and Switzerland declined to sign the pact but indicated they would construct monitoring stations the following year.

Great Britain, which was often cited as being the major source of the Norwegian acid rain, also declined to sign the agreement and did not promise to comply later. Spokesmen for the British Central Electricity Generating Board had denied its plants were a major cause of the acid rain, it was reported Jan. 17. They also had said most of the pollutants in question came from Norway itself and criticized British environmental authorities for not challenging Norwegian statements about the pollution.

Car pollution deadline extended. A bill delaying stiffer clean-air controls on automobile emissions was cleared by Congress Aug. 4, 1977 and signed by President Carter Aug. 8.

U.S. carmakers had threatened to shut down production lines for the 1978 models, which were just beginning their production year, claiming they could not meet the emissions control standards required by existing law.

Under the bill, the stricter controls were scheduled to go into effect for the 1980 model year. Originally, the standards were to have gone into effect in 1975. This marked the fourth relaxation of the deadline by Congress.

"The automobile industry now has a firm timetable for meeting strict but achievable emission reductions," Carter said in signing the bill. "This timetable will be enforced."

Since the bill continued other clean-air provisions that were controversial, agreement on a compromise version by Senate-House conferees took eight days of bargaining and a final seven-hour session. Final passage in the Senate then was delayed for a time by a threatened filibuster by Sen. Jake Garn (R, Utah).

Garn, and Sen. Orrin Hatch (R, Utah), protested that a provision to limit factory building in rural areas having clean air might restrict industrial growth in their state.

A filibuster effort by Garn at the end of the 1976 session had stymied the clean-air legislation. Senate leaders had let it be known they would fight the filibuster this time, a situation that could have delayed the vacation recess of Congress.

The final version of the bill kept the ban against new sources of pollution in areas having air cleaner than federal health standards required, although a variance would be permitted for temporary pollution, up to 18 days a year. The variance could be obtained from a state's governor only after hearings, however. If the U.S. interior secretary disagreed, the matter would be sent to the president for a decision.

In areas where the air was dirtier than federal standards allowed, new pollution sources would be admitted only if pollution from existing sources was reduced on an offsetting basis. The deadlines for compliance with federal standards would be 1982 for states, 1987 for cities with problems.

Pollution sources required to convert to coal from oil or natural gas would have until the end of 1980 to comply with clean-air standards with additional delays possible. The deadline for nonferrous smelters would be 1983, also with five additional years available.

States would be permitted to adopt California's standards for automobile emissions, which were stricter than the federal ones. These states would have to give two years' advance notice.

The bill retained for two more years the emission standards for 1977-model cars. These restricted tailpipe emissions to 1.5 grams a mile of hydrocarbons, 15 grams a mile of carbon monoxide and two grams a mile of nitrogen oxides.

For the 1980 models, the limits would be reduced to .41 gram a mile of hydrocarbons and seven grams a mile of carbon monoxide (nitrogen oxide emissions remaining the same).

For the 1981 model year, the standards would be 3.4 grams a mile of carbon monoxide and one gram a mile of nitrogen oxides (hydrocarbons unchanged). By then, the standards for all three pollutants would have reached the targets originally set under the 1970 Clean Air Act, but delayed since.

There were further easements possible under the new law. The Environmental Protection Agency would be allowed to grant, upon application by the manufacturer, a two-year postponement of the final carbon monoxide goal. It also would be permitted to ease the one-gram nitrogen oxide rule for diesels or other variant engines. A special temporary waiver was granted the American Motors Corp. from the final oxides rule.

EPA's Sulfur Dioxide Rules Upheld. Federal standards curbing sulfur dioxide pollution by industry in Ohio were upheld by the U.S. Sixth Circuit Court of Appeals in Cincinnati Feb. 13, 1978.

The standards, determined by the U.S. Environmental Protection Agency, were based on a formula that took into account the capacities of individual plants on a smokestack-by-smokestack basis and assumed that the plants operated 24 hours a day at full capacity.

Sulfur dioxide was a byproduct of coal burning.

The standards had been challenged by 32 companies which argued it was unrealistic to assume the plants operated at full capacity.

The 32 companies were joined in their suit against the standards by the Ohio Environmental Protection Agency.

The appeals court ruled unanimously that the formula reflected a rational choice within the discretion of the EPA.

The issue had evoked protest in Ohio because coal mined in the state had a high sulfur content in comparison with coal mined in the West.

Coal miners protested that the regulations would ruin the market for Ohio coal and put them out of work.

The EPA July 6 denied a request that it grant a moratorium for Ohio power plants in meeting federal clean-air standards. The request had been made by Ohio Gov. James Rhodes.

Rhodes said the utilities in the state, which used high-sulfur local coal, would either have to install expensive "scrubbers" to meet the standards or switch to low-sulfur Western coal. Importing coal would be harmful to Ohio's miners and mining companies, Rhodes protested.

The scrubbers eliminated 90% of the harmful sulfur dioxide emissions produced from burning coal and were "a workable technology," the EPA said in rejecting the request. It did not deny that the technique was expensive. Use of scrubbers could lead to a 4%-8% increase in consumer electric bills, the agency estimated.

The EPA pointed out that the standards were being met in many parts of the country and that Ohio was lagging three years behind the federal deadline for meeting sulfur dioxide clean-air standards.

Further delay, EPA Administrator Douglas Costle said, would hurt Ohio residents and could undermine clean-air efforts in neighboring states.

Ohio coal ruling—Federal District Judge H. David Hermansdorfer in Catlettsburg, Ky. upheld the constitutionality of the federal clean-air law May 7, 1979.

Specifically, he upheld Section 125 of the Clean Air Act Amendments of 1977, which gave the Environmental Protection Agency authority to require utilities, or other major coal users, to buy "regionally available coal" if buying the coal elsewhere would cause "significant" local unemployment.

The provision had been written by Sen. Howard Metzenbaum (D, Ohio) to prevent the state's electric companies from forsaking Ohio's high-sulfur coal for low-sulfur coal mined elsewhere, such as Kentucky.

Use of high-sulfur coal required utilities to install expensive anti-pollution equipment, so expensive that it was cheaper for Ohio's utilities to comply with EPA sulfur-emission rules by importing coal rather than using the local variety.

The case in Kentucky was brought by McCoy Elkhorn Coal Corp. of Lexington, Ky., a subsidiary of General Energy Corp. Joined by Ohio Edison Co., a utility based in Akron, Ohio, McCoy Elkhorn contended that the law deprived the company of the right to engage in interstate commerce for economic gain. That right could not be impaired by geographical boundaries, the suit said.

Hermansdorfer rejected that. He said, "Congress has the power to define a region about which it is concerned in terms of a state's boundaries or upon any other rational basis regardless of the size of the region."

The court did say the plaintiffs could "address themselves to the political process, not to the judiciary, for remedy."

Another suit in the Ohio coal controversy, filed by Cleveland Electric Illuminating Co., was pending in federal district court in Cleveland.

Still another, filed in Columbus, Ohio in March by the Consolidation Coal Co., claimed the EPA's sulfur rules were too stringent.

Consolidation Coal, a coal-mining subsidiary of Continental Oil Co., was a major supplier of coal to utilities in Ohio and elsewhere. The company had received cancellations of orders from utilities because of its high-sulfur coal.

The suit charged that the way the standards were set, by action of the Environmental Protection Agency, was an unconstitutional use of legislative power by an agency of the executive branch.

The suit charged in particular that the EPA's sulfur dioxide standards were "inaccurate and outdated" and more stringent than the Clean Air Act required.

EPA eases Ohio rule—The EPA proposed June 6, 1979 to ease air standards for two Cleveland Electric Illuminating Co. power plants.

The decision was announced by President Carter.

The plants involved were the Eastlake and Avon Lake facilities, one east and one west of Cleveland.

The relaxation of the rule would permit the plants to emit more than six pounds of sulfur dioxide per million British Thermal Units of coal burned. The existing rule permitted no more than 1.2 pounds of sulfur dioxide emission.

The current rule was "too stringent," the agency said, "given the unique lakefront nature of the plants." Air pollution dispersed more rapidly in rural areas.

What the EPA did in this case, actually, was change the basis of its rule for the two plants from an "urban modeling" to a rural model, where higher amounts of pollution were allowed because of the rapid dispersal.

Without the change, the EPA was facing a decision to order the plants to continue to use local coal, which had a high sulfur content. In which case, the utilities would have had to install expensive scrubbers to meet air-emission standards.

A switch of the utilities to low sulfur coal from the West would have cost mining jobs in Ohio, and, under a provision of the Clean Air Act, the EPA could order utilities to use local coal to avoid unemployment and economic disruption in the state.

Cleveland Electric had objected to installing the costly scrubbing equipment. Ohio coal miners had objected to any switch to out-of-state coal.

The EPA's relaxation of standards avoided both complaints, and "pleased" the President, he said, because it saved mining jobs and "will neither sacrifice public health nor cause higher utility bills for Ohio's consumers."

It did not please the Environmental Defense Fund, whose spokesman, Robert Rauch, called it "a quick fix that was dreamed up at the last minute to get the White House off the hot seat."

"It may save miners' jobs, but it sure doesn't protect the environment," Rauch said. "They could have done both by requiring scrubbers."

Sen. Howard Metzenbaum (D, Ohio), also praised the decision as far as the jobs were concerned. But he expressed concern about the environmental effect. Using "a rural standard," he observed, "will surprise Cleveland's farmers."

103 Areas Violate Air Rules. A report released Feb. 23, 1978 by the Environmental Protection Agency listed 103 of 105 major urban areas—those with populations exceeding 200,000 people—as violators of at least one of the five federal standards for air quality.

The only two areas that met the standards were Honolulu and Spokane, Wash.

The standards were set to curb pollution by particulate matter, sulfur dioxide, carbon monoxide, photochemical "smog" and nitrogen dioxide.

Three of the areas—Los Angeles/Long Beach, Calif., Chicago and Aurora/Elgin, Ill.—had pollution exceeding the federal limits in all five categories.

Twenty areas, including Cleveland, St. Louis, San Diego and Denver, were in violation on four of the five pollutants.

Only 20 of the major metropolitan areas were clear on four out of five of the pollutants. Miami, New Orleans and Little Rock were in this category. In all 20 of these areas, smog was the remaining problem.

Rules for Sulfur, Lime, Paper Plants. The Environmental Protection Agency set pollution curbs March 22, 1978 for sulfur-recovery plants, lime-manufacturing plants and kraft pulp mills.

The rules, which were effective immediately, applied to new facilities and not to existing plants unless they were modified in a way that increased pollution.

The standards were devised to reduce sulfur dioxide emissions from sulfur-recovery plants by 55,000 tons annually, on a national scale, by 1980. Sulfur-recovery plants were used by petroleum refiners to control sulfur dioxide emissions produced by combustion of fuel gases in the refining process.

The rules for new lime plants were expected to reduce emissions of dust and smoke by more than 10,600 tons annually by 1987.

For kraft pulp mills, the goal was to lessen emissions of smoke and dust, as well as sulfur compounds producing a "rotten egg" smell. The mills processed wood chips into pulp for the production of paper products.

Smog Control Standard Eased. The Environmental Protection Agency June 13, 1978 proposed a modification of its clean-air standard for smog control.

The modification, sought by business as a cost saver, was justified by a review of medical and scientific evidence, according to the agency.

The level of ozone, the EPA's term for smog, in the air did not harmfully affect joggers or cyclists, it was found, until it reached a concentration of .15 part per million.

Therefore, the agency eased the smog regulation to .1 part per million from .08 part, which was still within the "margin of safety" required by law.

In another move affected by the cost factor, the EPA June 13 issued final regulations on the "prevention of significant deterioration" of air quality.

The regulations actually tightened clean-air rules for new plants in areas where the air was relatively pollution free. The rules required installation of the best available pollution-control technology.

The agency originally wanted to increase the coverage of the regulations to about 4,000 facilities a year from the 165 cases handled under existing regulations. The cases involved detailed pre-construction reviews.

But Administration economists, specifically the President's Council of Economic Advisers and his Council on Wage Price Stability, recommended scaling back the coverage considerably in order to minimize "delay costs" for the industries involved.

The EPA found that it could exempt 2,400 relatively minor polluters accounting for less than 2% of the estimated newsource pollution.

It aimed the new regulations, therefore, at the 1,600 new businesses that would account for almost all the new pollution.

Half a year later the Environmental Protection Agency relaxed its limit on smog concentration Jan. 26, 1979 after "a careful reevaluation of medical and scientific evidence."

The new standard permitted a 50% increase in the allowable amount of ozone, a major component of smog, to .12 parts per million of air from the level of .08 parts per million established in 1971. This was slightly higher than the level of .1 part per million proposed by the agency in June 1978.

EPA Administrator Douglas Costle said the change was decided after new research by the agency indicated that even persons suffering from asthma and other chronic respiratory diseases could safely tolerate a .15 level of ozone per million parts of air.

The agency estimated that the cost of compliance with the new rule, as compared with the old one, would be $1.5 billion less a year.

Of the 105 major urban areas monitored for air quality, only Honolulu and Spokane, Wash. currently met the .08 ozone standard.

The new standard was immediately attacked by environmental and health groups as too lenient and by the American Petroleum Institute as too stringent. Automobile exhaust was the chief source of smog.

Utilities Get Clean-Air Proposal. The Environmental Protection Agency issued a proposal Sept. 11, 1978 that would require new power plants burning coal to install "scrubbers" to reduce sulfur dioxide emissions by 85%.

Standards for new plants were required by the 1977 Clean Air Act.

EPA Administrator Douglas Costle stressed, in presenting the proposal, that it was "not final and that all the options under discussion will continue to receive serious consideration."

The agency's proposal was considered by most observers to be at the strict end of the range of alternatives. Calling for use of what was known as the "full-scrubbing" method, the proposal would require all coal, regardless of sulfur content, to be scrubbed. Full-scrubbing, a costly operation, was favored by most environmentalists.

Industry, and the Energy Department, favored an alternative. This would be to have a sliding scale for allowable emissions and to permit "partial scrubbing," or a minimum level of scrubbing for all coal and additional scrubbing for coal with high sulfur content.

According to the EPA's estimates, based on the expectation that roughly 200 new power plants would be built by 1990, the agency's proposal would cost the industry $10 billion by 1990.

More Flexible Air Rules Proposed. The Environmental Protection Agency Dec. 21 offered a flexible plan for companies to meet clean-air requirements.

Under the current system, state enforcement agencies set limits for each pollution source in an industrial complex.

The EPA, under a so-called "bubble concept," proposed to permit trade-offs among the various sources in each complex, so long as the total pollution from the complex did not increase.

Each plant complex would be treated as if it were encased in a bubble. Regulation of air pollution, instead of being on a source-by-source basis, would be based on the total amount of pollution within the bubble.

The plan had been devised to encourage innovation in meeting clean-air standards and to allow companies the choice of a less expensive method whenever that option was available.

The agency imposed some conditions for using the new method. Trade-offs of some cancer-causing pollutants would not be permitted. The trade-offs in general would be allowed only if the pollutants being traded were comparable in nature and in their effect on public health.

TVA Accepts Accord. Tennessee Valley Authority directors Dec. 14, 1978 approved settlement of suits requiring the agency to clean up air pollution from its power plants.

The suits had been brought against TVA by the Environmental Protection Agency and several citizens' and environmental groups.

Suits were filed in federal courts in Knoxville, Memphis, Nashville and Chattanooga in Tennessee; Birmingham, Ala. and Paducah, Ky. against 10 of the TVA's 12 coal-fired electrical generating plants.

The coalition charged the TVA with responsibility for 16% of all sulfur dioxide emissions in the country and 38% of those in the Tennessee Valley.

Among the environmental groups in the coalition were the Sierra Club and the Natural Resources Defense Council.

The settlement actually had been negotiated in March by TVA Chairman S. David Freeman, then a director. Approval was voted following the appointment of Richard Freeman as a director, which gave the three-man board a quorum.

Under the settlement, the authority agreed to reduce emissions of sulfur dioxide and dust, or particulate matter, from its power plants. The goal was to reduce the pollution to about half its current levels.

The authority, the largest electric utility in the U.S., planned to burn higher quality coal and to design and build pollution-control facilities. The facilities were expected to cost about $1 billion.

The utility estimated that the annual capital and operating costs would be $447 million, plus any inflation cost.

Council Cites Clean Up Gains. The White House Council on Environmental Quality Jan. 25, 1979 cited many gains in the nation's effort to clean up its air and water.

The council, releasing its annual report, also contended that the economic benefits deriving from federal air-pollution regulations far outweighed the costs of compliance.

The cost of meeting federal standards in 1978, figuring public and private spending, was estimated by the council to be $13.1 billion.

The federal standards were saving the nation about $22 billion a year in damages that would have been caused by air pollution, the council said, based on preliminary results of a new study it was having conducted.

The council concluded that "the overall trend in most areas is towards continued improvement" in air quality, although most major cities had not as yet met federal standards in all five categories of pollutants—ozone, dust, sulfur dioxide, carbon monoxide and nitrogen dioxide.

The council reported there had been significant improvement from 1973 through 1976 in urban areas that had the most severe problems with smog and carbon monoxide.

All of the 43 major cities surveyed in the report had a least 27 or more days in 1976 when the air quality was found to have an official "unhealthy" rating.

In four cities—Los Angeles, Denver, Cleveland and St. Louis—the air was considered unhealthy on at least half of the days in 1976.

One favorable finding was that in 16 major cities, the number of days of unhealthy air declined 8% in the 1973 to 1976 period.

In another environmental category, the council reported there was "evidence of improvement" in the nation's water quality, although "we are a very long way from our goals."

A negative finding was reported concerning farm land. The report warned that prime farm land was being lost to residential and commercial development at the "disproportionate rate" of nearly four square miles a day.

The turnover, which the council considered damaging to the farm economy and the environment, was particularly noticeable in the Northeast, it said.

New Pollution Penalty Proposed. The Environmental Protection Agency proposed March 21, 1979 that polluting firms pay fines equal to the amount of money they saved by failing to install and operate anti-pollution equipment.

"In many instances, the economic savings resulting from noncompliance have encouraged environmental footdragging by violating industries," said EPA Administrator Douglas M. Costle.

"Sources violating the law by failing to install and operate necessary pollution control devices have long enjoyed an economic advantage over those that did what the law required."

The amount of the penalty would be determined by use of a congressionally mandated formula incorporating savings in capital, labor, material, energy costs and "any additional economic value" deriving from failure to follow the law.

Companies that were penalized would have 45 days to present a challenge.

Exemptions from penalties would be permitted under certain circumstances—if the violation was "insignificant and of short duration" and if noncompliance derived from strikes, fires or natural disasters or energy crisis.

Aircraft Emission Rules Revised. The Environmental Protection Agency March 27, 1978 revised air-pollution regulations for airlines.

Deadlines for controls on gaseous emissions would be delayed from two to five years, primarily because technology had not yet been developed that would enable the airlines to comply with the earlier standards.

Standards scheduled to take effect in 1979 for engines used in big jetliners, such as the 707 and 747 and DC-8, would be delayed until 1981 for hydrocarbons and carbon monoxide and until 1984 for oxides of nitrogen.

The 1981 standards for newly certified aircraft engines in commercial service would be delayed to 1984 for hydrocarbons and carbon monoxide. The standards would be eased for oxide of nitrogen.

All emission limits would be eliminated for small turbine and piston engines used extensively in private and business aircraft.

However, when the anti-pollution regulations did go into effect, they would be stricter and cover more planes than had the previous rules.

Under the earlier rules, only new 727 and 737 engines and DC9 engines would be covered by the standards. The latest version would extend the standards to old engines as well.

Truck Exhaust Rule Tightened. The Environmental Protection Agency proposed a further tightening of its exhaust standards for new buses and large trucks Feb. 15, 1979, effective in 1983.

The new rule would limit hydrocarbon emissions to 1.4 grams per brake horsepower hour and carbon monoxide emissions to 14.7 grams.

The current standard, set in 1977, was 1.5 grams for hydrocarbons and 25 grams for carbon monoxide.

GM, EPA Settle Emissions Dispute. The U.S. attorney's office in Detroit announced an out-of-court settlement June 5, 1979 of an auto-emissions dispute between the government and General Motors Corp.

The federal government had been investigating whether the company had tampered with auto emission-control equipment to enable certain cars to pass a clean-air inspection by the federal Environmental Protection Agency.

General Motors denied the charges. When the EPA undertook to probe the matter, GM sought to stop it with a lawsuit charging it was an unauthorized criminal investigation.

The company also challenged the EPA's authority to conduct its routine emissions inspections.

Eventually, U.S. Attorney James Robinson announced the Detroit office was entering the case to see if there were "criminal violations" by GM.

In the settlement announced June 5, the investigation was dropped. "It was determined that criminal prosecution was not appropriate," Robinson said.

For its part of the consent agreement, GM admitted no guilt but agreed to pay a civil penalty of $90,000.

The company dropped its challenges against the government, and it agreed to "certify" that it would not attempt to interfere with the integrity of the EPA's spot-checks of its production processes in the future.

SST, Other Ozone Threats & Skin Cancer

SST health link disputed. The debate over development of America's controversial supersonic transport (SST) assumed a new dimension March 17, 1971 as one of its Senate critics and the White House disputed whether the plane could cause a rise in the incidence of skin cancer.

Sen. William E. Proxmire (D, Wis.), who had led the campaign against the SST in the Senate, introduced publicly three scientists who supported a theory that fleets of SSTs could significantly increase the incidence of skin cancer. This could happen, Proxmire said, from a thinning of the layers of ozone in the stratosphere that shielded the earth from the sun's ultraviolet radiations.

The White House described Proxmire's SST-cancer link as "a shocking attempt to create fear about something that is simply not the fact." Later, White House Press Secretary Ronald L. Ziegler conceded that "some questions" had been raised, and that the Administration had no plans to move the SST into a full production if studies showed it would be a health hazard. Ziegler said, however, that "nothing would be gained by interrupting the development of the prototype" at the present time.

Proxmire also charged the Nixon Administration with seeking to "gag" Dr. Gio Gori, a government scientist, whom he said had confirmed the skin cancer hazard.

The White House denied the allegation. Gori himself said "I was not muzzled by the Administration—I don't think I was." Gori was an associate scientific director at the National Cancer Institute.

Proxmire referred to a paper prepared by Gori estimating that fulltime operations by a fleet of 800 SSTs would result in 23,000–103,000 new cases of skin cancer each year. Gori added that the 103,000 figure could be "a very conservative estimate."

In introducing the three scientists at a news conference, Proxmire said they represented a contingent of 21 others who also backed the skin cancer theory. He released written statements from the 21, many of whom suggested that one scientist's projection of 10,000 SST-related skin cancer cases each year in the U.S. was too conservative.

The skin cancer theory was first outlined in the fall of 1970 by Dr. James E. McDonald, an atmospheric physicist at the University of Arizona. McDonald presented his views to a closed-door session of the Transportation Department, which was responsible for the SST. Shortly afterwards, Transportation Secretary John A. Volpe said the SST-cancer link could be dismissed "categorically."

McDonald repeated his views March 2 to members of the House Appropriations Committee, which was holding hearings on the Administration request for SST funds.

Congress votes to end SST. A bill containing $97.3 million to terminate the project to develop a commercial supersonic transport plane (SST) was cleared by Congress May 24, 1971 and signed by President Nixon May 25. The funds were part of a second supplemental appropriations bill (HR8190) for fiscal 1971 which was approved by the House May 20 by a 264–28 vote, and by the Senate May 21 by a 27–25 vote. A final vote in the Senate was taken May 24 to reconsider the bill as reported by the House-Senate conference, but the move was rejected 34–21.

The SST was defeated largely on the basis of its cost and environmental effect—noise and air pollution. Proponents of the plane cited the U.S.' purported need for such an aircraft to maintain the nation's international position in aviation as well as the income and additional jobs (about 150,000) they said the program would generate.

The Nixon Administration's support of the project had been restated Aug. 27, 1970 at a hearing of the Senate Transportation Subcommittee of the Appropriations Committee. William M. Magruder, head of the government's SST program, presented the Administration's case. Magruder Sept. 16 had released a Transportation Department report to the White House Council on Environmental Quality. The report had rated the SST's effects on the environment as from "insignificant" to "trivial."

Executives of the British Aircraft Corp. and the Boeing Co. held a joint news conference in London Feb. 10, 1971 on the U.S. SST and on the Concorde, the joint British-French rival. They said that aircraft caused less than 1% of the world's industrial air pollution, and the SST would contribute only 1/5 of that. "In pollution terms," Dr. W. J. Strang, a British aircraft director concluded, the SST "would be a good thing."

The aerospace industry and the machinists' union Feb. 22 announced a $350,000 advertising campaign to counter the arguments of environmentalists and stress the importance of the SST to the national economy.

William D. Ruckelshaus, director of the Environmental Protection Agency, told the House Appropriations Committee March 1 that further planned research on the plane's exhaust system, which was the focal point of many of the environmentalists' attacks, would have answered the "critical environmental questions" that prompted the debate.

Transportation Secretary John A. Volpe later told the panel that many of the SST's opponents were guilty of "hysterical sloganeering." He said the SST held out the promise of long-range economic benefits. At present, Volpe said, 13,000 men and women were working on the prototypes; and if full-scale production were ordered the number would rise to 50,000. Counting the "multiplier effect" of industrial employment, the plane's economic impact had been linked with a reported 150,000 jobs.

Scientists warn vs. SST. A scientific panel warned Feb. 11, 1973 that large numbers of supersonic aircraft presented possible grave risks to the environment.

The panel, an ad hoc committee of the National Academy of Science's-National Research Council, said, "sufficient knowledge is at hand to warrant utmost concern."

Cited were increased amounts of ultraviolet radiation that might reach the earth's surface from the sun as result of nitric oxides emitted in jet exhausts. The oxides would degrade the ozone in the stratosphere, which served as an umbrella shield against harmful ultraviolet rays.

The report said excessive amounts of ultraviolet rays were harmful to both animal and plant life. "The formation of this protective shield of ozone in prehistoric time was most likely a prerequisite for the evolution of terrestrial life."

SST-ozone studies. The Transportation Department Jan. 21, 1975 made public a report finding that operation of the 30 supersonic transports (SSTs) currently flying or scheduled for service caused climate effects that were "much smaller than minimally detectable." It cautioned, however, that expansion of SST service should be monitored because the ozone shield in the stratosphere could be weakened by SST exhaust if the fleet were enlarged without reduction of current engine emissions.

A study issued March 31 by the National Academy of Sciences' National Research Council said that supersonic and subsonic flights in the stratosphere (altitudes above 40,000 feet) would increase the risk of skin cancer among people on the ground, particularly those in the Northern Hemisphere where most such flights took place.

The panel calculated that a 10% decrease in the stratospheric ozone layer would permit enough excess ultraviolet radiation to reach the earth to raise skin cancer incidence by at least 20%. They said engine exhaust emissions from a fleet of some 300–400 supersonic transports (SSTs) of the type once considered in the U.S. would have caused such an ozone depletion.

The scientists called for redesign of current jet engines and estimated it might take ten years and $100-million to develop engines with acceptably low emission levels.

Dispute over Concorde. The issue of noise pollution was the major factor in a dispute over whether the U.S. should allow the Concorde airliner, a French-British supersonic jet, to make flights to the U.S.

Transportation Secretary William T. Coleman Nov. 13, 1975 made public an environmental impact statement by the Federal Aviation Administration concluding that even the limited number of flights planned—four a day to Kennedy International Airport in New York and two a day to Dulles International Airport near Washington—would have "adverse environmental effects."

The FAA statement also said there could be "some" damage to the earth's protective ozone layer because of the Concorde's stratospheric emissions. Such damage could open the way to the earth's surface for more ultraviolet radiation from the sun, which could cause an increase in skin cancer. Coleman estimated that the number of nonfatal cases of skin cancer from the planned Concorde flights at 200 a year, a .1% rise in the annual U.S. rate of 250,000 cases.

As for other air pollution from the Concorde emissions, the FAA said it would be increased but without "significant off-airport" consequences.

Coleman stressed that he had an "open mind" on the matter and indicated that the noise factor might not be the determining one. Pointing out that the wide-bodied jets were noisier than the old propeller planes, he questioned whether it was reasonable to "prevent new technology" merely because of noise.

Coleman Feb. 4, 1976 announced his decision to allow limited Concorde service to Washington and New York on a 16-month trial basis.

Excluding noise, Coleman said he did not consider the environmental consequences of the limited service "to be substantial."

His decision also would enable continued development of a cleaner, quieter SST and would indicate, Coleman said, whether such a carrier would be a "sound capital investment."

The Concorde flights to Dulles International Airport outside Washington, D.C. were begun May 24.

Legal challenges to Coleman's ruling on the flights had been cleared just before the first flights were made. His decision was adjudged to be legal and reasonable May 19 by a three-judge panel of the U.S. Court of Appeals in the District of Columbia. The suit was brought by the Environmental Defense Fund and joined by New York State and others. A bid to pursue the case further by Virginia's Fairfax County, where Dulles was located, was rejected May 22 by Chief Justice Warren E. Burger.

Corcorde service into Kennedy had been barred March 11 by the Port Authority of New York and New Jersey, operator of Kennedy, until at least a six-month evaluation of Concorde operations elsewhere.

Carter backs Concorde trial flights. President Carter had sent messages to British and French leaders affirming his Administration's support of trial flights to the U.S. for the Concorde, the Anglo-French supersonic transport (SST), Jody Powell, presidential press secretary, said Feb. 16, 1977. But in answer to a query, Powell said Carter stood behind campaign statements in which he had called the Ford Administration's approval of the trial program a "mistake." According to Powell, the President believed "it wouldn't be wise to terminate the trial" because it was well underway.

Carter's messages were in response to communications he had received from British Prime Minister James Callaghan and French President Valery Giscard d'Estaing. They had expressed "concern" over a Feb. 3 action by the Port Authority of New York and New Jersey to delay until at least March 10 any decision on whether to allow Concorde flights to New York City's Kennedy International Airport.

The messages from Carter indicated that he wished to "approach this matter in a way that reflected the close friendship between our countries."

British Prime Minister James Callaghan discussed the Concorde with President Carter during a visit to Washington March 10–11. Callaghan disclosed March 11 that, contrary to expectation, he had not attempted to pressure the President on the SST furor.

French Foreign Minister Louis de Guiringaud March 8 called the Concorde issue "the first serious test of French-American relations" under the Carter Administration, and warned that a decision to ban the Concorde from New York City would affect trade relations between the U.S. and France.

White House Press Secretary Jody Powell March 9 said Carter believed the plane should be permitted into Kennedy Airport for the duration of the federally approved trial period.

Appeals court backs JFK Concorde ban—A three-judge panel of the 2nd U.S. Circuit Court of Appeals in New York City June 14 overturned a lower court order that would have allowed the Concorde to land at Kennedy International Airport.

The appeals court reversed a decision by U.S. District Court Judge Milton Pollack lifting a ban on Concorde operations at Kennedy imposed by the Port Authority of New York and New Jersey. The panel, in an opinion written by Chief Judge Irving R. Kaufman, said the Port Authority had the power to ban noisy aircraft as long as the ban was based on "fair, reasonable and nondiscriminatory" standards. The two other members of the panel, Judges Walter R. Mansfield and Ellsworth A. Van Graafeiland, concurred with Kaufman's opinion.

Aerosols & ozone threat. Two separate studies reported Sept. 26–27, 1974 that inert gases used as propellants in widely-used aerosol sprays were chemically broken down by sunlight and acted as a catalyst in destruction of the stratospheric ozone layer, which serves as a shield against harmful ultraviolet rays. The destructive action by these chlorofluoromethane gases added to concern about the essential ozone layer, which was also said to be threatened by nitric oxides from nuclear explosions and supersonic aircraft.

The New York Times reported Sept. 26 that Harvard University scientists had calculated that even if use of such gases (widely known under the trade name Freon) were halted as soon as practicable, the lingering effects would cause a 5% depletion of ozone by 1990. If use of the gases continued to increase at the present rate, the ozone level would be down 7% by 1984 and 30% by 1994.

In a study reported in the Sept. 27 issue of Science magazine, three University of Michigan scientists said chlorine derived from Freon gases could become the dominant factor in ozone breakdown within 10 or 15 years. The report stated that if emissions were halted immediately, ozone destruction would peak around 1990 and remain "significant" for several decades afterwards.

The report noted that its calculations could be understated, since they were based on the effect of the release of only the first chlorine atom, while actually all four potentially destructive atoms might be freed.

(In addition to use in aerosols, Freon was also widely used as a refrigerant.)

A federal panel said June 12, 1975 that aerosol sprays using fluorocarbons as propellants should be banned by January, 1978 unless new evidence proved that they did not dilute the protective ozone layer in the stratosphere.

The theory that aerosols depleted ozone in the stratosphere was "legitimate cause for concern," the panel said.

The task force, from 14 federal agencies, suggested some steps to be taken immediately: consideration of a labeling requirement for all aerosol products using fluorocarbons to identify the suspected gases, which were used in more than half the three billion aerosol cans sold annually; enactment of legislation to control toxic substances, which would enhance federal authority to require safeguards for commercial and auto airconditioners, for example, that used fluorocarbons as refrigerants; publicizing the potential hazard internationally, since the U.S. accounted for about 50% of total world output of fluorocarbons.

The Consumer Product Safety Commission July 14 rejected a petition to ban aerosol sprays. The petition had been filed by the National Resources Defense Council.

A National Academy of Sciences committee said in a report issued Sept. 13, 1976 that fluorcarbon use would almost certainly have to be regulated at some point to prevent weakening of the atmosphere's ozone layer.

"Selective regulation of fluorocarbon uses and releases is almost certain to be necessary at some time and to some degree of completeness," the report said. "Neither the needed timing nor the needed severity can be reasonably specified today."

It recommended a waiting period of no more than two years before regulatory action was taken. During the waiting period further studies would be made and more data gathered.

The Food & Drug Administration said April 26, 1977 that, effective Oct. 31, it would require that all food, drug and cosmetic containers that used chlorofluorocarbon propellants and were shipped in interstate commerce to be labeled with the following warning:

"Warning: contains chlorofluorocarbons and may harm the public health and environment by reducing ozone in the upper atmosphere."

The action was intended as a first step toward the eventual elimination of virtually all such containers.

Oregon curbs sprays—Gov. Robert Straub signed into law June 16, 1975 a bill making Oregon the first state to ban aerosol cans using fluorocarbons, effective March 1, 1977.

Fluorocarbon Spray Products Banned. A federal ban against the use of fluorocarbon gas in almost all aerosol sprays was announced March 15, 1978 in an action to prevent damage to the Earth's atmosphere.

Fluorocarbons floating into the atmosphere caused a depletion of the ozone layer, which protected the planet from harmful effects of the Sun's ultraviolet rays, according to scientific reports.

Without the protection, scientists warned, a higher incidence of skin cancer was possible, as well as changes in climate and harm to plant and other animal life.

The ban, issued by the Food and Drug Administration, the Environmental Protection Agency and the Consumer Product Safety Commission, would cut off manufacture of aerosol products using fluorocarbons after Dec. 15, 1978.

Entry of the products into the market would be prohibited after April 15, 1979.

The ban applied to 97% to 98% of all aerosols using fluorocarbon gas as a propellant. It would cover such products as deodorants, hair sprays, household cleaners and some pesticides.

The 2% to 3% of products exempted from the ban were those "for which no acceptable substitutes" existed. These included certain insecticides, respiratory drugs, contraceptive foams and cleaning sprays for electrical and aircraft equipment.

The ban covered what the agencies considered "all nonessential uses" of fluorocarbons in sprays. Most of the products involved were expected to be able to convert to use of mechanical sprayers or other propellants such as carbon dioxide or hydrocarbons.

Since the scientific finding of ozone depletion, and under the preliminary curbs ordered by the federal agencies, use of fluorocarbons in aerosols had dropped about 40% in the last three years.

The regulatory agencies estimated the regulations could cost the aerosol industry between $169 million and $267 million a year for four years, beginning in the fall of 1978.

Danger in Food & Drink & Other Every-Day Items

The Delaney Clause: All Food Carcinogens Banned

In 1958 the Food, Drug & Cosmetic Act was modified by an amendment stating that "no [food] additive shall be deemed to be safe if it is found to induce cancer when ingested by man or animal, or if it is found, after tests which are appropriate for the evaluation of the safety of food additives, to induce cancer in man or animal. . . ."

This so-called Delaney Clause, under which a variety of food additives have since been outlawed for sale in the U.S., was introduced by Rep. James J. Delaney (D, N.Y.). It has been a subject of dispute for years. Many activists in the consumer-protection movement argue that the clause protects the public from serious environmental danger. Opponents, including food-industry spokesmen, assert that the clause has led to bans on useful additives that protect health and have not been proven to cause cancer in people—even if they are found capable of causing cancer in test animals.

Scientists back additive curb. An informal conference of about 100 scientists and lawyers in New York agreed overwhelmingly that the 1958 Delaney Clause of the Food and Drug Act, which barred all food additives which could in any quantity induce cancer in men or animals, be retained for the present, it was reported Jan. 21, 1973.

The two-day conference, sponsored by the New York Academy of Sciences, was planned after Food and Drug Administration (FDA) Commissioner Charles C. Edwards joined industry critics of the clause. Edwards and other critics, testifying in September 1972 before the Senate Select Committee on Nutrition and Human Needs, said the clause was unscientific in allowing absolutely no qualifications, since current test methods could reveal traces of carcinogens so minute as not to be a health problem. They also argued that the clause could be interpreted as banning an additive if one cancer developed in one test animal. Edwards said the clause was difficult to enforce because of "conflicting, inconclusive" data.

Most conference participants reportedly said it would be impossible at present to determine safe levels of carcinogens, especially since the resulting cancer could be delayed as much as 20 years.

Some scientific support for the Delaney Clause had also been presented to the U.S. Surgeon General April 22, 1970 in a report by the Ad Hoc Committee on the Evaluation of Low Levels of Environmental

Chemical Carcinogens. Among recommendations and findings of the report:

In full consideration of the past and present states of carcinogenesis investigation this Committee offers the following recommendations:

1.a. Any substance which is shown conclusively to cause tumors in animals should be considered carcinogenic and therefore a potential cancer hazard for man. Exceptions should be considered only where the carcinogenic effect is clearly shown to result from physical, rather than chemical, induction, or where the route of administration is shown to be grossly inappropriate in terms of conceivable human exposure.

b. Data on carcinogenic effects in man are only acceptable when they represent critically evaluated results of adequately conducted epidemiologic studies.

2. No level of exposure to a chemical carcinogen should be considered toxicologically insignificant for man. For carcinogenic agents a "safe level for man" cannot be established by application of our present knowledge. The concept of "socially acceptable risk" represents a more realistic notion.

3. The statement made in 1969 by the Food Protection Committee, National Research Council (see Appendix II) that natural or synthetic substances can be considered safe without undergoing biological assay should be recognized as scientifically unacceptable.

4. No chemical substance should be assumed safe for human consumption without proper negative lifetime biological assays of adequate size. The minimum requirements for carcinogenesis bioassays should provide for: adequate numbers of animals of at least two species and both sexes with adequate controls, subjected for their lifetime to the administration of a suitable dose range, including the highest tolerated dose, of the test material by routes of administration that include those by which man is exposed. Adequate documentation of the test conditions and pathologic standards employed are essential.

5. Evidence of negative results, under the conditions of the test used, should be considered superseded by positive findings in other tests. Evidence of positive results should remain definitive, unless and until new evidence conclusively proves that the prior results were not causally related to the exposure.

6. The implication of potential carcinogenicity should be drawn both from tests resulting in the induction of benign tumors and those resulting in tumors which are more obviously malignant.

7. The principle of a zero tolerance for carcinogenic exposures should be retained in all areas of legislation presently covered by it and should be extended to cover other exposures as well. Only in the cases where contamination of an environmental source by a carcinogen has been proven to be unavoidable should exception be made to the principle of zero tolerance. Exceptions should be made only after the most extraordinary justification, including extensive documentation of chemical and biological analyses and a specific statement of the estimated risk for man, are presented. All efforts should be made to reduce the level of contamination to the minimum. Periodic review of the degree of contamination and the estimated risk should be made mandatory.

8. A basic distinction should be made between intentional and unintentional exposures.

a. No substance developed primarily for uses involving exposure to man should be allowed for wide-spread human intake without having been properly tested for carcinogenicity and found negative.

b. Any substance developed for use not primarily involving exposure in man but nevertheless resulting in such exposure, if found to be carcinogenic, should be either prevented from entering the environment or if it already exists in the environment, progressively eliminated.

• • •

The effects of carcinogens on tissues appear irreversible. Exposure to small doses of carcinogen over a period of time results in a summation or potentiation of effects. The fundamental characteristic which distinguishes the carcinogenic effect from other toxic effects is that the tissues affected do not seem to return to their normal condition. This summation of effects in time and the long interval (latent period) which passes after tumor induction before the tumor becomes clinically manifest demonstrate that cancer can develop in man and in animals long after the causative agent has been in contact and disappeared.

It is, therefore, important to realize that incidences of cancer in man today reflect exposure of 15 or more years ago; similarly, any increase of carcinogenic contaminants in man's enviroment today will reveal its carcinogenic effect some 15 or more years from now. For this reason it is urgent that every effort be made to detect and control sources of carcinogenic contamination of the environment well before damaging effects become evident in man. Similar concepts may apply to the needs for evaluation of other cronic toxicity hazards. Environmental cancer remains one of the major disease problems of modern man.

• • •

Physical factors are known to cause cancers in man and animals. For example, ultraviolet radiation causes skin cancer, and ionizing radiation cancer of various organs (e.g. leukemias, lung cancer, bone sarcomas, skin cancer). Exposure to a "background level" has been widely considered as unavoidable and, in the case of ultraviolet light, even necessary as an integral part of our natural environment. Strong epidemiologic and experimental evidence indicates the existence of a direct dose-response relationship between exposure to radiation and carcinogenic effects. Tolerance levels have been suggested for various forms of radiation and health benefits have been realized from their application. ...

Chemicals of many classes produce cancer in a large number of organ sites in animals. Cancers in man are known to be caused by several individual chemicals and by materials composed of mixtures of chemicals. Chemical carcinogens have been shown to act by surface contact with skin or mucosae, by inhalation, by ingestion, and occasionally by injection or implantation (medical or accidental). Chemicals may induce cancer at the site of initial contact (e.g. skin cancer from polynuclear hydrocarbons), the site of selective localization (e.g. bone cancer radionuclides), the site of metabolism and detoxification (e.g. liver or kidney cancer from aflatoxin or nitrosamines), or the site of excretion (e.g. urinary bladder cancer from aromatic amines). A complex and often uneven approach to the problem of preventing exposure to chemical carcinogens has developed over the years. It has become increasingly obvious that the hazard from a single chemical carcinogen cannot be evaluated out of context of the total environmental exposure. Estimation of the "cumulative carcinogenic dose" resulting from all possible chemical carcinogens or even from all sources of a single type or class of chemical carcinogens is presently impossible.

Prevention of exposure to known carcinogenic chemicals depends largely on man's ability to control their entry into the environment. Certain chemical carcinogens are natural products (e.g. metabolites of the amino acid trytophan) or naturally occurring contaminants (e.g. mycotoxins). Others are formed in the processing of natural products. Many, such as polynuclear hydrocarbons (e.g. benzo[a]pyrene), occur almost ubiquitously in our modern industrialized environment. They derive from most sources of organic combusion. A class of very potent carcinogens discovered only in recent years, the N-nitrosamines, include compounds that may be formed in the environment from nitrites and secondary amines. Many other known chemical carcinogens have been introduced as synthetic materials or by-products into man's present environment through a wide range of newly-developed industrial processes. Some of these, such as food additives, medicinal products, cosmetics, and certain household products or pesticides, were developed for human use. Several carcinogens derive from products such as tobacco smoke, developed exclusively for human use. In other cases chemical carcinogens not intended primarily for human exposure are introduced into the general environment and eventually come in contact with its inhabitants; many substances (certain polynuclear hydrocarbons, pesticides, metals, dusts, and fumes, etc.) gain widespread environmental distribution, thereby becoming pollutants of the air, soil, water, and food. Prevention of exposure to this broad spectrum of chemical carcinogens must take a variety of forms.

The productions of chemicals recognized as carcinogens for uses involving intentional human exposure can be identified and effectively eliminated. Exceptions to this approach should be made for substances that involve a well-defined health benefit (e.g. certain chemotherapeutic drugs). Use of such substances should be accepted on the basis of extraordinary evidence that their health benefit outweighs their risk.

The production of specific carcinogenic chemicals for uses that do not primarily involve an intentional exposure of man, but which result in such environmental contamination that extensive human exposure becomes inevitable, must also be controlled. The most effective prevention of exposure in man is the elimination of carcinogen production, or control of entry into the environment.

• • •

It is impossible to establish any absolutely safe level of exposure to a carcinogen for man. The concept of "toxicologically insignificant" levels (as advanced by the Food Protection Committee of the NAS/NRC in 1969; see Appendix II), of dubious merit in any life science, has absolutely no validity in the field of carcinogenesis. Society must be willing to accept some finite risk as the price of using any carcinogenic material in whatever quantity. The best that science can do is to estimate the upper probable limit of that risk. For this reason, the concept of "safe level for man", as applied to carcinogenic agents, should be replaced by that of a "socially acceptable level of risk".

While science can provide quantitative information regarding maximum risk levels, the task ultimately selecting socially acceptable levels of human risk rests with society and its political leaders. The evaluation of the balance of benefits and risks required for such a decision by society, should not be the result of uninformed guesswork but should be reached on the basis of complete and pertinent data, social as well as scientific.

• • •

Appendix II—Comments on 1969 Report of the Food Protection Committee

This Committee has examined a report entitled "Guidelines for Estimating Toxicologically Insignificant Levels of Chemicals in Food" published in 1969 by the Food Protection Committee—Food and Nutrition Board of the National Academy of Sciences—National Research Council. It records its strong objections to the principles expressed in that report, which states that natural or synthetic substances can be considered safe without experimental support under certain vaguely-stated conditions.

The Food Protection Committee Report assumes that " . . . a level of insignificance may be determined if: (1) There are available adequate scientific studies that establish safe levels of similar magnitude for at least two analogous substances. (2) the acute or subacute toxicity of the new substance and two analogous substances is of the same nature and degree." For "Chemicals in Commercial Production" it recommends that: "If a chemical has been in commercial production for a substantial period, e.g. 5 years or more, without evidence of toxicological hazard incident to its production or use, if it not a heavy metal or a compound of a heavy metal and, and if it is not intended for use because of its biological activity, it is consistent with sound toxicological judgment to conclude that a level of 0.1 ppm of the chemical in the diet of man is toxicologically insignificant."

To assume (a) that a 5-year period of use has any meaning for the evaluation of chronic toxicity in man, (b) that any chemical may be considered safe simply because two "analogous substances" are "safe", and (c) that acute or subacute toxicity are reliable guidelines for evaluating long-term toxicity is to display a lack of understanding and appreciation of factors involved in chronic toxicity, particularly of the irreversible and delayed toxic effects which occur in carcinogenesis.

Since the purpose of the report is to recommend guidelines and priorities for selecting chemicals for human use without direct experimental toxicological evaluation, the lack of consideration of irreversible long-term toxic effects (which would not be ruled out by the suggested criteria) makes the suggested approach practically inapplicable and potentially dangerous.

MEMBERS OF THE AD HOC COMMITTEE ON THE EVALUATION OF LOW LEVELS OF ENVIRONMENTAL CHEMICAL CARCINOGENS

(Ad Hoc Committee on the Evaluation of Low Levels of Environmental Chemical Carcinogens, National Cancer Institute, Bethesda, Md.)

Umberto, Saffiotti, Chairman, Associate Scientific Director for Carcinogenesis, Etiology, National Cancer Institute, Building 37, Room 3A21, Bethesda, Md.

Hans L. Falk, Associate Director for Laboratory Research, National Institute of Environmental Health Sciences, Research Triangle Park, N.C.

Paul Kotin, Director, National Institute of Environmental Health Sciences, Research Triangle Park, N.C.

William Lijinsky, Professor of Biochemistry, The Eppley Institute for Research on Cancer, University of Nebraska, College of Medicine, Omaha, Neb.

Marvin Schneiderman, Associate Chief, Biometry Branch, National Cancer Institute, Wisconsin Building, Room 5C10, Bethesda, Md.

Philippe Shubik, Director, The Eppley Institute for Research on Cancer, University of Nebraska, College of Medicine, Omaha, Neb.

Sidney Weinhouse, Director, Fels Research Institute, Temple University, School of Medicine, Philadelphia, Pa.

Gerald Wogan, Professor of Food Toxicology, Massachusetts Institute of Technology, 77 Massachusetts Avenue, Cambridge, Mass.

Staff Members: John A. Cooper, Executive Secretary, Richard R. Bates, James A Peters, Howard R. Rosenberg, Elizabeth K. Weisburger, John H. Weisburger.

Sen. Gaylord Nelson (D, Wis.) noted in the Senate Sept. 14, 1977 that two other "major conferences on food safety and the Delaney Clause"—a 1973 symposium by the New York Academy of Sciences and a 1974 forum by the National Academy of Sciences—had also failed to conclude that the Delaney Clause should be repealed. Nelson said:

At the 1973 Delaney conference in New York, no scientist, including those affiliated with industry, advocated weakening the Delaney clause.

At the 1974 National Academy of Sciences forum, scientists reached no consensus on modification of Delaney.

In other words, the most imminent scientists studying the issue do not believe that a safe level of a cancer-causing substance can be established for humans, which would support a change in the Delaney anticancer clause.

Dr. Philip Handler, President of the National Academy of Sciences, in a summary of the forum proceedings said:

For my part, I begin to view that [Delaney] clause as a great red herring rather than as a problem in our society. Certainly, on its face, all other things being equal, it is a perfectly rational guide to desirable societal behavior. No one in his right mind wants to put carcinogens into anything intended for human consumption. We should be perfectly willing to accept that guideline until the day when we find ourselves in the position of banning as a carcinogen some chemical entity which also offers great benefit. Until that time comes, we will not have to test the validity of the Delaney principle. When it does, we will have no recourse but to test the validity of the principle in a real life situation.

Dr. Handler continues:

* * * It has been said that the great harm of the Delaney clause is its deterrence to those who might otherwise be exploring new and important food additives. No such real case in point is known to me. (Academy proceedings, p. 175–6).

In testimony in May 1974 before the House Appropriations Subcommittee for Agriculture, former FDA Commissioner Alexander Schmidt, M.D., stated:

On the basis of the information, expert opinion and conclusions contained in the compilation, we are not prepared to state that the Delaney clause has had a deleterious effect, to date, upon the food supply, nor could we suggest any particular change in the anti-cancer clauses.

He said that "the growth of knowledge in carcinogenesis may eventually permit safe levels of carcinogenic additives to be determined, but that day is not yet here." The Commissioner also testified:

The evidence at hand does not indicate that the Delaney clause has barred public utilization of food additives of such importance that their prohibition has not been in the public interest. The question remains, however, as to whether the mere existence of the Delaney clause has had such a profound influence upon the FDA that action against carcinogenic substances, that might not have been taken otherwise, has been taken under the more general safety provisions of the FD&C Act. This question has no real answer, but it is clear from the history of the FD&C Act and anti-cancer legislation that the public wishes to have its food supply protected against the addition of "unsafe" food chemicals.

Academy Advises on Food-Safety Laws. The National Academy of Sciences recommended in a report March 2, 1979 that Congress significantly revise the nation's food-safety laws, including elimination of the automatic ban on any substance found to cause cancer in animals or humans. The academy report was ordered by Congress in 1977

Under the academy's proposals, the Food and Drug Administration would for the first time receive the power to classify substances by how risky they were and to regulate each classification differently. It could identify hazardous substances as high-risk, moderate-risk or low-risk. It could restrict sale or use, require warning labels or require public-education campaigns.

Another recommendation by the academy would permit government regulators to take into account questions of economic costs of banning a substance, as well as potential health hazards to the public.

The majority of the panel said the FDA should have "regulatory discretion," since "safety cannot be defined entirely by scientific processes." Dissenting members of the panel issued a strongly worded minority statement that insisted there was no "scientifically defensible way to divide carcinogens" into different risk categories since "the ability of science to quantify human risk" safely was still primitive.

The panel said saccharin could be determined "low-risk" or "moderate-risk," dependent upon FDA interpretation of animal tests and incidence of human cancers. The FDA could ban the sweetener "in whole or in part," or place a warning label on foods and drinks containing it. It could selectively ban it from schools. Decisions regarding nitrites used as preservatives in cured meats would be handled similarly.

FDA Commissioner Donald Kennedy told Congress that if he were given discretion to allow certain carcinogens into the food supply, he wanted very specific guidelines on how to make those decisions. Overly broad authority would leave the FDA commissioner "virtually the only target of special interests," he said.

Kennedy added that he was still required to ban saccharin by the 1958 Delaney Clause when an eighteenth-month congressional moratorium on the ban expired in May. He said he would seek to have saccharin removed from the nation's foods and beverages in any event, no matter what the laws said, because agency scientists remained convinced it may cause cancer.

'Threshold Dose' Theory. A longstanding controversy has flared within the scientific community over assertions that there is (or is not) a "threshold dose" below which a carcinogen would be harmless. Rep. David R. Obey (D, Wis.) presented data on the dispute July 27, 1979 in a statement in the Congressional Record:

One side in this controversy has argued that chemicals proven to cause

cancer in heavy dosages do not necessarily cause cancer at more typical low-dose levels, and that for many or perhaps all cancer causing chemicals there is a level of exposure low enough to pose no risk to human beings or in other words a "safety threshold." This would mean that requiring industry to reduce exposure to known carcinogens to the lowest possible level would be placing an unnecessary burden on industry. The regulation would be more severe than needed to protect the health of consumers or workers and that would be a strong argument to require regulatory agencies to establish safe threshold levels with each chemical proven to be cancer causing at high exposure levels.

Others have argued that any chemical that causes cancer at one level of exposure can be expected to pose some risk of cancer causation at any level. If millions of Americans are exposed to an air pollutant or food additive in only trace amounts we have only two ways to estimate whether significant harm is being done—either test a number of animals equal to the number of people exposed at precisely the same exposure level or test a small number of animals at a considerably higher exposure level. Since the first alternative would use all of the Nation's laboratories, toxic chemical researchers, and test animals for conducting a test on a single chemical, it really is not practical at all. So currently there is potentially only one way to identify such a hazard, feed it in heavy doses to a relatively small number of test animals and then make the assumption that a risk exists at lower exposure levels. It is precisely such tests and precisely that assumption that has been at the root of all the controversy.

The National Center for Toxicological Research, under the Food and Drug Administration, has recently conducted a massive and unprecedented experiment to examine the validity of the "threshold" and "no threshold" theories. A report on that experiment was printed in the June 28, 1979, "Occupational Safety and Health Reporter."

According to the report:

The theory that there is no "threshold dose level" below which a carcinogenic substance would be safe was supported by a recently completed carcinogenesis study using more than 24,000 mice.

• • •

Acting NCTR Director Thomas Cairns was quoted as saying:

"Explanation of the dose-response relationship at low doses is fundamental to the regulatory agencies' posture that there is no threshold level below which a carcinogen cannot exert its carcinogenic effect.

• • •

The study, using the carcinogen 2-acetylaminofluorine (2-AAF), was designed to determine with precision the effects of a known carcinogen at low dose levels, according to NCTR.

Among significant findings of the study were the following:

No threshold response effect was found at the lowest dose level used in the study.

The mice in the study developed a significant number of liver tumors which did not appear until after 18 months, at which point many current bioassay tests are ended.

The incidence of bladder tumors in the dosed mice dropped substantially when feeding of 2-AAF was stopped after the first nine months of the study. However, liver tumors continued to develop after 18 months, even when dosage was ended at nine months.

• • •

The controversy arises from the standard practice of testing suspected carcinogens by administering massive doses of a substance to a relatively small number of test animals. The results of such experiments are extrapolated to predict the effect of very low exposure levels on human populations.

Such tests, Cairns said, "have been challenged on scientific grounds and are confused, even distrusted, by laymen who see only the differences between the experimental process and ordinary life situations."

"The '800 cans of diet soda' perception of toxicological research and its validity is undoubtedly a serious impediment to the credibility of our research and the regulatory decisions that may be based on it."

Danger in Sweeteners

Some of the strongest opposition to government curbs on carcinogens arises when the government acts against a substance or habit that the public doesn't want to give up—e.g., artificial sweeteners and cigarettes.

Cyclamates banned in all foods. The Food & Drug Administration Aug. 14, 1970 reinstated a total ban on the use of cyclamates, an artificial sweetener, in all foods, including those labeled "drugs" for diabetics or other persons needing to restrict intake of calories. The government had first banned cyclamates in October 1969, but had modified the order in February to exclude use of the sweetener as a drug.

The August 1970 order made it illegal to sell any food, drug or soft drink containing cyclamates as of Sept. 1, 1970. The agency said its Medical Advisory Group on Cyclamates had "reviewed its recommendation" and decided on a total ban of the chemical "in the light of scientific evidence available to date."

The new evidence showed that much smaller amounts of cyclamates than previously tested produced cancer in rats. The agency said use of the chemical at a safe level would result in an "insignificant caloric reduction having no practical value for the obese or the diabetic patient."

Dr. Charles C. Edwards, FDA commissioner, had conceded in testimony before a House committee June 10 that cyclamates should have been withdrawn sooner.

(The Department of Health, Education and Welfare [HEW] had removed the artificial sweetener from the government list of substances recognized as safe in foods Oct. 18, 1969.)

Edwards told Rep. L. H. Fountain (D, N. C.), chairman of the House Committee on Government Operations, that "there is no question that it should have been done earlier," when asked about the government's ban. Edwards declined to say how much earlier.

Another health official who appeared before the committee, William W. Goodrich, assistant HEW general counsel, said that the government's action had not been taken sooner because of lack of agreement in the scientific study groups that advised the FDA about cyclamates.

Saccharin reported safe. A special study group of the National Academy of Sciences-Research Council reported to the FDA July 23, 1970 that the synthetic sweetener saccharin posed no known hazard to its users. The panel said its findings were made "on the basis of available information."

But the eight-man study group recommended further laboratory tests of the sweetener despite an "80-year history of saccharin use by man without evidence of adverse effects."

The FDA had requested the study in March 1969 after a University of Wisconsin researcher had reported that combinations of saccharin and cholesterol injected in the urinary bladders of mice caused cancers of that organ in some of the mice.

Saccharin curbed. The FDA Jan. 28, 1972 removed saccharin from its list of food additives "generally recognized as safe" (GRAS). It did so on the basis of new tests in which mice fed large doses developed bladder tumors.

Edwards said the action limited use to current levels while research continued. If the tumors were found cancerous and attributed to saccharin, the government planned to outlaw saccharin. The Jan. 28 action required American food processors to list the saccharin content on package labels. The FDA, following National Research Council advice, recommended a maximum adult daily use of one gram, the equivalent of seven 12-ounce bottles of diet beverage or 60 small tablets.

The 1972 interim rules were extended by the FDA May 24, 1973.

The rules had been scheduled to expire June 30, when the FDA expected to act on a review by the National Academy of Sciences (NAS) of several studies of the cancer-causing properties of the artificial sweetener. The FDA said, however, that the NAS would be unable to meet the deadline.

The FDA had announced May 21 that a pathology report on a two-year rat feeding study showed "presumptive evidence" that saccharin caused cancerous bladder tumors on three of 48 rats fed saccharin as 7.5% of their diet.

The FDA reported Jan. 9, 1975 that its study had been unable to determine whether saccharin caused cancer in test animals.

The FDA said that in the interim saccharin would continue to be marketed under current limitations.

Saccharin had been in use in the U.S. for about 80 years. Americans consumed about five million pounds of the substance each year, according to the government. Saccharin was a staple of the diet-food industry, with low-calorie soft drinks accounting for three-quarters of the yearly consumption.

FDA bans saccharin. The FDA March 9, 1977 issued a proposed ban on saccharin, the only artificial sweetener still available in the U.S. The agency based its decision in part on laboratory tests conducted by Canadian scientists that showed rats fed high dosages of the sweetener developed malignant bladder tumors.

The FDA ban applied to all foods and beverages with saccharin additives. However, the agency indicated that existing inventories of saccharin products would not be recalled.

Action draws protests—The FDA ban on saccharin drew angry protests from consumers and representatives of the food industry March 9–10.

William P. Inman, a vice president of Sherwin-Williams Co. of Cleveland, the only U.S. manufacturer of saccharin, March 9 said his firm had not "seen anything that even [came] close to conclusively proving that saccharin [was] a health hazard." Inman's contention was supported the same day by a spokesman for Abbott Laboratories in Chicago, maker of a popular saccharin-based sweetener, Sucaryl. The spokesman said that "a number of other well-controlled studies" in addition to the Canadian experiments had "shown no harmful effects from saccharin used in equally high doses."

(The FDA, in announcing the ban, had admitted that a human would have to drink 800 12-ounce soft drinks sweetened with saccharin every day for a lifetime to match the doses given to the rats in the Canadian tests.)

Robert M. Kellen, president of the Atlanta-based Calorie Control Council March 9 criticized the FDA decision as "an example of colossal government overregulation in disregard of science and the needs and wants of consumers." Kellen charged that the results of the Canadian tests were inconclusive and that the risk to human health was minimal. He called for an international investigation of the issue.

The executive vice president of Cumberland Packing Corp., maker of the nation's most widely used saccharin sweetener, Sweet 'n Low, March 9 called the ban "an outrageous and harmful action." Marvin Eisenstadt said the government, in effect, was telling diabetics they "can't taste anything sweet anymore."

Cumberland Packing March 10 announced plans to halt production for the immediate future and lay off 500 workers in New York City, 100 in Miami and 100 in Los Angeles. Sweet 'n Low was the company's sole product.

Both Coca-Cola Co. and PepsiCo Inc. March 10 said they probably would market diet soft drinks with sugar derivatives in the future.

A spokesman for the American Diabetes Association March 10 warned that the lack of sugar substitutes could have "very grave" effects for America's 10 million diabetics. Doctors considered diet control essential in the treatment of the disease. Most diabetics used an artificial sweetener as a substitute for natural sugar products.

Canada sets saccharin ban—The Canadian government March 9 announced that a broad ban on saccharin would take effect in that country June 1. As in the case of the U.S. action, the Canadian decision was based largely on the results of tests conducted by Canadian scientists that linked saccharin to cancer.

The Canadian ban would be more extensive than that of the U.S. The Ottawa government said saccharin would be forbidden in practically all its current applications. Beverages containing the substance would be outlawed after July 1. Drugs containing saccharin as a non medicinal ingredient would not be permitted after Dec. 31, 1978, with the exception of some "life-saving" drugs. Cosmetics, toothpaste and mouthwash containing saccharin would not be allowed after Dec. 31, 1979.

Trading reactions—Rumors of the impending U.S. and Canadian bans caused the common stocks of soft-drink manufacturers to drop sharply March 9. (The governments' announcements had been made after the close of trading in New York.) On the New York Stock Exchange composite tape, Coca-Cola Co. common stock fell $3 to $73 on a volume of 152,200 shares. PepsiCo Inc. common stock fell $2.62 to $68 on a volume of 50,600 shares.

World prices of raw sugar showed little response March 9. On the New York Coffee and Sugar Exchange, contracts with a May delivery date rose only three-hundredths of a cent per pound to close at 9¢, at least 3¢ below the cost of production.

Sugar futures showed only a moderate gain March 10, surprising many traders, who had expected the prices to rise sharply because of the saccharin bans.

Saccharin ban modified. The FDA April 14, 1977 modified the saccharin ban to allow saccharin to remain on sale for limited use as a nonprescription drug. Under the new proposal, saccharin could be sold in tablet, powder or liquid form in pharmacies, food stores and restaurants, but its use still would be prohibited in commercially prepared foods and beverages. (Commercially prepared foods and beverages currently accounted for 90% of saccharin use.)

The new proposal would ban the use of saccharin in cosmetics likely to be ingested, such as lipstick, and in nonmedical additives used to make prescription drugs taste better. It also would allow the sweetener to be labeled as an over-the-counter drug. This would circumvent the legal ban on cancer-causing food additives—the Delaney Clause added in 1958 to the Food, Drug & Cosmetic Act. The proposed drug classification would force manufacturers to show that saccharin was both safe and effective for the medical purpose for which it was intended, pursuant to the 1962 Harris-Kefauver amendments to the act.

Finally, the FDA proposal would require that packages containing saccharin be labeled: "Warning: saccharin causes bladder cancer in animals. Use of saccharin may increase your risk of cancer. For use as a non-caloric sweetener when sugar-restricted diets are medically indicated, as in patients with diabetes."

In the midst of a continuing furor over the proposed ban, FDA Commissioner Dr. Donald Kennedy defended the FDA action April 14, saying, "Our scientists now calculate that a moderate use of saccharin, the amount present in one large diet soft drink, if ingested daily over a lifetime by every American, might lead to 1,200 additional cases of bladder cancer per year."

The FDA announcement said:

Many of the 16,000 consumers who have written FDA since March 9 have worried that the Canadian rat study involved such high doses of saccharin that the results were unrealistic. There is an impression that almost any substance fed in such high doses would cause cancer.

Neither of these views is correct.

The exposure of test animals to high doses is the most valid way we know to predict whether a chemical may cause cancer in people. Such tests are both realistic and reliable.

They are, in fact, essential to predict rare occurrences—for example, to seek out and identify a substance that can cause cancer in only one out of every 20,000 Americans. That may be a rare occurrence statistically but it's still more than 10,000 people in our population.

It is essential that we use test animals to help us identify early enough to do something about them the suspicious chemicals to which we may be exposed in the foods we eat, the drugs we use, the water we drink and the air we breathe.

It's fairly easy for reasonable people to understand why we must use animals to try to predict which chemicals will and which will not be likely to hurt people. It is harder to understand why science must test these animals with doses far larger than humans are ever likely to receive. The first answer is practicality.

No one could breed, raise, sacrifice and examine test animals fast enough to find one case of cancer out of 20,000 animals. There aren't enough breeders, examiners, time or money.

Instead, we use fewer animals. And to compensate for that, we use high doses. And over the years we have established that the system works! Animal tests identical in principle to those used for saccharin have demonstrated cancer in animals for virtually all the chemicals known to cause cancer in people.

So, if a chemical tested in high doses on a limited number of animals causes cancer, we are concerned. We are concerned for two reasons: First, because science warns us that if a high dose of something causes cancer in a significant number of test animals, a low dose may cause cancer in some people; and, second, science reassures us that most chemicals do not cause cancer no matter how high the dose. It's simply not true, as many people believe, that too much of almost anything will cause cancer.

In fact, in 1969, the National Cancer Institute reported that of 120 pesticides and industrial compounds given to mice, only 11 were found definitely to induce tumors. And these chemicals were not randomly selected. Most were picked because there already was reason to suspect that they might cause cancer. Even so, the great majority of more than 100 suspicious chemicals did not cause cancer in animals when tested at high dose levels.

Recent experiments on saccharin conform to the requirements of good animal testing and good science. They tell us beyond reasonable doubt that saccharin is among the comparatively small number of substances that do cause cancer in test animals and, therefore, may be hazardous to humans.

We clearly cannot determine from animals exposed to high doses of a cancer-causing chemical precisely how many humans might get cancer from a lower dose. But there are methods for estimating the maximum number of people who might be so affected.

• • •

Since these early days of toxicology, the use of tests in laboratory animals to predict the long-term chronic effect of chemicals in man has been accepted by virtually all scientists and is today used by every technologically advanced country in the world. In the United States, many Federal agencies in addition to FDA, such as the Environmental Protection Agency and the National Cancer Institute, rely on these animal tests to assess the safety of a variety of compounds. In 1954, the National Academy of Sciences/National Research Council (the Academy) published a report entitled "Principles and Procedures for Evaluating the Safety of Intentional Chemical Additives in Foods." This report updated pamphlets published in 1951 and 1952 on the safe use of chemicals in foods. The 1954 report and subsequent publications by the Academy describe the widely accepted approach of animal tests for evaluating the safety of chemicals added to foods. The World Health Organization has also espoused the use of animal tests to assess the safety of food ingredients.

WHO finds no proven human risk—The World Health Organization May 13 said that to date, there was no proven evidence that saccharin caused bladder cancer in humans. The U.N. agency had carried out epidemiological studies, primarily among diabetics, that indicated no increased risk of bladder cancer.

A special committee of experts compiled the saccharin report on behalf of member nations who had requested information on the substance following U.S. and Canadian actions to restrict its use.

OTA panel affirms cancer risk—A scientific panel named by the Office of Technology Assessment to review the saccharin controversy for Congress reported June 7 that the artificial sweetener was a weak carcinogen that should not be considered safe for human consumption. The group was unable to definitively measure saccharin's potential to cause cancer in humans but cited studies showing it had caused bladder cancer in rats.

Dutch put limit on saccharin—The Netherlands' Health Ministry announced May 9 that saccharin would be banned from Dutch foodstuffs and drinks. Saccharin products for obese or diabetic persons would not be affected by the precaution, although labels would have to give the saccharin content of such products.

Saccharin linked to human cancer. A new Canadian study reported June 17, 1977 directly linked the use of artificial sweeteners to bladder cancer in humans. As a result, the U.S. Food and Drug Administration June 20 extended the comment period on its proposed saccharin ban by up to 60 days (until Aug. 31) to evaluate the study. The delay ensured that the ban would not go into effect before Oct. 1.

The as yet unpublished survey, conducted by the National Cancer Institute of Canada in conjunction with four Canadian universities, found that men who used saccharin or cyclamates had a 60% higher chance of developing bladder cancer than those who did not. The study showed no increased cancer risk among women who used artificial sweteners.

Previous concern about saccharin as a carcinogen had been based on evidence that it caused cancer in rats. The new study was the first to associate saccharin with human cancer. The survey, which involved 630 bladder cancer patients, also found that smoking was eight times more important as a determinant of bladder cancer than the use of non-nutritive artificial sweeteners.

FDA Commissioner Donald Kennedy said June 27 that the new study "raises serious questions about the wisdom of our present proposal," which would allow saccharin to remain on the market as a nonprescription drug. The recent findings raised doubts as to "whether saccharin should remain available for any purpose," Kennedy said.

Saccharin ban deferred. Legislation delaying a proposed Food and Drug Administration ban on saccharin cleared Congress Nov. 4, 1977, and President Jimmy Carter signed it Nov. 23.

The bill delayed implementation of the proposed ban for 18 months, during which time new scientific studies would be conducted. The bill mandated two studies: one of saccharin in particular, and another investigating the cancer-causing properties of food additives in general.

The bill also required a health warning label for food containing saccharin. The label would read: "Use of this product may be hazardous to your health. This product contains saccharin, which has been determined to cause cancer in laboratory animals."

(The label requirement applied only to food products introduced in interstate commerce 90 days after enactment of the bill.)

The bill also required retail stores that sold saccharin-containing items to post health warnings.

The House of Representatives gave final approval to the bill Nov. 3, and the Senate cleared it Nov. 4. Both chambers acted by voice vote.

Sen. Gaylord Nelson (D, Wis.) pointed out to the Senate Sept. 14 that the debate on the saccharin ban involved "very important issues." He said the issues are:

Public policy to protect human health and safety—how much protection people want versus the right to choose;

Whether the testing criteria on which public health policy decisions are made are valid;

The extent to which small amounts of cancer causing agents in the food supply is considered a human risk;

Whether benefits-versus-risks should be considered when making safety decisions for food.

The FDA's action was taken pursuant to the 1958 food additives safety law, which requires that foods be free of harm or any significant risk of harm and free of potential cancer-causing agents—the Delaney clause, section 409(c)(3)(A), Food Drug and Cosmetic Act. The law prohibits approval of a food additive—

> If a fair evaluation of the data before the Secretary (a) fails to establish that the proposed use of the food additive, under the conditions of use to be specified in the regulation will be safe. . . . (Sec. 409(c)(3)(A)).

Saccharin fails both the Delaney anticancer and general safety provisions of the statute.

Therefore, the FDA proposed the ban, pursuant to the law based on compelling scientific evidence that saccharin is a carcinogen in both man and animals.

Opponents of the proposed saccharin ban claim that:

First, it violates freedom of choice;

Second, it is not warranted by the scientific evidence, which is not conclusive respecting the potential for cancer in humans from saccharin use;

Third, the animal test methodology—using high doses—is an unrealistic predictor of harm for humans;

Fourth, there are many benefits to humans, which outweigh the small risk of cancer; and

Fifth, the Delaney anticancer law is too inflexible in light of modern technology, which allows detection of minute amounts of substances in parts-per-trillion.

Arguments for the ban are:

First, freedom of choice to allow widespread exposure to cancer-causing substances affects more than one individual, impacting on the entire society in terms of costs and the inability of most people to make adequately informed decisions in scientific and technical matters;

Second, the proposed ban is based on a valid law, which is designed to protect the public health from unsafe food additives;

Third, the scientific evidence for potential harm to humans is valid, based on retrospective epidemiology, statistical studies of humans exposed to saccharin over a long period of time;

Fourth, the animal studies are scientifically valid as predictors for humans, and have proven out the theory that virtually every carcinogen known to cause cancer in animals also does so in humans;

Fifth, there are no scientifically supported benefits to saccharin;

Sixth, the Delaney clause is based on a general consensus among scientists that no safe threshold for a carcinogen has been established;

Seventh, overturning the FDA's proposal sets a dangerous precedent for legislating on a substance-by-substance basis, with respect to the extent to which Congress intervenes in regulatory decisionmaking in response to interest-group pressures.

• • •

Dr. Donald S. Fredrickson, Director of the National Institutes of Health, testified to the Senate Health Subcommittee, June 7, 1977:

One must assume that until proven otherwise, materials shown to cause cancer in animals also cause it in human beings. It will be extremely difficult to prove that saccharin is an exception to this rule. When the animal data are carried over to man in the conventional way, they indicate that two or three percent of the 30,000 new cases of bladder cancer each year could be due to saccharin in the low doses now used by the American population.

Sen. Edward M. Kennedy (D, Mass.) told the Senate Sept. 15 that "the American people" had "reacted with shock and disbelief" to the FDA's decision to ban saccharin. The scientific community and medical profession were "divided" and the public "skeptical" over FDA Commissioner Donald Kennedy's "valiant effort to explain its [the FDA's] decision," he added. Sen. Kennedy said:

How reliably can we predict whether chemicals have the potential to cause cancer in man? If a substance causes cancer in animals, does it cause cancer in man? Can we extrapolate the degree of human risk from animal studies? Should carcinogens be automatically removed from the market or should there be an analysis of benefits and risks? If a substance has both benefits and risks, who should decide whether the risk should be taken—the Federal Government or the individual? What is the appropriate role of a Federal health regulatory agency? Is it to provide individuals with sufficient information to enable them to make their own judgments, or is it to protect individuals on the basis of its best scientific evaluation? Can consumers be provided with sufficient information to make informed judgments on their own in public health matters? When is it appropriate for a regulatory agency to provide information and allow individual assumption of risk? When is it appropriate for the regulatory agency to act on behalf of the individual? What is meant by the term "safe"? Is there absolute safety? If not, how does the risk-benefit decision get made and by whom?

The saccharin controversy raises all these questions. The Senate Health and Scientific Research Subcommittee has carefully examined these questions. On the basis of that review, I have reached the following understanding of the facts:

First. Saccharin causes cancer in rats.

Second. Most substances which cause cancer in rats cause cancer in humans. The degree of risk is impossible to predict.

Third. One Canadian study concludes that saccharin increases the human risk of bladder cancer from a lifetime risk of 1 in 100 to 1.6 in 100. By contrast, cigarette smoking increases the risk of developing lung cancer by 800 to 1,000 percent, and the risk of bladder cancer by 12 to 20 percent.

Fourth. According to that same Canadian study, approximately 7 percent of bladder cancer cases in Canada may be attributed to saccharin use. If those figures were to hold for the United States, saccharin use would account for 1,500 to 2,000 cases of bladder cancer per year.

Fifth. Two additional studies in progress in the United States by Dr. Ernst Wynder of the American Health Foundation and Dr. Irving Kessler of Johns

Hopkins Medical School do not show a correlation between saccharin use and bladder cancer.

Sixth. The Canadian study indicates only males are at risk from bladder cancer. There are 30,000 cases of bladder cancer in the United States each year, 22,000 of which are in males.

Seventh. As many as 40 million Americans may benefit from the use of saccharin. This figure includes diabetics, hypertensives, obese people, and those suffering from heart disease, not to mention the less significant benefits from reduced dental cavities.

Eighth. Although no formal studies of health benefits have been made, eminent scientists and physicians believe the benefit to saccharin use outweighs the risks. These include:

Antonio M. Giotto, professor and chairman of the department of internal medicine at Baylor College of Medicine;

Dr. Harriett Dustin, president of the American Heart Association;

Dr. Kurt J. Isselbacher, professor of medicine and chairman of medicine at Harvard Medical School;

Dr. Albert J. Stunkard, professor, department of psychiatry, Philadelphia General Hospital; and

Donnell Etzwiler, M.D., president of the American Diabetes Association.

Ninth. Reservations about the saccharin ban were also expressed by two prestigious medical journals: The New England Journal of Medicine and the Lancet. . . .

. . .

. . . Tenth. There is no unanimity of opinion among scientists. This division was also reflected in the opinions of the expert panel assembled by the Office of Technology Assessment to review the saccharin controversy. Approximately half the members of the OTA panel expressed the opinion that saccharin should not be banned because of its potential health benefits, while the other half supported the decision of the Food and Drug Administration.

Eleventh. The decision of the Food and Drug Administration to remove saccharin from the market was dictated by the provisions of the Food, Drug and Cosmetic Act. That act provided no discretion for the Commissioner. It does not allow for the weighing of benefits versus risks.

. . . I yield to no man in the U.S. Senate in my determination to reduce the risk of cancer. I know first hand of the ravaging impact that that disease can have on its victim and on the victim's family. But those who try to portray the saccharin controversy as a litmus test of whether one is for or against cancer do a grave disservice to the American people. Cancer kills—but so does heart disease—so does hypertension—so does obesity—and the victim is just as dead no matter what the cause. The real question is whether there are health benefits to saccharin to outweigh the potential health risks of saccharin.

When the chairman of the department of medicine at Harvard University School of Medicine and the chairman of the department of medicine at the Baylor School of Medicine believe that more harm would be done by removing saccharin from the market than by leaving it on the market, I believe it should be clear to everyone that some of the best medical minds in this country do not subscribe to the theory that saccharin represents an unacceptable health risk. Mr. President, even the former director of the National Cancer Institute has questioned the wisdom of FDA's banning of saccharin.

Given the division of scientific opinion, given the incomplete nature of the scientific evidence, it is wrong to allow the FDA to make a definitive decision on saccharin now. More needs to be known. The risks need to be more precisely defined, the benefits need to be scientifically demonstrated.

Mr. President, when the scientific community is evenly divided about what course of action to follow; when the medical profession is evenly divided about what course to follow; when the American Diabetes Association, the American Medical Association, the American Heart Association, the Juvenile Diabetes Foundation all argue to leave saccharin on the market; when other consumer groups such as the Health Research Group take a contrary opinion, then I believe the individual is in the best position to decide for himself or herself whether they want to expose themselves or their children to saccharin use.

Sen. Nelson Sept. 15 denied that saccharin was necessary for diabetics or for victims of other ailments in which heavy sugar use was harmful. He said:

What is being argued here on the floor is that to satisfy a sweet tooth we are going to expose 200 million people in this country to a cancer agent, millions of them involuntarily because they will not know it or do not believe the tests showing that it is cancerous.

We have the best food and drug law in the world. And the mandate in that law is to protect the safety of the food chain. What is the public question at stake here? Do you know what the public question is? The public question is, should we continue to corrupt the food chain of this country with a proven carcinogenic agent in order to sell soda pop? That is what it is all about. Soda pop.

Oh, you say that is not what it is all about. No, not quite all, but almost all. Three-quarters of the question is soda pop. What does that say about our value standards in this society? We will medicate every one so that someone can have the convenience of a diet soda while exposing millions of people to this cancer causing agent. We are going to have thousands of people, who are going to die from cancer for the convenience of being able to get a bottle of soda pop. And we are making a fundamental attack on the best food and drug law in any country in the world. It shocks me.

As I said soda pop is three-quarters of the problem we are talking about. People are using it in their homes. That is their choice. Among some of the most distinguished diabetologists in this country there is the opinion that there is no necessity for saccharin at all. It is true scientists are divided. The medical society is divided all the time....

When the OTA science panel appeared before our Health Subcommittee I asked the question of Dr. Frederickson. Dr. Frederickson is the Director of the National Institutes of Health. . . . I wanted to know whether there was any proven scientific need for saccharin. So, I asked Dr. Frederickson:

Are there any conclusive tests that have been done that demonstrate an important need for saccharin for diebetics, overweight, or heart patients? None have come to my attention.

Dr. Frederickson responds:

The answer is no, Senator Nelson. There is no test that is available that demonstrates a specific need for saccharin by such patients.

. . .

Now let us see what some of the distinguished diabetologists have to say about saccharin. Let us take Dr. Max Miller, who was the director of the 10-year university group diabetes program involving 13 clinical centers treating diabetics. He certainly ranks as a distinguished authority on diabetes....

Dr. Miller told us:

There is no role for saccharin in the regimes (diets) of obese patients we are treating. We have never included saccharin in instructions to diabetics. From the practical point of view, diabetics don't use much sugar anyway. Their diets can be arranged to allow some sugar intake in food, restricting calories and balancing carbohydrates. Sweeteners mask taste. I am amazed at how little sugar my diabetic patients take.

Now let us hear what Dr. P. J. Palumbo of the Mayo Clinic Medical School, assistant professor of medicine and diabetologist in one of the most distinuished medical clinics in the world whose program treats about 6,000 diabetic patients a year, told us. Let us hear what he said:

Saccharin is not—

I repeat:

Saccharin is not essential in diet management of diabetics. We can manage their diet satisfactorily without it.

Saccharin ban opposed by public. By mid-1978 it had become clear that a ban on saccharin would be widely unpopular.

A report on the cancer risk posed by saccharin, by the FDA's National Center for Toxicological Research July 19, advised the FDA that scientists would have to have more persuasive evidence and improved risk estimates before the public would accept a ban on the artificial sweetener. The report said that the health hazards of saccharin might be outweighed by possible benefits. (A Baltimore study by two doctors published in the July 28 issue of the Journal of the American Medical Association concluded that "neither saccharin nor cyclamate is likely to be carcinogenic in man, at least at the moderate dietary ingestion levels reported.")

Cyclamate ban continued. The artificial sweetener cyclamate was too dangerous to allow back on the market, the FDA ruled Oct. 4, 1976.

Abbott Laboratories, which originally developed and marketed cyclamates, had filed a petition in 1973 declaring that the chemical had "no cancer-producing or other adverse effects."

The FDA formally rejected the petition. It had announced May 11 that it would not lift the ban because of "unresolved" safety questions.

A scientific panel that reviewed the issue for the agency said the cancer-causing potential of cyclamate had not been established. The panel said, however, that it could not reach a conclusion on the safety of cyclamates for human consumption because of some incidence of cancer in cyclamate-fed animals.

Danger from Nitrite

Nitrite salts have been used for centuries to cure meat and other foods, and they have been found useful to protect foods from botulism. Small amounts of nitrite have always been a natural constituent of human food. In the 1960s, however, there began to be increasing concern that nitrite additives sometimes combined with amines and contaminated food with compounds called nitrosamines, some of which had been implicated as causes of cancer. Some studies indicated that nitrosamines might form in the digestive tracts of people who had eaten large quantities of nitrite- and amine-containing foods. But food-industry spokesmen opposed Food & Drug Administration plans to curb nitrite. According to industry assertions, this would be action against a supposed culprit that had not been proven guilty.

Additive suit filed. Ralph Nader's Center for the Study of Responsive Law filed suit in U.S. district court in Washington, D.C. May 3, 1972 to bar use of nitrates and nitrites as food coloring additives in cured meat products, after the Agriculture Department had rejected a petition seeking a ban.

The additive, which Agriculture authorities said was an effective preservative and antibotulism agent, had been known to combine with amines in foods to produce small amounts of nitrosamine, known to cause cancer in animals. Other evidence suggested that the additives could affect the brain, or lead to anemia in infants and aged persons if consumed in large quantities.

Labeling ordered—The Agriculture Department Aug. 23 ordered that both nitrates and nitrites be listed on labels of cured meat packages, pending determination of safe and necessary levels.

Nitrite rule scored. Four major consumer and public interest organizations submitted a statement to the FDA protesting its decision against an immediate ban on the use of sodium nitrate and nitrite as color and shelf life preservatives of cured meats and other foods, it was reported Jan. 6, 1973.

Consumers Union, the Environmental Defense Fund, the Center for the Study of Responsive Law and the Consumer Federation of America said the chemicals were not needed to prevent botulism, and could help produce a cancer-producing substance in the stomach.

Experts urge curbs. A panel of experts commissioned by the Agriculture Department recommended Sept. 9, 1974 that because of cancer-causing potential, sodium nitrates and nitrites should be either banned from use in processed meat products or severely restricted.

The panel said nitrates should be banned from most foods but recommended a temporary exemption for certain sausages and dried, cured products pending completion of further research. Nitrites would be permitted in most products, but only at levels necessary for botulism protection.

Meat industry gets ultimatum. The Agriculture Department Oct. 18, 1977 ordered the meat industry to prove that bacon and other meats cured with nitrates did not cause cancer when cooked. The industry was given until Jan. 16, 1978 to present data on the use of nitrates and nitrites in meat and to show that such use posed no harm to the health of consumers.

The Agriculture Department order followed a similar action by the Food and Drug Administration. The FDA Aug. 31 had given the meat industry 60 days to present data on the use of nitrates and nitrites in poultry.

Nitrites curbed in curing bacon. The Agriculture Department May 15, 1978 issued regulations requiring a cut in the amount of nitrites that could be used in curing bacon. Nitrosamines were formed when bacon cured with nitrites was crisply fried. A still lower nitrites requirement, for use along with other preservatives, was proposed for a year later.

It was estimated that about 90% of the bacon marketed already met the temporary standard, but smaller companies that did not use vacuum packaging systems encountered problems meeting the requirements.

The May 15 regulations (which were effective June 15) called for a reduction in the amount of sodium nitrite to 120 parts per million and required that it be used only in combination with 550 parts per million of sodium erythrobate or sodium ascorbate agents used to block nitrosamine formation.

Regulations to take effect in May 1979 called for 40 parts per million of nitrite in combination with 0.26 parts per million of another preservative, potassium sorbate. Bacon would not be permitted to contain more than 5 parts per billion of nitrosamines.

Nitrite link to cancer. Sodium nitrite was found to cause lymph cancer in laboratory rats, a joint statement by the Food and Drug Administration and the Agriculture Department said Aug. 11, 1978.

The finding came as the result of an FDA-sponsored study by the Massachussetts Institute of Technology that for the first time identified sodium nitrite, alone, as a chemical carcinogen. Until this study, it had been thought that nitrites were a threat only when combined with amines to form nitrosamines, which were known to cause cancer.

The report was generally described as the "Newberne Report on the Effect of Dietary Nitrite in the Rat." The MIT study was directed by Dr. Paul M. Newberne.

The four-year, $500,000 research study found that 13% of the rats fed sodium nitrite developed lymphoma, and 8% of those not receiving nitrites contracted cancer. The causative factor was said to be clearly distinct from that of nitrosamines. The difference in the cancer rates was considered "significant."

The FDA said that the statement was issued so that the MIT study would be placed on the public record as a "red flag."

The danger in the continued use of nitrites presented the FDA with the need to balance risks, since nitrites inhibited growth of the bacterium that caused botulism.

After weighing the hazards of botulism against the hazards of cancer, the FDA concluded that the risk of botulism was greater, and said Aug. 31 that it would be irresponsible for the government to immediately ban nitrites from all the processed foods in which they were used.

A phasing out of nitrites was proposed, starting with products in which nitrites were not needed to prevent botulism and progressing to a "goal" of "total" phase-out as other safe preserving methods were perfected. (Two-thirds of all pork and one-tenth of all beef was treated with nitrites.) It was believed that it would be impossible to remove nitrites from some products, such as canned hams and some lunch meats.

Nitrites also naturally occurred in drinking water and many foods, especially leafy and root vegetables. They were present in 7% of the U.S. food supply, according to the FDA.

The Newberne report was criticized by various industry, scientific and Congressional sources. Rep. William C. Wampler (R, Va.) held a press conference in the House Agriculture Committee room Oct. 4 to present scientific criticism of the report. He inserted in the Congressional Record a report on the scientists' views. Excerpts from this report:

According to Richard V. Lechowich of Virginia Polytechnic Institute and State University, "the fact is that if nitrite were banned, consumers would be presented with new products that would not look, smell, or taste like the cured products now known. Without nitrite, there would be no frankfurters or wieners, no Vienna sausage, no bacon, no corned beef, no deviled ham, no pastrami, no canned ham, no chopped luncheon meats, no cold cuts. Also eliminated would be all kosher cured meat products."

Lechowich headed two different task forces of scientists appointed by the Council for Agricultural Science and Technology (CAST) to evaluate the nitrite issue. CAST is an association of 25 food and agricultural science societies.

"... Current evidence indicates that no more than 2% of the nitrite to which the body is exposed is due to cured meats. Almost all of the remainder is produced in the body by normal body processes. Obviously, then," he says, "there is little we can do to reduce our exposure to nitrite by eliminating the use of sodium nitrite in meat curing."

Nitrite is a very reactive ion. Most of the nitrite absorbed by the blood stream from the digestive tract probably reacts with hemoglobin and changes it to methemoglobin, which does not carry oxygen to the body (the hemoglobin is eventually regenerated). But some, according to Phillip Issenberg of the Eppley Cancer Institute at the University of Nebraska Medical Center, may react with certain organic nitrogen compounds to produce N-nitroso compounds. "N-nitroso compounds as a class," says Issenberg, "are highly potent carcinogens in experimental animals and are presumed similarly carcinogenic in humans although there is currently no evidence that any human cancer in the United States has resulted from exposure of the human population to such compounds in food and other environmental sources."

Issenberg points out that "In addition to preformed N-nitroso compounds (including nitrosamines) that are inhaled from the air, ingested in the food, and derived from other environmental sources, there is probably some synthesis of these compounds in the human body from the nitrite normally produced in the digestive tract. With by far the major part of the nitrite being produced in the digestive tract, most of the exposure to N-nitroso compounds as well as nitrite may well be due to formation of these compounds in the body.

"We have no knowledge of the significance of nitrite as a cause of human cancer," says Issenberg, "but we must raise an objection to the estimates of human cancer risk developed on the basis of Newberne's data by FDA and USDA for consumption of nitrite in cured meats. The FDA–USDA estimates are of very dubious validity because some of them are considerably higher than the incidence of all cancers from all causes that arise in the lymph system in the human population in the United States. If we take into account the information that less than one-fiftieth of the total exposure of the human body to nitrite is due to cured meats, and if nitrite from all sources contributes equally to the incidence of cancers in the lymph system, the FDA–USDA estimates are 10 to 450 or more times higher than the estimate we derive from human data on the assumption that all cancers arising in the lymph system are caused by nitrite."

Danger from Food Colors

Violet No. 1 banned. The FDA April 5, 1973 announced a ban on further use of Violet No. 1, the food coloring used by the Department of Agriculture for grade labels on meats, and by industry in a variety of food products, because of preliminary Japanese studies indicating that large quantities of Violet No. 1 may have been carcinogenic in laboratory rats.

The substance had been used for 22 years, and had been confirmed as safe by an independent panel nominated by the National Academy of Sciences in 1972. The Agriculture Department said April 5 it would switch to yellow, orange and green stamping colors.

FDA attacked on food dye problem. A General Accounting Office report issued Oct. 24, 1975 suggested that the Food & Drug Administration "act promptly to establish the safety of red dye No. 2 or prevent its use in foods, drugs and cosmetics." The report, requested by Sen. Gaylord Nelson (D, Wis.), said continued use of the dye without a finding on its safety "exposes the public to unnecessary risk."

The report cited studies linking the dye, the most widely used food coloring in the country, to harmful effects on test animals, such as cancer, birth defects, miscarriages and genetic damage.

The GAO noted that the FDA had postponed a decision on the dye's safety 14 times since 1963 after requests from the food or cosmetics industry.

FDA bans Red No. 2 dye. The most widely-used dye in foods, drugs and cosmetics, Red No. 2, was banned by the FDA Jan. 19, 1976.

An FDA study had found that Red No. 2 in high doses caused a statistically significant increase in cancer among test animals. A review of the study by the agency concluded that while the danger of the dye might be questionable its safety could not be established.

FDA Commissioner Alexander M. Schmidt, in announcing the ban, said, "Clearly, the burden of proof belongs not with the government or the consumer but with those who claim that Red No. 2 has a safe and useful purpose in the food supply and in our drugs and cosmetics."

Schmidt said there was no evidence of a public health hazard from products already on the market and they were not being recalled. Use of the dye had averaged more than one million pounds annually in recent years. A petroleum derivative, it had been used in such products as lipsticks, pill coatings, liquid medicine, noncola soft drinks, candy bars, gelatin desserts, syrups, baked goods, breakfast cereals, frankfurters and cold meats, corn chips and canned fruit.

The ban on manufacturing Red No. 2 went into effect Feb. 12 while a court challenge against it continued.

The challenge was filed by the Certified Color Manufacturers Association, an industry trade group; Warner-Jenkinson of St. Louis and H. Kohnstamm & Co. of New York, both color manufacturers; and Monarch Nugrape of Doraville, Ga., a soft drink concentrate manufacturer.

The ban had originally been scheduled to become effective as of Jan. 27, but U.S. Judge Aubrey Robinson Jr. of Washington, D.C. imposed a temporary delay Jan. 27 and set a hearing date to determine a procedural question about the ban. The ban was upheld at the hearing Feb. 6; Robinson held that it was up to the manufacturer to prove the dye was safe and that the FDA did not have to establish the reverse before the ban.

The U.S. court of appeals stayed the ban Feb. 9. It then lifted the stay Feb. 11, without explanation, and set a hearing for April on the merits of the industry's appeal. Further appeal was made to Chief Justice Warren E. Burger, but he refused Feb. 13 to postpone the ban.

The ban was upheld by a three-judge panel of the U.S. Court of Appeals in Washington July 6.

Danger from DES in Livestock

The synthetic steroid diethylstilbestrol (DES), which for years had been used as a growth stimulant in livestock, came under attack after it was reported to be implicated in cancer in animals and in human beings.

Ban on DES proposed. Sen. William Proxmire (D, Wis.) Nov. 8, 1971 submitted legislation to ban the use of DES in feeding cattle and sheep. DES was used by livestock producers to fatten their animals before slaughter.

According to the Agriculture Department, a ban on DES would increase the price of beef by 3½ cents a pound. In introducing his bill, Proxmire said that "cheap beef or lamb is a very bad bargain indeed if it brings with it the threat of poor health."

A similar bill was introduced in the House Nov. 9 by Rep. Ogden R. Reid (R, N.Y.). Reid's bill carried with it criminal penalties for anyone who "knowingly" dealt in interstate commerce with beef, lamb or food products from animals treated with DES.

Use in animals limited. The Agriculture Department Jan. 4, 1972 announced new regulations for the use of DES as a growth hormone in food animals.

Starting Jan. 8, no DES could be fed cattle or sheep within seven days of slaughter, compared with two days under the old rule, and animals brought to slaughter would now require certification of compliance. Large doses of DES had been found to induce cancer in test animals.

The Food & Drug Administration later banned the use of DES in liquid form in cattle and sheep feed, it was reported March 10, 1972.

The action was taken after tests uncovered DES residues in nearly 1% of sample animals, twice the level found in 1971, although stricter rules had been in effect since Jan. 8. Further tests showed that liquid DES had adhered to feed processing equipment, contaminating later batches of feed supposedly free of the chemical, which could not lawfully be fed to animals within seven days of slaughter.

The FDA warned it would ban all use of the substance, which had produced cancers in laboratory animals, if residues continued to appear.

Court actions begin—The FDA said May 31 it had filed a criminal complaint in U.S. district court in Salt Lake City against Parnell Green of the Green Livestock Co. at Layton, Utah, for marketing cattle in which traces of DES were found. It was the first criminal action involving DES.

The Agriculture Department reported June 9 that two more cases of DES residue in cattle livers had been discovered, bringing to 24 the total number of cases since January, when tougher DES regulations had been put into effect.

The next day, Department of Agriculture inspectors reported they had found residues of DES in 1.9% of 1972 samples of beef and lamb liver, up from .5% in 1971, before new regulations on DES took effect. A rise in the rate of contamination to 2.27% was reported by the Agriculture Department July 20.

Ban tightened. The FDA Aug. 2, 1972 banned all further production of DES for use as a growth hormone in cattle feeds, but it allowed cattlemen to continue using DES in feeds until Jan. 1, 1973.

FDA Commissioner Charles C. Edwards said he acted under requirements of the 1968 Delaney amendment to the Food, Drug and Cosmetic Act, which banned all substances in foods that caused cancer in humans or animals, although, he said, "no human harm has been demonstrated in over 17 years of use."

The order permitted continued implanting of DES pellets in cattle and sheep. The pellets, which contained one-thirtieth the amount of DES in direct feed supplements, had not been known to leave detectible residues.

Secretary of Agriculture Earl L. Butz said Aug. 2 he regretted the FDA decision, which he said could add 3½¢ a pound to consumer beef prices.

A subcommittee of the Senate Health Committee approved an immediate ban on DES in feed and pellets Aug. 3. Edwards had opposed the bill in a July 21 hearing of the subcommittee. The FDA, he said, believed "piecemeal legislation directed at any given substance" was not "appropriate for making regulatory decisions that are to be based on scientific evidence," since "DES will not be the only substance to generate these kinds of issues."

Sen. Edward M. Kennedy (D, Mass), who chaired the hearing, noted that 21 countries, including Argentina and Australia, the leading beef producers, had banned DES.

Edwards had announced June 16 a formal proposal for a DES ban, in order to set in motion machinery for a public hearing, but at that time he repeated his belief that the hormone was "safe when used as directed." The FDA announcement noted that a ban would ultimately cost consumers $300 million–460 million in meat prices, because of increased feed requirements.

Such a ban was announced by the FDA April 23, 1973 (but federal courts later overturned the ban on the ground that hearings had not been offered to manufacturers as required by the law).

In a July 10 Washington Post interview, National Cancer Institute Director Frank J. Rauscher asked for a complete ban, saying "anything that increases the carcinogenic burden to man ought to be eliminated from the envirnoment if at all possible, and in this case it is possible."

Ban voided—The U.S. Court of Appeals ruled in Washington Jan. 24, 1974 that the FDA had acted illegally in 1972 and 1973 in banning DES. The court said the drug could be marketed again until the FDA held the required hearings or the secretary of health, education and welfare concluded that "such marketing constitutes an imminent hazard to public health."

The court said the FDA had used "scare tactics" instead of sound regulatory procedures in banning the drug without hearings. Noting that "most drugs are unsafe in some degree," the court said that in light of the "acknowledged value" of DES in enhancing meat production, the FDA should consider the possibility of "meaningful restrictions" on the consumption of DES residues rather than an outright ban of the drug.

The FDA said Jan. 28 that it would not appeal the decision but would set hearings to consider the possibility of new restrictions.

Canada curbs imports. The Canadian government announced regulations, effective April 9, 1974, to limit meat and livestock imports. The curbs were instituted to aid Canada's depressed cattle market, but DES was also involved.

The new import rules, disclosed by Agriculture Minister Eugene Whelan, required certification by the federal authorities of the exporting country that the animals shipped to Canada had not been given DES. Use of diethylstilbesterol as a livestock feed additive was illegal in Canada.

Canada's Cabinet June 20 rejected a U.S. proposal to end the curbs.

U.S. Secretary of Agriculture Earl Butz had warned that day: "If the Canadian market is not opened, I am prepared to recommend more drastic action and we have retaliatory actions we can take."

The U.S. had offered a compromise plan under which American feeders and veterinarians would have been required to certify that cattle exported to Canada had not been fed with DES. In rejecting the U.S. proposal, the Canadian government reiterated its insistence that the U.S. Department of Agriculture (USDA) itself conduct the certification program. The USDA charged June 21 that the DES-ban was in reality a non-tariff barrier erected to protect the domestic Canadian market.

The Toronto Globe and Mail June 22 reported that the Cabinet had been split in reaching its June 20 decision. Health Minister Marc Lalonde, it said, had favored the U.S. proposal, while Agriculture Minister Eugene Whelan had argued successfully to continue the embargo, demanding a more rigorous certification plan.

Ban ended—The Canadian regime lifted its ban on U.S. meat Aug. 2, announcing that Ottawa and Washington had agreed on a certification system that would assure that no cattle fed with DES would enter Canada.

Ban fails in Congress. The U.S. Senate Sept. 9, 1975 voted, 61–29, to end the use of DES as a growth stimulant for livestock. The measure, however, failed to win House approval. The bill would have prohibited the administration of DES to livestock, as a feed additive or as a pellet implant, until the Department of Health, Education and Welfare determined that it was "safe and presents no scientific health hazard and doesn't contribute unreasonably to man's carcinogenic burden."

The measure also contained a provision concerning the use of DES as a morning-after contraceptive by women. It would require a warning that DES might cause cancer and that it should not be taken as a contraceptive except in cases of rape and incest.

Ban sought anew. The FDA Jan. 9, 1976 again proposed a ban on DES in animal feed because traces of the drug continued to be found in the livers of animals after slaughter.

New ban ordered. The FDA announced June 28, 1979 that it was banning the use of DES as a growth stimulant fed to cattle and sheep. The manufacture and shipment of DES as an animal drug was ordered halted by July 13, and its use in livestock was ordered ended by July 20.

The ban would affect the four leading makers of DES: American Home Products Corp., New York; Dawes Laboratories Inc., Chicago; Vineland Laboratories Inc., Needham, Mass., and the Hess & Clark division of Rhodia Inc., New York.

The ban would not affect the use of DES as a human drug. DES could still be used as treatment for certain types of cancer, as an emergency morning-after contraceptive, and could also be given to women during menopause.

PBB Case

Michigan PBB Contamination. Several scientific studies had concluded that an accidental contamination of cattle feed with a highly toxic chemical had spread through the food chain to most of the population of Michigan, according to a Wall Street Journal article Oct. 9, 1978.

The article, based in part on a study reported in a current issue of The Lancet, a British medical journal, said investigators had interpreted studies as indicating that eight million of Michigan's 9.1 million residents were carrying polybrominated biphenyls, or PBBs, in their bodies.

The PBBs had devastated cattle herds in the state and had been found to cause liver cancer in rats.

Dairy cattle in Michigan had been accidentally contaminated in 1973 and 1974 by a packaging and shipping error that resulted in several hundred pounds of PBBs being substituted for magnesium oxide, a dairy-cattle nutritional supplement.

PBBs were flame retardants used at the time by the plastics industry.

The contaminated feed was distributed throughout Michigan, and cattle began exhibiting drastic symptoms that often led to death. The symptoms included loss of appetite and weight loss. Milk production went down and miscarriages increased.

When the trouble was traced to PBBs, steps were taken to re-stock the herds with uncontaminated cattle. Tests were begun to determine the effects, if any, on people.

The level of toxicity or safety for humans from PBB contamination, if any, was not known.

It was assumed that human exposure to PBBs would be focused on the farm workers at the contaminated farms, plus workers in the production process of the chemicals. There were an estimated 10,-000 to 12,500 people living on the contaminated farms.

Because PBBs were fat soluble, and breast milk from mothers was 4% fat, testing was done on breast milk. PBB residues were discovered.

The testing was extended after it was found in June 1976, from an unrelated survey of pesticide residues, that milk from four mothers who were not from the contaminated farms contained PBBs.

A study of 53 mothers who gave birth in August 1976 found that 51, or 96%, had PBBs. The concentrations ranged from .05 parts per million parts of milk to one part PBBs per million parts of milk.

Early in 1978, a test of blood and of fat tissue from men and women found that 98% of the samples contained PBBs.

Dr. Irving Selikoff of the Mt. Sinai School of Medicine in New York, who conducted the test, said his findings corroborated those of the breast-milk studies.

By projection, investigators concluded that eight million of Michigan's residents were carrying PBBs.

Although the contamination was thought to have been halted, and little or no recontamination was expected, the people carrying the PBBs were expected to carry them the rest of their lives.

The passing of the chemicals from the body through lactation was the only known way of excreting the chemicals. There was no known way for males to excrete PBB residues.

Suit dismissed—Judge William Peterson of Wexford County Court in Cadillac, Mich. Oct. 27, 1978 dismissed a suit by farmers seeking damages for the PBB poisoning of their dairy cattle.

The suit in Cadillac was brought by Roy M. and Marilyn Tacoma, dairy farmers of Falmouth, Mich. The defendants were Michigan Chemical Co., which accidentally shipped the PBBs, and the Michigan Farm Bureau Services Inc., which unknowingly mixed PBBs with dairy feed and distributed it to farmers.

Michigan Chemical Co. later merged into Velsicol, a subsidiary of Northwest Industries Inc. The farm bureau agency was a unit of the Michigan Farm Bureau.

In dismissing the case after a 14-month trial without jury, Peterson said there was no evidence that PBB contamination had necessitated the forced slaughter of the Tacomas' dairy herd.

Peterson further said it had not been shown that PBB in small quantities was toxic to cattle.

The greatest tragedy in the case, Peterson said, was the "needless destruction of animals exposed to low levels of polybrominated biphenyl and even of animals that never received any PBB."

An estimated two million farm animals had been destroyed by design after cattle sicknesses and deaths multiplied and the PBB contamination became known, which was not until May 1974.

The chemical firm, which admitted responsibility, eventually paid some $40 million to 670 Michigan farmers to settle out of court.

The Tacoma case was the first of the PBB cases to come to trial. Unlike many of the settled claims, in which the PBB level in the cattle was relatively high, the Tacoma case involved a herd that was considered to have a low-level of contamination.

The Tacomas had not used the original batches of wrongly mixed feed. They claimed their cattle had been harmed by feed contaminated by PBB residue in the farm agency's mixing equipment.

Danger in Drinking Water

Water found impure. The results of a report released Aug. 17, 1970 by the Department of Health, Education and Welfare indicated that millions of Americans were drinking potentially hazardous water or water of inferior quality. In some cases, the contaminants were suspected carcinogens.

According to a water quality survey, conducted in 1969 by the Bureau of Water Hygiene, of 18.2 million persons served by the systems sampled, 5% drank water rated potentially hazardous—exceeding Public Health Service mandatory limits of chemical or bacteriological contamination—and another 11% drank water that was safe but of inferior quality—having a bad taste, odor or appearance.

The survey covered 969 public water systems in nine regions: the state of Vermont and the metropolitan regions of New York City, Charleston, W. Va., Cincinnati, Charleston, S. C., Kansas City, Mo., New Orleans, Pueblo, Colo., and San Bernardino, Calif. In a statement accompanying those documents of the report released to newsmen, Water Hygiene Bureau Director James H. McDermott said that while the water systems examined were not selected to "provide a perfect random sample . . . the results are reasonably representative of the status of the water supply industry in the United States."

McDermott said most of the poor quality water came from relatively small water systems, those serving communities of less than 100,000 persons. He said: "Some of the very small communities were even drinking water on a day-to-day basis that exceeded one or more of the dangerous chemical limits, such as selenium, arsenic or lead."

The report found that 56% of the systems tested had deficiencies in facilities—inadequate source protection and disinfection and deficiencies in pressure in the distribution system. Most of these deficiencies were also found in the smaller systems. The survey also found that 77% of water system plant operators were poorly trained and 79% of the systems sampled had not been inspected for a year prior to the survey.

Charles C. Johnson Jr., assistant surgeon general and administrator of the Consumer Protection and Environmental Health Service, said in a foreword to the report that the "overwhelming majority of people in the U.S. can be assured that the water they drink today is safe," but that "clearly there is an immediate need, in many localities, for upgrading present water treatment and distribution practices." He said the survey findings "are not reassuring with regard to the future."

Water quality bill passed. A bill dealing with oil spills and water pollution—the Water Quality Improvement Act of 1970 (HR4148)—was passed by unanimous votes of the Senate March 24, 1970 and House March 25 and was signed by President Nixon April 3.

The bill made the owner or operator of a vessel or offshore or onshore facility liable for the cleanup costs of an oil spill —up to $14 million for a vessel, or $100 per gross ton, whichever was less, and up to $8 million for a facility. Exceptions were provided if the spill resulted from an act of God, an act of war, federal negligence or an act by a third party.

The owner was subject to absolute liability if found guilty of willful negligence or misconduct. Penalties were established also for failure to notify authorities of an oil slick. A $35 million fund was authorized to finance federal cleanup of oil spills.

The legislation had been approved by both houses in 1969—by the House April 16 and Senate Oct. 8—but had been delayed in conference by a dispute over the liability issue. The original House version called for proof of liability that the owner "willfully or negligently" discharged the oil. The Senate conferees held out for absolute liability with financial limits.

In other areas, the final bill provided for (a) establishment of an Office of Environmental Quality in the executive office of the President, (b) pollution control of the Great Lakes and clean lakes research; (c) a study of the effects of pesticides on the environment; (d) a pledge of compliance with state water-pollution standards prior to federal licensing of a nuclear power plant; and (e) establishment of standards for control of pollution from sanitation facilities on ships and pleasure craft.

Dumping curbed. President Nixon Dec. 23, 1970 issued an executive order requiring industries to obtain a federal permit before dumping wastes into U.S. waterways. Russell E. Train, chairman of the Council on Environmental Quality, described the President's action as "the single most important step to improvement of water quality that this country has taken."

The new procedures made use of the 1899 Refuse Act, originally intended to keep navigable waters free of obstuctions. Environmentalists had urged the government to use the measure to fight pollution, and the new order would outlaw all discharges unless industries received permits from the Army Corps of Engineers. The act applied only to industries, but Nixon, in issuing the order, said the government would "continue to vigorously employ other authorities for dealing with violations of water quality standards by municipalities."

Under the procedures announced by Nixon, industries would receive permits only if they received state and interstate certification that the discharges met water quality standards. In addition the permits would have to be approved by the Environmental Protection Agency (EPA).

EPA drops dumping standards—EPA Administrator William Ruckelshaus said July 20, 1971 that the EPA would not try to establish national industrial dumping standards envisioned in Nixon's plan.

Ruckelshaus said regional officials would use their own judgement in issuing permits to discharge waste in U.S. waterways.

Under the program announced by the President, an estimated 40,000 industries would have had to apply for permits by July 1 to discharge waste under the 1899 Refuse Act. (The deadline passed with thousands of applications not filed.) Permits were to be issued under guidelines established by the EPA. The EPA admitted that without the guidelines, regional officials could impose specific discharge limits on only "a selected minority" of the permits.

Ruckelshaus said the attempt to write guidelines for 18 "critical industry groups" demonstrated "the complexity of trying to set national base-level standards across an industry." An EPA July 15 memo told regional officials to concentrate on "the most seriously polluted waters" and the "major sources of pollution" and that the permits "should also reflect availability of completed modeling studies and other data."

Cancer-link focus in water study. The Environmental Protection Agency Nov. 8, 1974 issued a report stating that 66 organic chemicals, some suspected of being carcinogenic (cancer-causing), were present in treated Mississippi River water used by New Orleans and nearby communities. EPA Administrator Russell E. Train simultaneously ordered an immediate nationwide study of chemical contaminants in drinking water to examine the extent and seriousness of the situation.

Among the chemical agents cited in the report were two chlorine compounds, chloroform and carbon tetrachloride, which had known cancer-causing potential in some animal species. Train said the EPA had been taking a closer look at water chlorination, the process by which drinking water was purified in the U.S., to determine if some of the suspected chemicals were being produced in reaction with the chlorine, which of itself was not carcinogenic. An EPA spokesman said, however, that the agency was "in no case . . . urging that the chlorination process be stopped." Government studies had found further traces of the chemicals in the chlorinated drinking water of Cincinnati.

A private Washington-based group, the Environmental Defense Fund (EDF), criticized the planned EPA study, saying that immediate steps should be taken to apply alternate purification methods. The EDF had issued a report Nov. 7 demonstrating a "highly suggestive" link between Mississippi River water and high cancer death rates in Louisiana communities that depended on the river for their water supply. It also noted that carcinogenic compounds had been identified in the drinking water of San Francisco, Washington, D.C. and Evansville, Ind., in addition to New Orleans and Cincinnati.

Neither the EPA nor the EDF report alleged that the relationship between cancer and drinking water had been proven.

Following later studies, however, the EPA reported April 18, 1975 that measurable amounts of chemical substances that might cause cancer had been found in all 79 of the nation's drinking water systems it had tested. Administrator Russell Train said the basic conclusion from the survey was "that the problem of organic chemicals in public water supply systems exists throughout the country." All 79 water supplies investigated contained some chloroform, which was being studied by the National Institutes of Health as a possible carcinogen.

In special studies of certain areas, dieldrin, a pesticide identified as carcinogenic by the EPA, was found in water supplies of four of five areas tested, and water in the fifth area was found to contain vinyl chloride, another carcinogen. Asbestos fibers were found in water for several areas.

Drinking water bill enacted. A $156 million, three-year program to safeguard drinking water was cleared by Congress Dec. 3, 1974 and was signed by President Ford Dec. 16. Under the new law, national standards for safe drinking water were to be set at the federal level by the Environmental Protection Agency (EPA), which could seek compliance by court action if the primary enforcement, assigned to the states, were neglected. The bill also permitted citizen suits against public water systems to gain compliance with the standards. Each state was guaranteed eligibility for at least 1% of the federal grants authorized under the program.

Maximum permissible levels were set for specific contaminants and for turbidity of the water.

The EPA issued its proposed standards March 15, 1975, effective in June.

Progress on water pollution. The Environmental Protection Agency reported Feb. 21, 1975 that 95% of 3,000 major industrial water polluters had agreed to compliance schedules to use the "best practical" technology to clean up their operations by July 1, 1977 and the "best available" technology by July 1, 1983. "Very strong progress" was reported in cleaning up the nation's lakes and rivers under the program, which began in December 1970.

There were delays, however. Industry and local communities were running behind schedule in meeting the deadlines of the Water Pollution Control Act of 1972, according to a draft report made available Sept. 5 by the staff of the National Commission on Water Quality.

Under the 1972 Act, industry was to have the "best practicable" clean-up equipment installed by 1977, and the "best available" treatment methods by 1983. Communities were to have secondary, or two-stage, sewage treatment operating by 1977. By 1985, there was to be "zero discharge" of pollutants in waterways.

The report estimated the costs of meeting the goals: for industry's first-stage goal, "best practicable" equipment by 1977, $25 to $40 billion; 1983 goal, $20 billion more. A substantial part of these outlays, 85%, was projected to clean up only five industries—metal finishing, chemicals, pulp and paper, electric power and mining.

No major price increases for products was foreseen as a result of the clean-up, except in the metal finishing industry, where prices were expected to increase an average of 5% for the first phase and 10% for the second.

The clean-up costs for municipalities were estimated at $40 billion. Despite federal spending of billions to meet 75% of the cost of municipal sewage-treatment plants, however, the goal of secondary-treatment by 1977 was running six years behind schedule, at current spending rates.

The report also estimated some benefits to be derived from meeting the clean-up goals—$6 billion annually by 1985 from opening more beaches, $21.3 billion from improving commercial and recreational fishing.

Drinking water standards proposed. The Environmental Protection Agency proposed initial standards for the nation's drinking water March 15, 1975. The rules were to take effect in June after a period of public comment. Permanent standards were to take effect in December, 1976.

Maximum permissible levels were set for specific contaminants and for turbidity of the water.

Exemption overturned. U.S. Judge Thomas A. Flannery March 24, 1975 ruled against a decision of the Environmental Protection Agency to exempt certain possible water pollution sources from its permit requirement. The agency granted the exemptions—for storm sewers, many animal confinement facilities and feedlots, forestry activities and some irrigation return flows—with the claim it did not have enough manpower to regulate all possible pollution sources.

Citing the water act, Flannery said "such difficulties must not stand in the way of Congress' mandate" that a comprehensive permit program covering all sources be established.

EPA authority upheld. The Supreme Court Feb. 23, 1977, unanimously upheld the EPA's authority to issue uniform curbs on an industrywide basis to curb pollution of the nation's waterways.

A challenge to the EPA's authority was brought by eight chemical companies. They contended that the guidelines, issued under the Federal Water Pollution Control Act amendments of 1972, should be on a plant-by-plant basis.

The Fourth Circuit Court of Appeals had rejected the companies' argument but characterized the EPA's broad guidelines as only "presumptively applicable" to individual plants.

The Supreme Court's opinion, written by Justice John Paul Stevens, said that the plant-by-plant application sought by the companies "would place an impossible burden on EPA" that Congress had not intended.

The high court held that some allowance must be made for variations in individual plants, except for new plants, where Congress intended to impose "absolute prohibitions" on pollution.

Stevens asked the EPA, however, to "give individual consideration to the circumstances of each of the more than 42,000 dischargers who have applied for permits." This would allow time, Stevens said, for industry to install the necessary pollution control equipment.

FMC plant shut under court order. FMC Corp.'s Charleston, W. Va. plant was shut under court order March 9, 1977 for discharging carbon tetrachloride into drinking-water supplies of communities along the Kanawha and Ohio rivers.

A temporary restraining order, barring production of carbon tetrachloride at the plant, was issued by U.S. Judge District Charles H. Haden 2d in Petersburg, W. Va. The Environmental Protection Agency, which sought the order, said the plant had been responsible for at least 20 spills of the chemical into the water supplies in the last two years. The latest spill had been detected March 8.

The chemical, used in cleaning agents, was said by the EPA to be a cause of liver damage in human beings.

The production ban, which extended until March 19, was the first such legal action ever taken under emergency provisions of the Federal Water Pollution Control Act and the Safe Drinking Water Act, according to the EPA.

Agreement reached with EPA—Judge Haden lifted the production ban March 15 after the company and the Environmental Protection Agency reached an agreement for monitoring of the carbon-tetrachloride production and installation of equipment to contain spills.

Until then, the company was to maintain around-the-clock surveillance of production. More sophisticated equipment for containment was scheduled to be installed by Jan. 1, 1978.

Toxic chemicals in Hudson River. The Hudson River contained "a complex spectrum" of toxic and cancer-causing chemicals, according to a report issued Sept. 28, 1977 by the Environmental Defense Fund and New York Public Interest Research Group.

The report, based on a two-year study of water samples from upper and middle stretches of the river, cautioned that area residents who drank water from the Hudson could be "victims of an unnecessarily high exposure to environmental carcinogens."

Drinking water was withdrawn from the Hudson River drainage basin in at least seven areas.

EPA Seeks Anti-Cancer Water Filtration. The Environmental Protection Agency Jan. 25, 1978 proposed rules to guard against the presence of cancer-causing chemicals in municipal drinking water systems.

The regulations would protect specifically against the presence of trihalomethanes, which were formed when chlorine was added to water to kill bacteria. Trihalomethanes included chloroform, which was a known carcinogen.

The EPA proposal would require large water systems to limit the presence of trihalomethanes to no more than 100 parts per billion parts of water.

The regulations also sought control against the entry of organic chemicals into drinking water sources by pollution.

Special filtering processes would be required to remove the toxic chemicals. The EPA estimated that implementation of the new rules would cost $350 million to $450 million over the next three to five years.

The standards would apply to water systems serving more than 75,000 people.

Systems serving between 10,000 and 75,000 people would be required only to monitor their water for presence of the chemicals.

Water Pollution Rules Set. Final regulations issued by the Environmental Protection Agency June 20, 1978 required industries to remove toxic substances from waste water discharged into municipal sewer systems.

The regulations, covering about 40,000 plants in 21 major industries, required installation of the "best available technology economically achievable" to remove 65 toxic substances.

Enforcement programs would be handled primarily by local water-treatment agencies, which would receive financial help from the federal government.

The enforcement programs were to be in place by 1983 for industries using treatment plants with capacity of 5 million gallons or more of water a day.

The regulations were issued under legislation enacted in 1977. Specific standards for the different industries would be issued later.

EPA to Ease Clean Water Rules. The Environmental Protection Agency proposed Aug. 10, 1978 to ease water pollution rules for certain industries. The effort was part of the agency's campaign to reduce the inflationary impact of its rules.

The rules to be eased concerned only organic debris and dirt, not toxic pollutants. The industries involved were only those throwing off such so-called conventional pollutants.

Of 93 industries in this category, the EPA determined that the current water pollution controls for 18 of the industries appeared to be "unreasonable" and could be eased without significant adverse impact on water quality.

The agency proposed to suspend the controls in another 18 industries pending further review.

Many of the industries to be exempted were in the food processing business—fruit and vegetable canners, seafood processors, slaughter houses and packing houses.

Glass producers and certain metal producers also were to be exempted.

The specific requirement to be relaxed was that plants must install the best available pollution-control equipment by mid-1984.

Cigarette Smoking

By the end of the 1950s it had become widely accepted that cigarette smoking was a serious environmental health hazard—and probably a cause of lung cancer. The evidence against the cigarette has grown increasingly damning.

Lung-cancer connection. Dr. Leroy E. Burney, then surgeon general of the U.S. Public Health Service, had charged in an article in the Journal of the American Medical Association (made public Nov. 26, 1959) that (a) smoking was the "principal" cause of the U.S.' increase in lung cancer, (b) cigarettes apparently were three times worse than pipes and seven times worse that cigars as a lung-cancer cause and (c) no filter or tobacco treatment materially reduced or eliminated the hazard of lung cancer. Burney added that air pollution also apparently was a cause of the lung-cancer increase.

Dr. Oscar Auerbach, N.Y. Medical College associate professor and East Orange (N.J.) Veterans Administration Hospital scientist, reported at the AMA meeting in Dallas Dec. 4 that (a) lung tissue studies of 238 men smokers showed cell changes that "probably represent a change toward cancer" and (b) the extent of these changes "depend almost completely on the number of cigarettes smoked."

Both reports were challenged by the Tobacco Institute and the Tobacco Industry Research Committee as statistically unsound and ignoring contradictory evidence.

Dr. John H. Talbott, editor of the Journal of the American Medical Association, said editorially Dec. 11 that there was insufficient evidence to prove the case for either side.

Surgeon General's report. U.S. Surgeon General Luther L. Terry Jan. 11, 1964 released a federal report that described cigarette smoking as a definite "health hazard" that "far outweighs all other factors" as a cause of lung disease. The report, "Smoking and Health," noted that 70 million Americans were cigarette smokers during 1963.

The report was prepared by a federal advisory committee appointed by Terry Oct. 27, 1962 to evaluate and reprocess existing studies and statistics on the relationship between smoking and health. Terry served as the committee's chairman.

Chief concern of the committee was the rising death rate in the U.S. from lung cancer, arteriosclerotic (mainly coronary) heart disease and chronic bronchitis and emphysema.

The committee evaluated three kinds of evidence—animal experiments, clinical and autopsy studies and population data. Its conclusions were based primarily on the combined results of seven population studies involving men selected at random and observed until death. On the basis of an analysis of the deaths of 37,391 of the 1,123,000 men involved in the seven studies, the committee concluded that:

(1) The death rate, from all causes, was 68% higher for smokers than for nonsmokers. For coronary artery disease, the leading cause of death in the U.S., the death rate was 70% higher; for chronic bronchitis and emphysema, leading causes of severe disability, the rate was 500% higher; for cancer of the lungs, the most common site of cancer in men, nearly 1,000% higher. The death rate for cancer of the larynx and of the esophagus, for oral cancer, for peptic ulcer and for a group of circulatory diseases was also higher for smokers.

(2) The number of cigarettes smoked daily, the age at which the habit started and the degree of inhalation affected the death rate. Men who smoked fewer than 10 cigarettes daily had a death rate, from all causes, about 40% higher than nonsmokers. The death rate of those who smoked 10-19 cigarettes was about 79% higher; the rate for those who smoked 20-30, about 90% higher; the rate for those who smoked 40 or more, 120% higher. The death rate of those who started smoking before 20 years of age was higher than those who began after 25.

(3) Cigarette smoking was a much greater causative factor in lung cancer than air pollution or occupational exposure.

(4) There was no evidence that nicotine substantially caused disease. Certain components of tobacco smoke—polycyclic aromatic hydrocarbons—had been found to cause cancer in animals.

(5) There was no link between tobacco and cancer of the stomach.

Bill requires warning. Legislation requiring that cigarette packages, cartons and containers be labeled with health warnings was passed by Senate voice vote July 6, 1965 and 285-103 House vote July 13 and was signed by President Lyndon B. Johnson July 27.

The warning statement—"Caution: Cigarette Smoking May Be Hazardous to Your Health"—was required as of Jan. 1, 1966. It was to be put in a "conspicuous place" and be in "conspicuous and legible type." The bill barred, until July 1, 1969, any requirement of a health statement in cigarette advertising. It also barred the requirement of any other statement on cigarette packages.

Bill bars cigarette ads. After considerable controversy, Congress in March 1970 passed a compromise bill outlawing cigarette commercials on radio and TV starting Jan. 2, 1971. President Richard M. Nixon signed the measure April 1, 1970. The cut-off date was chosen to permit cigarette companies to broadcast commercials during the widely viewed telecasts of football bowl games.

The bill signed by Nixon would also strengthen the warning on cigarette packages to read: "Warning: The Surgeon General has determined that cigarette smoking is dangerous to your health." The bill also authorized the Federal Trade Commission to require warnings in other cigarette advertising after July 1, 1971, if it voted to do so.

Tobacco firms accept ad warnings—The Tobacco Institute, Inc., a trade association representing cigarette companies, said April 15, 1971 that 7 of the U.S.' nine cigarette manufacturers had agreed to display a health warning in advertisements of their products.

The agreement was widely viewed as a compromise measure designed to head off possible Congress or FTC action to require stiff health warnings in all cigarette advertisements.

Under the accord, the seven companies agreed to depict in all future newspaper, magazine and billboard ads their brands' packages "legibly showing the health warning that Congress requires on the packages."

The FTC announced Jan. 31, 1972 that the U.S.' six largest cigarette makers had agreed to an amplified warning in their cigarette advertisements.

The FTC had warned the companies in July 1971 that it would start court action unless they agreed to display the health warnings.

The six companies signing the consent agreement accounted for 99% of all cigarette production in the U.S. and virtually all the cigarette advertising.

They were American Brands, Inc.; the Brown & Williamson Tobacco Corp.; Liggett & Myers, Inc.; the Lorillard Division of Loews Corp.; Philip Morris, Inc.; and the R. J. Reynolds Tobacco Co.

During the past year, advertisements by all of the companies except American Brands had included pictures of cigarette packages which carried the statement: "Warning: the Surgeon General has determined that cigarette smoking is dangerous to your health."

FTC spokesmen had said that the warnings displayed voluntarily in the cigarette advertisements were not sufficiently conspicuous.

Under the consent order, the same warning had to be displayed in a black-bordered space at the bottom of each advertisement.

Larynx damage linked to smoking. Medical researchers at the Veterans Administration Hospital in East Orange, N.J. reported Jan. 10, 1970 that autopsy studies of 942 men had yielded further evidence linking cigarette smoking to the development of cancer in the larynx.

The studies also provided further evidence that smokers can recover from precancerous conditions once they stop smoking, the scientists said.

The senior researcher of the report, Dr. Oscar Auerbach, a pathologist, said "the analysis showed that the more a person smoked the more likely he was to have changes in his larynx cells that are believed to precede the development of cancer."

Two of Auerbach's co-workers said the autopsy studies had been an attempt "to zero in on the relationship between smoking and cancer through different approaches."

Auerbach said the autopsies had revealed these findings:

■Of 88 men autopsied who had never smoked regularly, three-fourths showed no typical changes in bronchial cells. The same was true of 116 men who had stopped smoking entirely.

■Among those who smoked more than two packs a day, 85% had advanced cell damage in the larynx.

■All of the 519 men who smoked at least one pack a day had some cell damage in the larynx.

Dogs develop lung cancer. Two cancer researchers reported Feb. 5, 1970 that 12 of 86 dogs that were trained to smoke cigarettes developed lung cancer after two and a half years of smoking. They said it was the first time malignant tumors had been produced in large animals by exposing the animals to cigarette smoke.

The scientists, Dr. E. Cuyler Hammond, an epidemiologist associated with the American Cancer Society, and Dr. Oscar Auerbach, a pathologist at a Veterans Administration hospital in New Jersey, revealed their findings in New York City.

The American Cancer Society said the findings "effectively refute contentions by cigarette manufacturing interests that there is no cigarette-cancer link, and any claims to the contrary were only 'statistical.' "

(A spokesman for the Tobacco Institute, an organization sponsored and funded by tobacco interests, said it was "impossible" to "draw a meaningful parallel between human smoking and dogs subjected to these more stressful laboratory conditions.")

Hammon and Auerbach said their study also found:

Cigarettes with filter tips that reduce the inhaled tar content of the smoke by at least 49% and reduce the nicotine content by at least 37% are "less harmful to smoke (in dogs) than non-filter cigarettes."

There was a "dramatic difference in the incidence of malignant tumors in the filter smoking, and non-filter smoking dogs."

British doctors condemn smoking. Great Britain's Royal College of Physicians, in a wide condemnation of cigarette smoking, said Jan. 5, 1971 that nearly 28,000 English men and women died prematurely each year as a result of smoking. The College, England's leading body of physicians, said smoking had created a "holocaust" and forecast that by the 1980s the death toll could rise to as many as 50,000 Britons.

The College called on the government to prohibit all forms of cigarette advertising, to ban vending machine sales of cigarettes in public places and to require the printing of warning statements on all cigarette packages. The physicians also urged the government to launch a permanent anti-smoking campaign.

The recommendations were included in a 148-page report, entitled "Smoking and Health Now." It was prepared by 13 of the College's members under the direction of Lord Rosenheim, a neurologist and the College's president. It was the second smoking report prepared by the 6,800-member body. The first, issued in 1962, discussed the reasons cigarettes should be viewed as a general health hazard.

The 1971 report said an average smoker could expect to lose five and a half years of his life compared with the non-smoker, that smokers were about twice as likely to die in middle age as were non-smokers and that two smokers out of every five were likely to die before 65, compared with one out of every five non-smokers.

The report asserted that "cigarette smoking is now as important a cause of death as were the great epidemic diseases . . . that affected previous generations in this country." The physicians said that the government, while saying that it accepted the evidence of the dangers of smoking, had "taken no effective action to curtail the habit." The document criticized British officials for spending nearly 10 times the sum for public education on road safety as on antismoking programs each year.

Japanese warned on smoking. A Japanese health official warned Jan. 11, 1971 that the annual death toll from lung cancer in Japan would double to more than 20,000 by 1977 unless the government took steps to discourage cigarette smoking.

The official, Dr. Takeski Hirayama of Japan's National Cancer Center, said his work has shown that the lung cancer death rate was 30% higher among smokers than non-smokers. Dr. Hirayama had been investigating smoking and lung cancer since 1965.

In 19 years—from 1950 through 1969—lung cancer deaths in Japan had increased tenfold. In 1950, 1,119 lung cancer deaths were reported. In 1969, the death toll rose to 10,130.

Women find smoking hard to give up. U.S. doctors and psychologists overseeing a government study on the behavioral patterns of smokers in San Diego, Calif. and Syracuse, N.Y. said Jan. 9, 1971 that early findings showed women to be less successful than men at breaking the cigarette habit. The study was sponsored by the U.S. Public Health Service.

The researchers said they were at a loss to explain what they described as "a consistent phenomenon" of women's resistance to giving up cigarettes and—among those women who do give it up—a "relapse" rate that was 38% higher than that of men.

(In the last 15 years the number of women smoking cigarettes had nearly doubled while the number of men who smoked dropped. Since 1966, the number of adult Americans who smoked cigarettes decreased by 4.5 million to a 1970 total of 44.7 million adult smokers. But that drop, however, was made up largely of men who stopped smoking. Women contributed little to the decrease.)

Smoking linked to cancer recurrence. Cigarette smokers who continued to smoke after being successfully treated for cancer faced a much greater risk of developing another malignancy than did smokers who stopped after treatment for cancer, according to a report by a physician with the University of Louisville Medical School.

Dr. Condict Moore published the results of his study Oct. 25, 1971 in the Journal of the American Medical Association.

In his study, Moore worked with 203 cigarette smokers who had been successfully treated for cancer by surgery or X-rays. Moore said that 40% who continued to smoke suffered a recurrence of cancer in their mouths, throats, voice boxes or lungs. Only 6% of those smokers who stopped developed new cancers in areas exposed to smoking.

Cigarettes also endanger nonsmokers. The U.S. surgeon general asserted Jan. 10, 1972 that those who do not smoke cigarettes faced some of the same health hazards of smoking that imperiled smokers.

The latest indictment of cigarette smoking was contained in Surgeon General Jesse L. Steinfeld's annual report to Congress.

Steinfeld placed new emphasis on carbon monoxide as a hazard in cigarette smoke. He said nonsmokers could be exposed to dangerous concentrations of carbon monoxide while sitting in a small, smoke-filled area. The 226-page report contended that the effects could be particularly hazardous for a person with heart or lung disease.

Steinfeld's report cited studies showing that the levels of carbon monoxide in a room or automobile with persons smoking could rise above the occupational guideline of 50 parts per million in effect in the U.S. For the first time he listed carbon monoxide among the "most likely" contributors to the hazards of cigarette smoking. Tar and nicotine had previously been listed as the others.

At a news conference in Washington, Steinfeld said that although most persons would not be exposed to such high concentrations of carbon monoxide for long periods of time, "the fact that such dangerous conditions can develop should sound a warning to us."

As he did in his 1971 report, Steinfeld recommended banning smoking in public places.

(The Tobacco Institute, which represented the major tobacco processors, released a statement Jan. 10 contending that Steinfeld's report "ignores" and "misrepresents" the work of researchers that cast doubt on the idea that smoking was a hazard to one's health.)

Steinfeld estimated that there were about 44 million smokers in the U.S., but said the figure would have been nearly 75 million had the government not campaigned against smoking.

Radiation in tobacco linked to cancer. A form of radiation found to develop from smoking tobacco had been linked to cancer of the lungs by a research project at Harvard University. In 1964 it had first been proposed that the radiation, known to be emitted from the element polonium found in most green plants, including tobacco, caused cancer.

Although radiation in large amounts was known to cause cancer, it had remained unproven as to whether the doses inhaled in tobacco were sufficient to cause the disease. However, experiments performed by the Harvard group showed that when an amount of polonium, similar to that inhaled by a smoker over a lifetime, was introduced into hamsters' throats a significant number developed lung cancer. The study was published in the journal, Science, a publication of the American Association for the Advancement of Science, and was reported in the Washington Post May 29, 1975.

It was calculated that a two-pack-a-day smoker received 20 rads of radiation during a 25 year period. (A rad was a unit of absorbed dose of ionizing radiation.) When hamsters received only 15 rads 13% developed lung cancer. In addition, one of the researchers, Dr. John B. Little, noted that when the hamsters were exposed to polonium as well as one or more of the other carcinogens found in tobacco "a much higher incidence of lung tumors" was found than if the carcinogens were acting alone.

Little said that if the research were verified, the polonium could actually be filtered out of the smoke. In fact, he explained, "many of the new [cigaret] filters are already doing just that."

Consumer unit bars cigarette ban role. The Consumer Product Safety Commission ruled May 17, 1974 that it lacked statutory authority to act on a petition by Sen. Frank Moss (D, Utah) calling on the commission to ban 27 brands of high tar cigarettes as hazardous substances.

Low-tar, low-nicotine cigarettes cut risk. The number of lung-cancer deaths among smokers of cigarettes with a reduced tar-and-nicotine content was 26% less than among comparable smokers of cigarettes with "high" levels of those substances, the American Cancer Society said Sept. 14, 1976. The ACS survey, the first large-scale attempt to analyze how levels of tar and nicotine affected smokers' mortality rates, involved more than one million men and women who had been studied over a 12-year period that ended in June 1972.

The study reconfirmed the link between smoking and disease, showing a 30% to 75% higher death rate among smokers of "low" tar and nicotine cigarettes than among persons who never had smoked regularly. It also supported previous findings that the lung-cancer death rate among pipe or cigar smokers was double that of nonsmokers. Death rates for pipe or cigar smokers from lip, tongue, mouth and esophageal cancer were as high or higher than for cigarette smokers.

For purposes of the study, researchers defined "high" tar levels as 25.8 to 35.7 milligrams and "low" as less than 17.6 milligrams. "High" nicotine levels were 2.0 to 2.7 milligrams and "low" levels were 1.2 milligrams or less.

Health official stresses reduced toxins—Smoking-related illness and death could be significantly reduced in several decades if the tobacco industry made a concerted effort to produce less hazardous cigarettes, an officer of the National Cancer Institute said Oct. 28. Dr. Gio B. Gori told a symposium on smoking and disease that it was currently impractical to abolish tobacco use or to anticipate a society of nonsmokers.

Given the available technology to remove toxic components from cigarettes, Gori considered the marketing of products with a reduced tar-and-nicotine content "the single most important and potentially successful disease prevention opportunity in contemporary society."

Gori noted that the current tar yield of cigarettes was about one-third of those manufactured in 1955 and that nicotine levels had been reduced by one-half.

'Tolerable' cigarettes debated—Some cigarettes "are so low in tar and other toxic substances as to cause no observable hazards," it was said later by Gori, deputy director of the National Cancer Institute's Causes-and-Prevention Division. This view, given Aug. 9, 1978, was based on the results of government-funded research intended to find a safer cigarette.

Researchers in the project had tested more than 150 modifications of the ordinary cigarette in efforts to reduce the hazards of smoking. They identified 27 cigarette brands containing what Gori described as "tolerable levels" of tar. (None of the 27 brands exceeded 10.3 mg of tar or 1.01 mg of nicotine.)

The "tolerable level" was the amount of tar contained in two pre-1960 cigarettes. Research had shown that persons who smoked no more than that had no higher death rate than did nonsmokers.

Gori said the toxic substances in the 27 brands were so low that in one case a smoker could smoke more than a pack a day without risk beyond that shared by a nonsmoker.

Tobacco companies had already gone a long way in weaning persons away from the old cigarettes. The Washington Post Aug. 14 cited data that showed that the cigarette lowest in tar and nicotine in 1954 had more of both than the cigarette that currently had the highest amounts.

Gori said he thought the present, less hazardous brands were only the "forerunners" of those that would be marketed in the future and added that "considerable improvement is still possible."

There was immediate reaction to Gori's use of the word "tolerable." The U.S. surgeon general, Dr. Julius Richmond, told smokers Aug. 10 not to be misled into thinking that there were "tolerable" levels of nicotine, tar and other toxic substances in some brands.

The directors of the National Cancer Institute and the National Heart, Lung and Blood Institute issued a joint statement Aug. 10: "We reject any inference that scientists now believe the use of less hazardous cigarettes may be considered 'tolerable' or safe."

Gori said the health leaders had misinterpreted his statements. He emphasized that he was not calling any cigarette safe, "The only cigarette that is safe is the cigarette that is not lit."

Filter cigarettes seem as less perilous—Precancerous cell changes in the lungs of men smoking lower tar, lower nicotine cigarettes in the 1970s were found less common than in men smoking the stronger cigarettes of the 1950s, scientists from the American Cancer Society and the Veterans Administration Medical Center, East Orange, N.J., reported in a study published Feb. 22, 1979 in the New England Journal of Medicine.

The new study was done on lung tissue specimens taken at autopsy from 445 men who died in 1970–77 of causes other than lung cancer. More than 20,000 sections were studied.

Among heavy smokers who died in the 1970s, the lung changes thought to be precancerous were 2.2%. Among roughly the same number of heavy smokers who died in the 1950s, the changes were found in 22.5%. The abnormalities were not found in nonsmokers.

An American Cancer Society spokesman called the new report "optimistic" and said it indeed suggested that smokers could reduce their lung cancer risk by switching to low tar and nicotine brands if they could not quit entirely. However, he pointed out that the study did not take into account deaths among smokers caused by heart disease, other lung diseases and other cancers. He said "the nation's guard against cigarette health hazards must not be allowed to relax."

There was no data on the precise brands of cigarettes smoked, but the scientists concluded that because of the changes in cigarettes since the 1950s "everyone who has been a habitual cigarette smoker for 25 years or longer must be smoking cigarettes with less tar and nicotine."

Anti-smoking drive announced. The American Cancer Society announced Oct. 15, 1976 a five-year campaign against cigarette smoking called "Target 5." The program's goals were to get 12.5 million of the 50 million adult smokers in the U.S. to quit, to persuade half the nation's nine million teenage smokers to quit and to persuade the U.S. government to halt its $60-million annual subsidies to various branches of the tobacco industry. The society voted to spend $1 million on the first year's objectives.

A tobacco-industry spokeman charged the society with engaging in propaganda rather than "the basic science research needed to prove whether its beliefs about smoking are right or wrong."

HEW campaign—Health, Education & Welfare Secretary Joseph A. Califano Jr. Jan. 11, 1978 announced a campaign to break the cigarette habit in the U.S. and to discourage young people from starting it.

Califano's proposed anti-smoking package supported the Civil Aeronautics Board proposed ban on cigarette smoking in airliners. It would restrict smoking in public areas of the 10,000 government buildings run by the General Services Administration and would raise, or graduate, the federal excise tax on cigarettes, based on the tar and nicotine content of the product. Califano said a joint HEW-Treasury Department task force would investigate "whether tax policy can influence decisions about smoking."

The HEW project would also target special "high-risk groups" by revising warning labels for persons particularly endangered by smoking.

As part of the consumer education-public interest effort, broadcast networks would be asked to step up the frequency of anti-smoking spot announcements, which had dropped sharply since cigarette advertising was banned from radio and television in 1971. Califano also announced that for fiscal 1979 (beginning Oct. 1), the newly created Office on Smoking and Health would have a total budget of $23 million, $6 million of which would be earmarked for education.

The program was announced on the anniversary of the Surgeon General's 1964 Report on Smoking and Health, the document that publicly linked smoking with lung cancer. Since then, 14 million Americans, mostly white males, had given up smoking. But enough teenagers, women and minorities had taken up the habit to keep the number of smokers relatively constant.

Lobby Groups Criticize HEW Plan—Dr. Sidney M. Wolfe, director of the Health Research Group (an affiliate of Ralph Nader's Public Citizen Inc.), criticized HEW's proposed anti-smoking campaign Jan. 11 for its failure to challenge the Agriculture Department's expenditure of $80 million annually to support the growing of tobacco and its price. Other anti-smoking lobbyists criticized the program for relying on voluntary cooperation, not compulsory compliance.

How Many Young Americans Smoke

A Half-Pack or More a Day

(By educational background of those no longer in school)

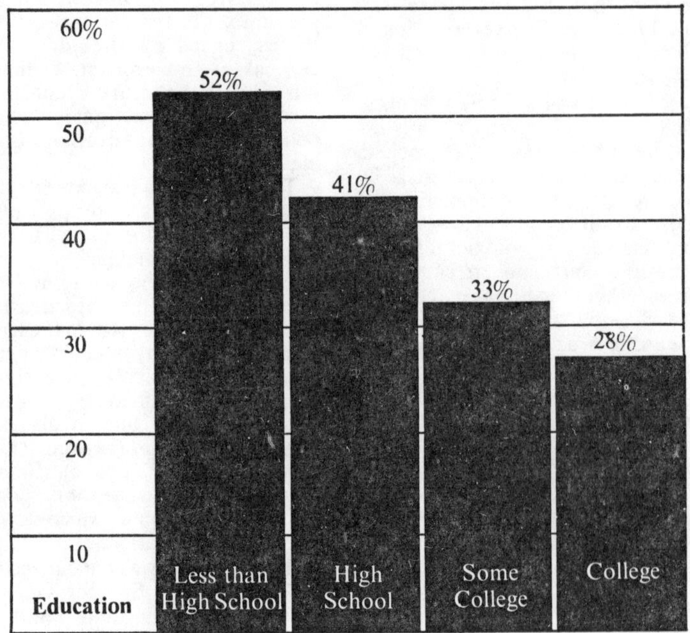

Source: American Council of Life Insurance

People's attitudes often differ from their behavior, and young Americans are no exception when it comes to matters of health care, says the Health Insurance Institute.

This was revealed by a survey of 2,284 American youths, ages 14 to 25. Ninety percent agreed cigarette smoking is one of the causes of lung cancer, but 35 percent admitted smoking daily.

Education seemed to influence their habits, the Institute said. Some 52 percent who left high school without a diploma said they smoked half a pack a day compared to 28 percent of college graduates.

A spokesman for the American Tobacco Institute said the plan "vastly oversimplified" the issues and was an intrusion on the civil liberties of Americans. Institute vice president William F. Dwyer called Califano's recommendations "the personal product of a prohibitionist mentality."

AMA Study Finds Smoking Harmful. Cigarette smoking was reported by the American Medical Association Aug. 5, 1978 in Chicago to cause lung and heart diseases and to contribute to many other maladies, including ulcers.

The findings were the result of a 14-year, $15-million study financed by the top U.S. tobacco companies and intended to refute the U.S. surgeon general's contention that cigarette smoking was hazardous to health.

Research into the cancer-causing properties of cigarettes was minimal as the researchers said that area had already been covered thoroughly, but they said they did find cancer-causing agents in nicotine.

The report concluded that "cigarette smoking plays an important role in the development of chronic, obstructive pulmonary diseases and constitutes a grave danger to individuals with pre-existing diseases of the coronary arteries."

In addition, it found that nicotine irritated the gastrointestinal tract, causing indigestion and even peptic ulcers. The study indicated that smoke inhibited bacteria-destroying organisms, making smokers more prone to infections.

Part of the report dealt with tobacco addiction. One factor among many contributing to addiction appeared to be nicotine. It was found that the number of cigarettes smoked by volunteers in the study decreased significantly when nicotine was given intravenously.

1979 Surgeon General's report. U.S. Surgeon General Julius B. Richmond Jan. 11, 1979 issued a 1,200-page report that reaffirmed and expanded earlier warnings about the health dangers of cigarettes. The report had been ordered by Secretary of Health, Education and Welfare Joseph A. Califano to coincide with the first anniversary of Califano's campaign against what he called "public health enemy number one."

Dr. Richmond labeled smoking "the single most important environmental factor contributing to early death" and said his report provided "overwhelming evidence" linking cigarette smoke to cancer, heart disease and numerous other illnesses. He concluded that women, industrial workers and young people ran special risks by smoking.

Although similar warnings had been issued before, the mass of statistics showed that smoking had risen markedly among young women over the last decade while overall among women there had been a slight decline in the number of smokers. Smoking among men had fallen significantly and the total proportion of adult smokers had fallen to 33% of the population from 41% in 1966.

Califano, commenting on the increase in female smokers, said, "Women who smoke like men die like men who smoke."

Califano promised a stepped-up campaign against smoking that would include more television advertisements, efforts to get more states to restrict smoking in public buildings, expanded anti-smoking projects in schools, and endeavors to have life insurance companies reduce premiums for nonsmokers.

Research and education within HEW rose to $29 million in fiscal 1979 from $19 million in 1978 and Califano said it would be still higher in 1980.

The Tobacco Institute, an industry association, Jan. 10 called the report "more rehash than research."

The report was also criticized Jan. 11 by an anti-smoking lobby group, Action on Smoking and Health. A spokesman for ASH termed the report "criminally deficient and misleading" and compared the health hazards of smoking to those of heroin addiction.

Cigarette Manufacture Increases. The output of U.S. cigarette manufacturers continued to increase despite cancer warnings, the Commerce Department reported Feb. 11, 1979.

The cigarette industry produced $6.1 billion worth of cigarettes in 1977, up from $3.6 billion during 1972. The industry employed 39,000 workers in 1971 with the majority located in Virginia (12,400) and North Carolina (17,900).

Anti-smoking laws rejected. At least two anti-smoking proposals failed to win enactment in 1979:

A bill banning smoking at all public meetings in Maine was vetoed March 13 by Gov. Joseph E. Brennan. The measure would have covered practically any gathering down to the village level and provided for a $50 fine. Brennan, a "reformed" smoker, said he believed making it a crime was bad public policy and the bill was an unnecessary intrusion into the affairs of local government.

A proposed ordinance that would have banned cigarette smoking in many public places was narrowly rejected by Dade County, Florida voters May 8.

The proposition, which was put on the ballot by petition, lost by only 820 votes, out of more than 190,000 cast (96,512 to 95,692).

The proposal, promoted by the Group Against Smokers' Pollution (GASP), would have restricted smoking in most "enclosed public places, places of employment, educational facilities and health facilities." Separate smoking and nonsmoking areas would have been required in these places.

Some indoor areas would have been exempted, such as factories, bars, homes, hotel rooms, pool halls and boxing and wrestling arenas.

An organized opposition to the proposal raised $964,161, at least two-thirds of which came from tobacco companies. GASP reported spending only $8,000.

Other Cancer Hazards

HEW study on alcoholism. A Department of Health, Education & Welfare report on alcohol and health made public July 11, 1974 indicated that alcohol abuse among high school students had risen sharply. The study, prepared by the National Institute on Alcohol Abuse and Alcoholism, also contained the finding that heavy drinkers ran far greater risk of getting certain kinds of cancer—of the mouth, throat region, esophagus and liver—than nondrinkers.

The report also cited international studies and concluded, "Cancers of the mouth, pharynx, larynx and esophagus and primary cancer of the liver appear to be definitely related to heavy alcohol consumption."

Nader group seeks TCE ban. Health Research Group, a public-interest group backed by consumerist Ralph Nader, requested June 25, 1975 that Food & Drug Administration ban the use of trichloroethylene (TCE) in food because it had been shown to cause cancer in animals. A recent National Institute of Cancer study found a 30%-40% incidence of tumors in mice fed TCE. The chemical was used in some processes for decaffeinating coffee.

FDA sets chloroform ban. The Food & Drug Administration April 6, 1976 proposed banning the use of chloroform in drugs and cosmetics because of a potential health risk.

The proposal was based on a report received in March from the National Cancer Institute finding that chloroform induced cancer in test animals.

Chloroform had been used in small amounts to flavor some cough medicines and toothpastes. It also had been used in liniments and as a solvent to make adhesives and resins for food packaging.

Plastic soft-drink bottle challenged. The Natural Resources Defense Council April 21, 1976 challenged Food & Drug Administration's interim approval of plastic soft-drink and beer bottles.

In a suit filed in U.S. District Court in the District of Columbia, the council cited a potential health risk from "migration" of chemicals from the plastic, particularly a substance known as acrylonitrile (ACN), to the contents of the bottle.

The council said that there was "some reason to doubt" the safety of the bottles, which were undergoing further study by the FDA. ACN was closely related chemically to vinyl chloride, which had been shown to produce cancer in test animals.

Plastic soft drink bottles were being test-marketed in several regions and were being considered by a beer producer.

Hamburgers questioned, fluoridation cleared. During 1978 studies indicated that pan-fried hamburgers might be carcinogenic, but water fluoridation was cleared as a potential cancer cause.

■ The possibility that pan-frying hamburgers might increase the risk of cancer was reported May 16 by a Washington University scientific research team. Tests showing mutagens developed in beef when cooked at high temperatures prompted the researchers to suggest that meat be eaten rare, or be cooked in a microwave oven or broiled to avoid the risk. The concern was with the heat, not the meat itself.

■ A federal study to investigate allegations that fluoridating water to prevent tooth decay increased cancer rates determined that there was no link and no adverse effect on overall health. The study of 46 cities, published May 18 in the New England Journal of Medicine, showed virtually no difference in the death rates. According to the survey, the death rate from cancer was 195 in the cities with fluoride and 197 in the cities without.

Hair dyes termed cancer-causing. The chemical substance 4 methoxy-m-phenylenediamine (4MMPD), an ingredient of many permanent hair dyes, was a potential carcinogen that could be absorbed through the scalp, a public interest group said Oct. 17, 1977. The Environmental Defense Fund (EDF) announced that a soon-to-be-released National Cancer Institute study, part of a project to detect cancer-causing agents, showed that laboratory rats and mice fed vast amounts of the chemical had developed malignant tumors.

The NCI had informed the Food and Drug Administration that the hair dye chemical was cancer-causing when ingested by animals. (Before the agency could take action, it had to determine whether the tests indicated a health hazard when the chemical was applied to the skin.)

A spokesman for the Cosmetic, Toiletry and Fragrance Association, the industry trade group, called the EDF's conclusions "not only hasty, but incorrect." The industry countered that the "unevaluated" NCI study was based on experiments in which the test animals consumed quantities of the chemical that were "equivalent to a woman drinking 25 bottles of hair dye a day every day of her life."

The EDF said 4MMPD was found in "a large proportion" of permanent hair dyes manufactured by Revlon Inc., Alberto-Culver Co., the Clairol division of Bristol-Meyers Co. and Cosmair Inc. The fund estimated that such products were used by 25–30 million women in the U.S. alone. The public interest group said that it had petitioned the FDA to require warning labels on products stating that 4MMPD "can enter your bloodstream through your scalp and has been shown to cause cancer in animals."

Non-permanent hair dyes or rinses, which washed out of the hair after several shampoos, did not contain the chemical and were not included in the safety dispute.

GAO cites hair dye risk—The assertion that some widely used hair dyes presented a potential health hazard was backed Dec. 14 by a General Accounting Office report urging the Food and Drug Administration to require warning labels for those products containing "colors known to cause or suspected of causing cancer."

The GAO study said that the chemicals 2,4-diaminoanisole and toluene-2,4-diamine were "used in all three types of coal tar hair dyes," (so-called because the chemicals, currently derived from petroleum or natural gas, were originally obtained from coal tar). On hair dye ingredient labels, 2,4-diaminoanisole was commonly called 4MMPD. Both chemicals cited by the GAO had been detected by a National Cancer Institute screening project.

The three basic types of dyes mentioned referred to temporary (rinses that washed out), semipermanent (preparations that gradually wore off after several washings) and permanent. The Environmental Defense Fund's warning had been limited to the permanent hair dyes.

The GAO also noted that coal tar colors derived from benzidine, a known carcinogen, were used in at least 26 semipermanent and temporary hair dye preparations. A Clairol spokesman responded that none of the benzidine dyes mentioned in the GAO report were used by any major manufacturer of hair coloring.

FDA bans coloring dyes. An order banning six coloring dyes used in soaps, lipsticks and other cosmetics was issued Dec. 12, 1977 by the Food & Drug Administration. Of the six dyes, five—Red Nos. 10, 11, 12 and 13 and Yellow No. 1—were believed to contain potentially carcinogenic substances. None had ever been approved for use in food.

The sixth color, Blue No. 6, was banned for all uses—except as an identifying color for surgical sutures—because the dye's manufacturers had failed to submit FDA-required safety data.

A recall of products containing the banned colors was not considered necessary, an FDA spokesman said.

Curbs vs. Two Other Chemicals Urged—The National Institute for Occupational Safety & Health Jan. 13, 1978 recommended safeguards against worker exposure to these other chemicals: 4-methoxy-m-phenylenediamine, found in many permanent dyes for hair, and tetrachloroethylene, used by many dry cleaners.

The Food and Drug Administration on Jan. 4 had proposed a label warning for dyes containing the hair-dye ingredient.

Medical Research, Treatment, Prevention & Hazards

War on Cancer

Nixon starts anti-cancer campaign. In his State of the Union Message Jan. 22, 1971, President Richard Nixon requested a $100 million appropriation for efforts to find a cancer cure. He called for total war on the disease. "The time has come in America," he said, "when the same kind of concentrated effort that split the atom and took man to the moon should be turned toward conquering this dread disease."

Anti-cancer drive unveiled. President Nixon's chief science adviser Feb. 13, 1971 explained the Administration strategy for its war on cancer. A feature of the program was Nixon's decision to give stewardship of the drive to the National Institutes of Health despite Congressional pressures for the establishment of a new, separate agency to head the effort.

Details of the program were announced by Dr. Edward E. David Jr., the White House science adviser, in a speech in Chicago to the Association of American Medical Colleges.

In an interview before his speech, David said the Administration expected resistance from some congressmen over Nixon's decision to put control of the drive in the hands of the Institutes of Health. He added, however, that it would not be sound policy to create a separate agency to oversee the drive.

In outlining the program, David said he expected the cancer problem to be solved piece by piece, perhaps over a number of years. He said the effort would permit researchers and scientists to pursue individual leads that looked the most promising at any given time, but with a flexibility that would allow new avenues to be explored in view of changing scientific data.

At the present time, medical authorities viewed two areas as possibly holding the key to solving the cancer puzzle. One was the search for proof that viruses may cause some cancers in humans. Another key area was believed to be understanding the basic mechanisms by which cells, normal and abormal, control their growth, multiplication and their production of substances used by the body.

An exact breakdown of how the funds earmarked for the cancer drive were to be spent was not available. In his state of the Union message, and in his proposed budget, President Nixon asked for an appropriation of $100 million, of which about $30 million would be used to get the anti-cancer program started. With the National Cancer Institute's $232 million request, the total effort would have a fund of more than $300 million.

Cancer Control Month, 1971

Proclamation 4039. ***March 29, 1971***

By the President of the United States of America a Proclamation

This Nation may stand on the threshold of one of the greatest triumphs in human history—the conquest of cancer. If we can now achieve that great goal, we will have lifted from the human family forever the pain, the suffering and the unbearable fear of that most dreaded of all diseases.

Decades of research have brought us at last to the moment when scientists can look with renewed hope toward victories in the prevention and treatment of cancer. This moment presents an opportunity that we dare not pass up. The lives of millions now living and countless more yet unborn can be touched—and saved—by what we do.

I have proposed a bold new effort to bring us closer to the goal we seek. I have asked for an additional $100 million this year to press toward the conquest of cancer. I know that money alone cannot guarantee victory in a struggle as complex and difficult as this. But I also know that this search can be quickened by great strides. When they occur, we must be ready to seize upon them and grasp, if we can, the prize that has been sought for so long.

Just as the whole world could benefit from this effort, the whole Nation must be behind it. The Congress, by joint resolution of March 28, 1938 (52 Stat. 148) requested that the President issue annually a proclamation setting aside the month of April as Cancer Control Month.

Now, Therefore, I, Richard Nixon, President of the United States of America, do hereby proclaim the month of April 1971 as Cancer Control Month, and I invite the Governors of the States and the Commonwealth of Puerto Rico, and the appropriate officials of all other areas under the United States flag to issue similar proclamations.

To give new emphasis to this serious problem, and to encourage the determination of the American people to resolve it, I also ask the medical and allied health professions, the communications industries, and all other interested persons and groups to unite during the appointed month in public reaffirmation of this Nation's efforts to

New cancer agency opposed. A Congressional proposal to give stewardship of the Nixon Administration's drive to conquer cancer to a new, separate federal agency ran into unexpected opposition March 9, 1971.

A Johnson Administration health official and spokesmen for two American science and medical organizations told a Senate subcommittee that while they endorsed the expanded effort against cancer, they believed establishment of a new health agency would probably be more of a hindrance than help.

They were joined in their criticism by officials of the Department of Health, Education and Welfare (HEW). The HEW officials told the Health Subcommittee of the Senate Labor and Public Welfare Committee that a new, separate cancer agency would be costly and of doubtful effectiveness and would tend to separate cancer research from the overall medical research effort.

The Nixon Administration had said in earlier statements that it planned to use the National Institutes of Health (NIH) and National Cancer Institute to oversee the cancer effort.

The proposal's new opponents indicated support for the idea of putting control of the cancer effort in the hands of the NIH. Dr. Howard A. Schneider of the University of North Carolina told the Senate panel that replacement of the National Cancer Institute by a new federal agency would herald the beginning of the ultimate destruction of the NIH centers.

Schneider, who represented the 11,000 member Federation of American Societies for Experimental Biology, said "we deplore" the possible erosion of the NIH responsibilities.

His observations were backed by Dr. Philip R. Lee, an HEW official in the Johnson Administration. Lee said, "We do not need more separation; we need more intimate interchange of ideas and interaction among investigators." Lee, chancellor of the University of California, San Francisco, said be believed it would be a mistake to begin to "dismantle NIH in favor of an untested approach."

Nixon to lead drive. President Nixon said May 11, 1971 that he would assume personal command of his Administration's war against cancer.

The President said he hoped his own direct leadership of his proposed national cancer program would bring closer the day when a cure was discovered for the disease.

Nixon said his program would be the sole research enterprise in the government's medical and health establishment that would be budgeted independently and be directly responsible to the White House.

In announcing that he would personally direct the program, Nixon did not make any specific request for funds. He said, however, that the effort would lack neither money nor organization. Nixon said that "to the extent money is needed it will be provided."

With Nixon at the time of the announcement was Elliot L. Richardson, secretary of health, education and welfare, who stressed that throughout the drive there would be close cooperation between personnel running the President's program and officials within the NIH. He said the groups would be "collaborators." Richardson said the Administration plan would absorb the National Cancer Institute into the new program.

In his statement, the President said that "success will test the very limits of our imagination and our resourcefulness. It will require a high sense of purpose and a strong sense of discipline."

Congress approves funds. Compromise legislation approved by Congress in December 1971 authorized the expenditure of $1.59 billion over three years for the federal anti-cancer program. The House of Representatives passed the bill by voice vote Dec. 9, and the Senate adopted it by 85–0 roll-call vote Dec. 10.

The legislation had been bottled up in Congress after the House and Senate had passed different versions of the legislation. At the center of the controversy was the question of whether a new agency would be set up to administer the expanded program or whether it should be controlled by the existing federal health apparatus.

The bill produced by Senate-House conferees left the stewardship of the program within the National Institutes of Health, as had the House version of the bill.

Shortly before the conferees agreed on the bill, President Nixon notified them that he was willing to work with either the House or Senate version.

The main thrust of the compromise bill was directed at cancer research rather than patient care. It did, however, re-establish some public health programs for cancer detection and other control measures. As part of clinical research studies, 15 centers were to be set up to treat cancer patients.

Under the legislation, President Nixon was to appoint a director of the National Cancer Institute, the existing government agency charged with overseeing the cancer research program. The agency's budget was to be prepared by the director and sent directly to the Office of Management and Budget.

Cancer drive detailed. Dr. Frank J. Rauscher Jr., selected by President Nixon to coordinate the nation's stepped-up war on cancer, said May 25, 1972 that his immediate goal as director of the National Cancer Institute was to carry to doctors throughout the U.S. details of known medical procedures that were successful in treating certain types of cancers.

(Rauscher, one of the Cancer Institute's leading scientists, had been appointed director of the institute May 5. In that post, he was responsible for direction of the research programs which drew funds from the institute's $377 million annual budget.)

To make available the details of known successful treatments, Rauscher said he would like to set up as many as 100 clinical cancer treatment centers across the country. There, local doctors could be trained in the latest treatment techniques by the doctors and scientists who pioneered them.

But explaining known treatments was seen by Rauscher as a short-term goal. He said the long-range objective was prevention. Rauscher said the primary goals in cancer work was to find solutions such as by vaccines, elimination of cancer-causing substances in the environment and to learn the answer about the basic biological process that turns healthy cells into cancerous ones.

New plan of attack prepared. A five-year plan aimed at accelerating research into the causes and treatment of cancer was made public by the White House Aug. 17, 1973.

The proposed program, prepared by 250 leading cancer specialists under the sponsorship of the National Cancer Institute, called for expenditures of $500 million in fiscal 1974, which were to increase to $852 million by fiscal 1978 and to $1.7 billion by fiscal 1982.

Dr. Frank J. Rauscher, the President's choice to direct the effort against cancer, had told the White House that in fiscal 1974 he required $640 million "to carry out the objectives the executive and members of Congress have often enunciated," the Washington Post reported July 28.

Reports of White House intentions to pare $140 million from the figure asked by Rauscher caused Senate Democrats Mike Mansfield (Mont.) and Warren G. Magnuson (Wash.) to charge that the publicized war against cancer was "more myth than reality." Both warned that budget restrictions would have an adverse impact on efforts against cancer and other diseases.

The Wall Street Journal reported Aug. 20 that the plan failed to resolve several fundamental issues that had divided the scientific community since the inception of the federal cancer fighting plan: it failed to provide clues to resolve the dilemma of how much should be invested in long-term research aimed at fundamental causes and how much should be funneled into immediate application of existing knowledge. Nor did the cancer plan relieve the distress felt over Administration policy aimed at elimination of direct training research grants. Moreover, the Journal said, the scientific community feared that the Cancer Institute and its layman bureaucracy, by virtue of control of the funds, would begin to assert themselves in purely scientific matters.

Cancer death rate up sharply. The cancer death rate rose in 1972 at a faster rate than in any year since 1951, the National Center for Health Statistics reported April 7, 1973.

The mortality rate was 166.8 per 1,000 deaths in 1972 versus 161.4 in 1971, a 3.3% increase.

A spokesman said much of the increase could be attributed to the increased proportion of the population over age 55, an age group more prone to the risks of cancer. He said the remainder of the increase could be blamed on increased rates of smoking and increases of other carcinogens in the environment. Examples of these were additives to food, growth stimulants for cattle, air and water pollutants, and asbestos at work sites.

Cancer institute reports show increasing survival rates. Two separate studies released by the National Cancer Institute in 1975 indicated improved survival rates for victims of cancer in the U.S. The first study, released July 17, compared the survival rates of white cancer patients diagnosed between 1960–71. The second, reported Aug. 28, compared treatment results of white and black and male and female patients.

The July 17 report, "Recent Trends in Survival of Cancer Patients 1960–71," measured one-year and five-year mortality rates of white patients suffering from 48 types of cancer. The report made use of 230,500 patients in the 1960s and 45,400 patients in 1970–71. NCI used an earlier report for its 1950s statistics.

Among the most encouraging results were the survival rates for sufferers of Hodgkins disease. Five-year survival rates for males went from 31% (1950s) to 38% (1960–64) and 52% (1965–69). For women, rates for the corresponding time intervals went from 38% to 46% and 56%.

One-year survival rates for acute leukemia in males under 15 years of age increased from 26% (1950s) to 40% (1960–64) and 60% (1965–69) and finally, 76% (1970–71). The rate in females went from 21% to 41% to 62% to 71%. However, the five-year survival rate progressed at a much slower rate, going from 1% (1950s) to 4% (1965–69) in males and from 1% to 7% for the corresponding time period in females.

Female breast cancer patients' five-year survival rates increased from 60% in the 1950s to 64% in the late 1960s. According to NCI, the upward trend reflected an increased proportion of early diagnosis of the cancer. (The World Health Organization disclosed that statistics covering the past half-century showed breast cancer as the third leading cause of death, after accidents and suicides, among women 35–54, it was reported Aug. 10.)

Upward survival rates were also recorded for prostate, testis, kidney, bladder, brain, thyroid, larynx and skin cancers. Little change, however, was shown in the survival rates of lymphosarcoma or reticulum cell sarcoma.

The second study, which used data from the same hospitals, found that between 1955–64 white cancer victims lived, on the average, 40% longer than blacks who got cancer. It was further discovered that white women had the best chance of survival, followed by black women, white men and black men.

NCI officials, who edited the report, said the study indicated that cancer in blacks was more likely to be fatal because it was usually discovered later than it was in whites. In the Aug. 28 Washington Post report of the findings, Dr. Paul Cornely, a Howard University professor emeritus and former public health official, blamed the high cancer mortality rates in blacks on the inaccesibility of medical care as well as the environmental hazards of the ghetto and low-paying jobs. He said he felt that the mortality rate was probably approximately the same among blacks and whites of the same economic status. However, NCI officials said that physiological reasons for blacks' poor survival "should be explored."

The longer survival rate among women has been attributed in large part to the defenses provided by their hormonal makeup. In addition, women generally went to doctors more often and had cancers more susceptible to cure. Of the 240,580 cases of cancer studied, if other causes of death were not taken into account, 42% of white women escaped cancer death after 10 years, 33% of black women, 25% of white men and 15% of black men.

WHO official cites gains in cancer treatment. Modern methods of treatment made it possible to cure 3 or 4 out of every 10 persons with cancer, according to Dr. Alexander S. Pavlov, a Russian who was assistant director general of the World Health Organization (WHO). However, in his Nov. 1, 1975 report, Pavlov still attributed to cancer over six million new cases annually and five million deaths in the world.

Pavlov said there were over 1½ million Soviet citizens still alive who had been cured of cancer five or more years ago. Worldwide, Pavlov cited "highly effective" treatment of cancer of the skin, lip, larynx and uterine cervix. He added that, with continued international cooperation in research, a cure for cancer was possible "within a few decades."

In the same report, another WHO official said it was suspected that toxic substances in the environment were the cause of 80% of all human cancers. As an example, the official cited a seven-year study which found a "strong correlation" between the food eaten in certain parts of Africa and the high number of liver cancer cases found in that region.

Cancer-agent clearinghouse planned. Dr. Frank Rauscher, director of the National Cancer Institute, announced plans March 29, 1976 to set up a national clearinghouse that would gather information about cancer-causing agents in the environment. Rauscher said that the clearinghouse would test substances and report findings to the public as the findings became available.

Cancer-frequency studies underway. The chief epidemiologist at the International Agency for Research on Cancer, an affiliate of the World Health Organization at Lyons, France, said in a New York Times interview June 3, 1976 that studies were underway to determine why certain forms of cancer occurred more frequently in some parts of the world than in others. Dr. Calum S. Muir said that among the types being probed in relation to a definite geographical region were cancer of the esophagus in Brittany and Normandy in France and along the southeast coast of the Caspian Sea in Iran, of the colon and rectum among beer-drinkers in Dublin and Copenhagen and of the breast among Japanese women living for many years in the U.S. Dr. Muir cited a form of cancer known as Burkitt's lymphoma, peculiar to Uganda, which attacked children there. He said that a study of all females in Iceland was underway to see if breast cancer and genetic factors were linked. The study was being partly funded by the National Cancer Institute.

The WHO agency said May 10, 1977 that it was starting a 7-year program to develop a worldwide cancer surveillance network that would relate environmental factors to the incidence of cancer in various populations. Scientists currently estimated that 80%-90% of all cancers were directly or indirectly caused by environmental agents.

Dr. John Higginson, the United Nations cancer agency's director, announced that after a preliminary two-year study, the agency would spend $1 million a year for five years to monitor suspected carcinogens in different cultures, with particular emphasis on Third World countries. The proposed network would collate data gathered by national cancer registries, when available, and would fund limited surveys in poorer countries, where the trend toward industrialization was viewed as a cancer threat.

After five years, scientists in the surveillance program would attempt to identify and evaluate the chemical, occupational and life-style factors that influenced cancer.

War on cancer evaluated. Dr. David Goldenberg, executive director of the Ephraim McDowell Community Cancer Network in Lexington, Ky., reported at the National Governors' Conference in Louisville, Ky. in July 1979 that:

Although 1,120 cancer patients die daily in the U.S., we are achieving a saving of 797 lives each day. This comes to 291,000 Americans being cured each year, which is 41.6% of the 700,000 new cases diagnosed annually. These lives saved each year are enough to populate such cities as Tampa, Spokane, and Lexington in Kentucky.

Since it has been imputed that each premature death due to cancer costs between $41,000 and $69,000, the lives saved each year are returning to the economy in the form of productive work, earnings, and taxes between 11 and 20 billion dollars, or more than has been spent on the entire federal cancer program since the establishment of the National Cancer Institute in 1937.

Goldenberg told the governors:

Although I cannot assure you that any amount of money in a single year will permit us to eradicate this dread disease, the National Cancer Program, although a modest effort in monetary terms, has had an impressive record of accomplishment.

Advances in cancer detection, diagnosis and therapy have had an important effect in reducing the mortality rate in a few kinds of cancer, such as the lymphomas, particularly Hodgkin's disease, childhood leukemia, thyroid cancer, bone cancer, testicular cancer, bladder cancer, and cancer of the uterus. In 1950, we were able to save 25 percent of cancer patients; today, over 41 percent. The American Cancer Society estimates that 3 million people in the U.S. are alive today although they have had cancer.

The best example of eradicating a cancer by improved early detection is that of cancer of the uterine cervix. The Pap test is capable of detecting not only early stages of cancer, but abnormal changes in the cervix 5 to 10 years before it may turn into cancer. Similar research is in progress for the early detection of other cancers, but under the current budget, only a fraction of the research deemed acceptable by scientific review can be funded; a fraction that was two-fifths of approved grants in 1978.

I remind you that this is what has been termed a "war on cancer." Since establishment of the National Cancer Institute in 1937, about 8 billion dollars have been invested in cancer research. For the 3 million Americans we have been able to save, we compute that each life saved cost us only $2,667.

How does this compare to the costs of each new cancer death? What is the impact of cancer on our nation's economy? The cost of all diseases in the U.S. in 1975 has been estimated at $245 billion, which includes hospital and physician and other direct costs, as well as indirect—although very real—expenses, such as lost earning power and productivity due to premature death.

Cancer makes up about 9 percent of this total cost, amounting to about $30 billion a year. Dividing this amount by the relative cancer occurrence figures for each state, the cancer economic burden by state in 1978 comes to $2.7 billion for California, $1.5 billion for Florida, Texas, or Illinois, $1.2 billion for New Jersey, $3 billion for New York, $1.8 billion for Pennsylvania, and $510 million for Kentucky.

An effective cancer control program, that is, the proper and rapid transfer of new technology and knowledge to the practice of medicine, must reach those who need attention most, at the local, community level. This can be done best by the states and the local communities themselves.

All segments of the public are rightfully impatient and demanding that money breed results, indeed, rapid returns, as measured by important "breakthroughs" and instant "cures," and the journalistic and political forces are easily persuaded that anything less than such accomplishments are failures on the part of science and medicine to fulfill the expectation that we win the so-called "war" on cancer.

The scientist approaches the complexity of cancer with a realization that it will take a long, sustained, stepwise effort to bring the more than 100 forms of cancer under control. The patients and their families are slowly learning that cancer is not a hopeless scourge imbued in secrecy and shame.

An opposing view was expressed by Ruth Rosenbaum in the Nov. 25, 1977 issue of New Times. She wrote:

The U.S. still holds the record for cancer incidence—50 percent more than the world average—while the chance for an American to survive a cancer invasion has not increased more than 1 percent since the late forties. And this, despite improvements in early diagnosis and refinements in surgery, chemotherapy and radiation therapy—the only hopes that the American Cancer Society and the National Cancer Institute dangle before the public.

It took Irving Rimer, ACS Vice President of Public Information, alone among the top ACS executives, to crack the cheeky new statistics riddle in ACS's 1975 annual report: "Cancer incidence," it teased, contradicting every other source on the subject, "has declined slightly in the last 25 years."

"You have to understand something," Rimer explained. "Somewhere around 1972 or '73, we stopped including in our calculations all skin cancers except melanoma, the only one that's fatal, and also in situ cervical cancers, because many experts don't consider these to be cancers at all. Since together they account for a large number of cases, that could be why the incidence has gone down."

Treatments & Controversies

Breast cancer surgery debate. Breast cancer surgery on Betty Ford, wife of President Ford, and on Margaretta Rockefeller, wife of Vice President-designate Nelson A. Rockefeller, resulted in widespread public discussion of the disease, which afflicted 90,000 U.S. women and resulted in the deaths of 30,000 others in 1973. New findings concerning treatment also increased public interest.

Mrs. Rockefeller, 48, underwent surgery for the removal of her left breast, 32 adjacent lymph nodes and part of the underlying chest muscle Oct. 17, 1974 after doctors at a New York City hospital had confirmed that one large and two small nodules in her breast were malignant.

In announcing the surgery on his wife, Rockefeller said she had been prompted to examine herself for possible malignant lumps because of the heightened "consciousness" that followed Mrs. Ford's operation.

Despite the high incidence of occurrence of breast cancer, its treatment remained in dispute. A study released by the National Cancer Institute Sept. 29 found that a radical mastectomy, the operation performed on Mrs. Ford, was unnecessary in many cases. The study also found that chemical therapy could "drastically" reduce the incidence of recurrence of breast cancer.

The institute was reporting the results of studies involving 1,700 women at 37 U.S. hospitals since 1971. The report showed that radical mastectomies, which prduced life-long pain, weakness and periodic swelling of the arm, were not required for patients whose lymph nodes were cancer-free. By changing normal procedures, surgeons could order immediate laboratory tests on the lymph nodes, the report said. If the tests failed to show malignancy in the nodes, the surgeons could limit treatment to the less disfiguring, less traumatic simple mastectomy—amputation of the breast only. (Normal procedure was to remove the lymph nodes and conduct tests afterward.) "I would estimate that well over half of those [undergoing breast cancer surgery] would be candidates for the less radical procedure," Dr. Frank J. Rauscher, director of the institute, said. Currently, 95% of all women undergoing breast cancer surgery received radical mastectomies.

(The almost universal use of the radical mastectomy had been criticized by some women's rights groups, who suggested that surgeons, most of whom were men, would be less likely to perform such a radical procedure to treat a comparable male affliction.)

The American Cancer Society Oct. 17 took a cautious view of the institute study, pointing out that it had three more years to run before anything definitive could be said about the relative effectiveness of the simple mastectomy. The society said it would continue to recommend radical mastectomy for most cases of breast cancer.

Another study, reported in the Oct. 14 issue of Time magazine, indicated that chemotherapy had been found effective in controlling and preventing cancerous tumors in the lymph nodes. Among 67 premenopausal women who had undergone surgery for breast cancer, only one of 30 given the oral drug L-phenylalanine mustard (L-PAM) had recurrence of cancer, while 11 of 37 women receiving no drug treatment had recurrences.

High rate of breast cancer discovered—A network of new breast cancer clinics across the U.S. had uncovered 2½ times the expected number of malignancies among the first 88,000 women screened, it was reported March 26, 1975. This very high detection rate was attributed to the fact that the women were being tested regardless of whether they showed signs of cancer, and detection had been much higher than if they depended on self-examination.

Thermography fails in breast cancer—Medical researchers at the University of Cincinnati concluded that thermography, a method of detecting malignant tumors (carcinomas) by measuring the excess heat they gave off, was proving useless in spotting early cases of breast cancer, the Wall Street Journal reported July 28, 1976.

Krebiozen ban upheld. The Supreme Court Oct. 15, 1973 let stand a ruling that the drug Krebiozen was not recognized as a safe and effective cure for cancer and therefore could be banned from the market.

Ban on laetrile continued. The importation and sale of laetrile, an alleged cure for cancer, would continue to be banned by the federal government, U.S. Food and Drug Administration chief Donald Kennedy said May 6, 1977. The ban was upheld by a Supreme Court ruling June 18, 1979.

Laetrile, also called vitamin B-17 and the chemical amygdalin, occurred naturally in the pits of apricots and peaches, in bitter almonds and other plants. It was available in 26 countries and was currently being smuggled into the U.S. from Canada and Mexico. Amygdalin contained small amounts of the poison cyanide.

Promoters of laetrile use claimed that it could prevent and cure cancer. They contended that since there was no evidence of the chemical being harmful, the ban on it should be lifted. However, the FDA noted that laetrile was the most tested of all potential cancer cures and that five studies by the National Cancer Institute alone had indicated that it was therapeutically worthless.

An FDA bulletin issued April 14 to physicians and other health professionals nationwide said supporters of laetrile use were "more vocal and better organized than in the past." The agency warned that early cancer patients who believed in laetrile's efficacy might be putting "their lives on the line" by failing to receive orthodox medical treatment.

Laetrile's background—It was in the days of Prohibition that a California doctor first used an apricot extract to improve the taste of moonshine whiskey. Later, the doctor experimented with the extract to treat tumors in animals. When the supposed anti-cancer agent did not prove effective, its use died out. But the San Francisco physician's son, Ernst Krebs Jr., isolated an alleged cancer-fighting substance from the apricot pit in 1949. He called the extract "laetrile." Since then laetrile has been a source of conflict in the field of medicine. Here is a chronology of the Laetrile controversy:

1920—The forerunner of laetrile was first used by Dr. Ernst T. Krebs Sr. in treatment of cancer.

1949—Dr. Krebs' son, biochemist Ernst T. Krebs Jr., isolated an extract from apricot pits and called it "laetrile."

1952—Biochemist Krebs claimed to have made laetrile safe for injection into humans.

1953—The California Medical Association's Cancer Commission investigated laetrile as a cancer treatment. The commission found it "completely ineffective" when used in large doses on cancer in laboratory animals.

Oct. 10, 1962—President John F. Kennedy signed into law the Drug Amendments of 1962. The law provided that the FDA has to certify new drugs to be effective as well as safe, thereby laying the legal basis for the ban on laetrile and other questionable cancer cures.

1962—Ernst T. Krebs Jr. and the John Beard Memorial Foundation pleaded guilty to violating the new drug provisions of Federal Food, Drug & Cosmetic act.

1963—The California State Department of Public Health issued a regulation prohibiting the use of laetrile in the state.

March 1963—The FDA reported no evidence that laetrile is effective in cancer treatment.

Aug. 2, 1965—Dr. Ernst T. Krebs Sr. agreed to a permanent court injunction against further distribution of laetrile.

Sept. 1965—Dr. Krebs pleaded guilty to criminal contempt of court for disobeying a restraining order prohibiting the shipment of laetrile.

Jan. 21, 1966—Dr. Krebs pleaded guilty to contempt of court for shipping Laetrile.

Feb. 3, 1966—Dr. Krebs was given a one-year suspended sentence by a U.S. District Court in California for failing to register as a producer of drugs.

April 20, 1970—FDA assigned an Investigative New Drug application number to the McNaughton Foundation on California for testing amygdalin-laetrile.

May 12, 1970—The application was terminated when the FDA found "serious preclinical and clinical deficiencies."

Sept. 1, 1971—FDA found "no acceptable evidence of therapeutic effect to justify clinical trials" of laetrile.

1976—Alaska became the first state to permit doctors to prescribe and administer laetrile.

Jan. 21, 1977—U.S. District Judge Gordon Thompson Jr. ruled in San Diego that terminally ill patients may import laetrile.

Courts grant access to laetrile—Under a ruling by federal District Court Judge Luther Bohanon of Oklahoma City, some cancer patients had been importing laetrile from Mexico legally, it was reported April 17, 1977. Bohanon initially had ruled in favor of one cancer patient who sought the alleged cancer remedy. He later expanded the ruling to include about 20 other terminally ill persons.

Judge Bohanon April 8 issued a list of conditions under which patients could have access to laetrile, stressing that he had made no attempt to determine the drug's ability to fight cancer. Bohanon's order stipulated that laetrile be made available to terminal cancer patients who had sworn statements from a doctor on their condition. The physician's statement had to include "evidence of a rapidly progressive malignancy" and specify that recognized forms of cancer treatment would be administered in conjunction with laetrile.

Federal district court judges in New York and California also had ordered that terminally ill cancer patients be allowed to import laetrile. In San Diego, Calif., U.S. District Court Judge Gordon Thompson Jr. had said Jan. 21 that to deny a patient freedom of choice in the absence of a known remedy for his illness "would be grossly paternalistic of this court." Three doctors who had certified that no cure was available for the patient in question also had approved his use of laetrile.

Sloan-Kettering finds laetrile useless—Researchers at Memorial Sloan-Kettering Cancer Center in New York City said at a press conference June 15 that laetrile did not possess preventative, tumor-regressing or curative anticancer powers. Their findings were based upon a four-year study of the chemical's effects upon cancerous tumors in animals. The scientists conceded that laetrile's alleged pain-relieving properties could not be evaluated by their study.

The Sloan-Kettering report stated that scientists had been unable to confirm experiments conducted by Dr. Kanematsu Sugiura in 1972–73 that had shown laetrile to be effective against lung cancer in mice. The authors of the report noted Sugiura's current contention that "laetrile is not a curative, but is a palliative agent."

AMA rejects laetrile proposal—A proposal by a special committee of the American Medical Association suggesting that laetrile be made available without a prescription was rejected June 21 by the AMA's policy-making body. The committee, which had not found any beneficial properties in laetrile, had recommended its over-the-counter sale in order to curtail the black market trade of the substance. It was estimated that laetrile smuggling had grown into a $20-million industry. Approximately 50,000 Americans were using laetrile as a cancer treatment.

Laetrile smugglers sentenced—Robert W. Bradford, 46, president of the Committee for Freedom of Choice in Cancer Therapy Inc., was fined $40,000 and put on 3 years' probation May 16, 1977 for smuggling laetrile into the U.S. from Mexico. Three co-defendants, Frank Salaman, Dr. John A. Richardson and Ralph S. Bowman, were also placed on probation and fined a total of $40,000.

All four defendants were sentenced by federal district court Judge William B. Enright in San Diego. Salaman, 52, was vice president of the Freedom of Choice committee, which claimed a membership of 35,000. Richardson, 54, was a physician whose medical license had been revoked in 1976 for treating cancer patients with laetrile, in violation of a 1969 California statute. Bowman, 52, was Richardson's business manager. Bradford and Richardson, like many of those in the laetrile movement, were members of the John Birch Society.

The convicted laetrile conspirators were the first of 19 defendants indicted on smuggling charges to stand trial. Andrew R. L. McNaughton, 60, a Canadian citizen living in Mexico, was described by investigators as the "kingpin" of the operation. McNaughton, who had been involved in several stock fraud cases in the U.S., admitted that his McNaughton Foundation in Tiajuana had once received $130,000 from Joseph Zicarelli, the alleged head of organized crime in Hudson County, N.J.

States authorize laetrile—The Indiana state legislature May 1, 1977 overrode a veto by Gov. Otis Bowen and made Indiana the first state to authorize the manufacture, sale and use of laetrile, which was banned from interstate commerce by the Food and Drug Administration. The bill, effective June 1, also legalized the use of the artificial sweetener saccharin.

The Florida state legislature approved a bill May 2 to allow doctors to administer laetrile when requested by a patient.

By June 23, with action by Louisiana, ten states had authorized the manufacture and sale of laetrile. Arizona, Nevada, Texas, Washington, Delaware and Oklahoma had taken such action by June 21.

Three more states had taken similar action by Jan. 10, 1978, when New Jersey Gov. Brendan Byrne signed a bill authorizing its intrastate sale and use.

New Jersey senators who supported the bill cited cancer victims' civil rights and freedom of choice as the major factor in casting their votes. Detractors of laetrile, such as Democratic State Senator Joseph L. McGahn, a physician, had told the 1976–77 legislature that should someone die because they chose to use laetrile over a more conventional cancer treatment, "that death will be on your head."

Laetrile Found To Enlarge Rat Tumors. Two researchers found that when they gave Laetrile to rats with cancerous tumors, the tumors grew larger and the rats died from cyanide poisoning, it was reported July 13, 1979.

Laetrile was found lethal to rats in studies by Dr. Janardan D. Khandekar and Harlan Edelman of the Evanston, Ill. Hospital and Northwestern University's medical school.

Khandekar's report in the Journal of the American Medical Association described the progressive increases in the size of tumors in rats given Laetrile as "realistic in terms of human ingestion." He also said that the study's findings raised serious questions about the use of Laetrile in clinical medicine "under any circumstances."

FDA approves cancer detection test. The Food & Drug Administration said Jan. 9, 1974 that it had approved plans by Hoffmann-LaRoche, Inc. to begin marketing for limited use a test to aid in the detection of cancer. The test would involve the use of radioactive materials in low dosages to measure the level of carcinoembryonic antigen (CEA) in the blood. CEA, a blood protein, was found in higher than normal concentrations in cancer victims.

While the test would not be a primary diagnostic tool because it gave false results in certain instances, it would be valuable for use among patients already treated for cancer, as it might indicate a relapse several months before other clinical signs had appeared.

Melanoma drug. The National Institutes of Health were reported May 5, 1975 to have approved a new drug to combat melanoma, a deadly form of skin cancer. After 3 years of trials, decarbazine, or imidazole carboxamide, generally known as DTIC was the only drug found effective in treating the cancer. The Institute said it wasn't certain how DTIC worked but that it had doubled the survival rate of patients with the disease.

Treatments & tests. Among other developments of 1975:

Dr. Isaac Djerassi, a Pennsylvania physician, reported March 24 the development of a drug therapy that could significantly improve the chances of survival of children suffering from osteogenic sarcoma, a highly lethal bone cancer. The treatment involved high doses of methotrexate, a drug that poisoned cells, followed by the use of citrovorum factor, a second drug which rescued normal cells but not the cancerous ones.

A means of destroying tumors by causing miniature atomic explosions within cancer cells, destroying them while having little effect on surrounding cells or skin tissue, was reported March 25 to have been used on a small group of patients. Dr. Morton Kligerman, director of the University of New Mexico's cancer center, and Dr. Malcolm Bagshaw, chairman of the department of radiology at Stanford University's School of Medicine, announced the new approach, called "pimeson," or "pion" therapy, at the American Cancer Society's seminar for science writers in San Diego, Calif. The treatment was considered a possible treatment for localized cancers.

Two major studies which suggested that tuberculosis vaccine BCG could protect against human leukemia were questioned in more recent studies based on the experience of thousands of persons in the U.S. and abroad, according to a report April 7 to a research conference at the National Cancer Institute. The original studies had alleged that those inoculated with BCG in Quebec, Canada, and in Chicago had lower leukemia rates than the rest of the population. However, a reanalysis of those studies cast doubt on the validity of the estimates.

Two new means of determining different forms of cancer were reported being developed. One was a simple blood test said to detect lung cancer in an early stage while the other made use of a laser system to identify cervical and vaginal cancer.

The blood test, developed by Drs. L. Fred Ayvazian and Rosalyn Yalwo, detected dangerous amounts of the hormone ACTH (adrenocorticotropic hormone), which was generally associated with lung cancer. According to the Aug. 19 report, the reliability of the tests was confirmed in over 150 tests on cancer and emphysema patients at the Veterans Hospital in East Orange, N.J.

Ayvazian noted, however, that although the cancer could often be found before it spread, certain types were still fatal. "But we believe," he concluded, "that with this method we can improve the curing rate."

Scientists from the Los Alamos Scientific Laboratory in New Mexico said they had developed a new laser system which could identify cancer cells of cervical and vaginal cancers. According to the Oct. 24 report, the method was faster and possibly more accurate than the familiar Pap test.

Neutron beam used. The neutron beam of the Naval Research Laboratory atom-smashing machine in Washington had been used since 1973 in an unconventional treatment of stomach and pancreas cancers, it was reported June 13, 1978. The treatments had been given by a team from Georgetown and George Washington universities. The researchers weren't claiming any cures but felt the treatment was worth more investigation as they had observed some shrinkage of tumors that would not have been expected with other treatment.

Cancer Diagnosis Seldom Secret. Most physicians, 97%, no longer kept the diagnosis of cancer secret from their patients, it was said Feb. 26, 1979 in the Journal of the American Medical Association.

The study, conducted by the University of Rochester Medical Center, used a questionnaire that was identical to one used in 1961. At that time, 90% of the responding physicians indicated a preference for not telling cancer patients the diagnosis.

Those responding to the new survey said they rarely made exceptions to the practice, saying "perhaps more patients are being told because more need to know."

It was also noted that many hospitals were clinical research centers where patients must be told their diagnosis to satisfy legal requirements of informed consent.

Pediatricians were the only specialized doctors who more often made exceptions about giving such information. Age, intelligence, emotional stability and relatives' wishes were most frequently cited as factors in deciding whether to inform the patient.

Danger in Medical Practice

Investigational drugs & the FDA. The main federal agency charged with regulating the trade in medicines is the Food & Drug Administration (FDA). Sen. Abraham A. Ribicoff (D, Conn.), chairman of the Senate Subcommittee on Executive Reorganization & Government Research, charged in the Senate Sept. 19, 1973 that the FDA had been lax in its regulation of "investigational new drugs—drugs approved for testing but not for public sale." These were drugs, he said, that "had been administered in clinical experiments to human subjects." Ribicoff made his charge on the basis of an investigation conducted on his orders by the Government Accounting Office (GAO), which found that the FDA did not always halt the use of suspected carcinogens. He said in a statement in the Congressional Record:

The GAO study discusses only 10 of the more than 6,000 drugs currently classified as investigational new drugs. But the results of the GAO study and the subcommittee staff findings strongly suggest that FDA regulation of investigational new drugs has been lax and has not adequately protected the patients who take these drugs. They also show a failure to adopt safe testing procedures by certain drug companies.

Specifically, the report found that in eight cases, FDA failed to halt human tests after receiving indications that the drugs were not safe. As a result, over 2,000 people were exposed to the hazard of unsafe drugs. GAO further found that the drug companies unnecessarily delayed reporting adverse drug effects to FDA and that once this data was received, FDA did not require necessary patient followup in six cases to protect the health of the people who had been given suspect or unsafe drugs.

Before an experimental drug may be administered to human beings, it must first be given to animals. Prior animal testing is required because there is often some correlation between the ability of a drug to produce adverse effects in animals and its ability to produce such effects in human beings. While the precise relationship between animal results and human results is often indeterminate, it is clear that a drug that has been shown to produce cancerous tumors in animals presents a greater potential risk to human beings than a drug that has shown no adverse health effects in animals.

Current FDA regulations require both substantial animal testing and substantial human testing before a drug is approved for general public sale, rather than investigational use.

The GAO survey showed a consistent pattern for FDA delay in reviewing the data submitted with the IND application. For Practolol, the delay was 3 months. For Triflocin, it was 8 months. In both cases, animals given the drugs developed cancerous conditions. For the other drugs reviewed, the delay ranged from 4 months to a full year. During this time, the drug companies routinely began human testing....

The most dramatic example of FDA's failure to halt human testing after notice of evidence of cancer in animal tests is the drug Practolol, sponsored by Ayerst Labs. When the test data was reviewed, the medical officer concluded that "this study is indefensible and unacceptable." On March 11, 1970, FDA recommended to the sponsor than human testing be discontinued. Testing continued. On April 8, FDA again advised the sponsor to discontinue testing, but the sponsor refused. At that time, the sponsor submitted to FDA the results of a study showing that cancerous tumors had been found in mice. (Ayerst had notice and substantial documentation of the results of this study on August 14, 1969, but had failed to provide it to FDA until nearly 8 months later. By contrast, the Canadian Food and Drug authorities had had possession of the study since August 27, 1969.) Still, FDA took no effective action to terminate testing on human subjects.

In January 1971, FDA tried for a third time to persuade the sponsor to discontinue tests on human beings. Ayerst not only refused to discontinue the tests, but also refused even to make the finding of the mouse study—indicating cancerous tumors—available to the doctors who were conducting the experiments. Those doctors thus had no way of evaluating the risks to which their patients were being subject. Finally, on August 27, 1971, fully 17 months after FDA had first advised the Ayerst to discontinue testing, and after a fourth request from FDA to discontinue, the tests were stopped.

This case is not unique. Another similar case history is that of Oxprenalol Hydrochloride, sponsored by Merrell-National Labs. In this case, it took the FDA 6 months and two requests to stop human testing after tumors had been found in mice....

The GAO found that the time lag between discovery of the effects of human and animal tests and reporting them to FDA ranged from 40 days to 19 months. The case of Triflocin, sponsored by Lederle Labs, was typical. There, the sponsor took 7 months to analyze the results of a study which eventually showed bladder cancer in rats. Meanwhile, human testing was in progress. FDA concluded that the delay was "not unjustified because such delays were apparently standard operating procedure for this company. FDA stated that it "did not consider the delay unusual." The fact that the delay was not unusual, rather than supporting a finding that it was justified, seems to point to the very opposite conclusion.

With respect to Practolol, sponsored by Ayerst Labs, the sponsor failed for 8 months to supply FDA with the results of a study showing cancerous tumors in mice.

In the case of MK-665, an oral contraceptive sponsored by Merck, Sharp and Dome Research, the sponsor waited over a month before notifying FDA that cancer had been found in dogs treated with the drug. The Justice Department declined to bring a criminal prosecution in this matter....

Ribicoff insisted that the FDA "should more closely monitor all human testing" and require test sponsors to perform follow-up checks on FDA orders. Companies that failed to perform proper follow-up tests should be disqualified as IND (investigational new drug) sponsors, Ribicoff declared. He said:

Several of the cases reported by GAO illustrate the need for these steps. One of them was MK-665, sponsored by Merck, Sharp and Dome, which was shown to cause breast cancer in dogs. Only about one-third of the patients who received the drug in clinical tests have been examined.

One of the most flagrant cases of a drug company's resistance to FDA with respect to followup is that of Cinanserin, sponsored by E. R. Squibb & Sons. Human testing had been discontinued in August 1969, because of the appearance of tumors in the livers of rats. In October 1969, Squibb informed FDA that it was not considering followup. According to a letter of July 30, 1970, from the FDA Commissioner Edwards to Squibb, the question of followup had been raised by FDA with Squibb in a telephone conversation of December 9, 1969, with Dr. Lawrence Marks, a Squibb vice president. According to the letter, "he—Marks—stated that he would investigate and call back in a week. There was no reply."

Squibb continued to resist FDA's suggested followup procedures. As a result of Squibb's refusal, FDA medical officers recommended a full evaluation of Squibb's qualifications to be a sponsor of any investigational new drugs, because of its failure to fulfill its responsibility to patients placed in jeopardy.

After several FDA letters had gone unanswered, FDA officials visited the Squibb facility in New Brunswick, N.J., on June 26, 1972. As of November 17, 1972, the FDA still considered Squibb's followup on Cinanserin inadequate. It is noteworthy, however, that throughout this protracted and sometimes heated disagreement, FDA relied exclusively on persuasion in attempting to require a followup. In the absence of regulations requiring followup, FDA apparently felt itself powerless to act more vigorously. FDA could have at any point, however, required followup as a condition of IND approval or required followup by regulation. Thus, the agency's inability to require followup was a direct result of its own inaction.

Realizing that its lack of followup regulations was leaving patients unprotected and that drug companies would not voluntarily perform adequate followup, FDA contracted with the National Academy of Sciences for a study to be conducted by an NAS committee. The committee was formed in April 1972. Its chairman was Dr. Lawrence Marks, the Squibb vice president who had participated in the controversy over followup on Cinanserin.

As mentioned previously, after receiving no reply to a series of letters asking Squibb to undertake further followup, on June 26, 1972, FDA officials visited the Squibb plant in New Brunswick, N.J. According to a memorandum dated June 29, 1972, by an FDA inspector, Dr. Marks telephoned the inspector from Squibb headquarters in Princeton while the inspector was at the New Brunswick plant. According to the memorandum, Dr. Marks advised the inspector of his position as chairman of the NAS committee studying the very question of followup. The memorandum continues:

> In view of this, Dr. Marks did not feel that as a representative of Squibb, he should commit the firm to a followup procedure until such a procedure is standard throughout the industry. He further supports this belief in that he feels that the FDA is not completely sure as to what followup should be made as evidenced by the fact that they set up the NAS Committee. Dr. Marks said that he had advised Dr. Marion Finkel (an FDA official) of his position several weeks ago and questioned the need for our assignment.

Dr. Marks confirmed to the subcommittee his conversation with Dr. Finkel and stated that he does not remember the conversation with the inspector. It was confirmed, however, by the two other FDA employees. At the time of the conversation, June 26, 1972, Dr. Marks was still Chairman of the NAS Committee. He subsequently resigned in August 1972, for reasons unrelated to the Cinanserin followup problem.

It was poor policy for FDA to tolerate a situation where the chairman of a committee established and financed by FDA for the purpose of recommending followup procedures is at the same time personally attempting, on behalf of his firm, to dissuade FDA from requiring followup examinations in a particular case. It is clear that responsible officials at the FDA were quite aware of Dr. Marks' dual role. . . .

DES linked to cancer in women. The Food & Drug Administration was accused Oct. 26, 1971 of sidestepping for four and a half months a decision on banning the use of synthetic estrogens by pregnant women.

A drug in the synthetic estrogen family—diethylstilbesterol (DES)—had been linked to several cases in which young women whose mothers had taken the drug during pregnancy had been afflicted with vaginal cancer.

According to an article in the Washington Post, the number of known cases tying vaginal cancer in young women to their mothers use of DES was 60.

The Post article said that the FDA was asked by the New York State Department of Health in June to "initiate immediate measures to ban the use of synthetic estrogens during pregnancy." The appeal was made after cancer researchers linked 13 cases of vaginal cancer to the drug. Dr. Hollis S. Ingraham, commissioner of health in New York, in a letter to the FDA commissioner, Dr. Charles Edwards, said his department had begun a program of "continuous surveillance and monitoring" to try to detect the disease as early as possible. Ingraham urged Edwards to initiate a similar program on a national basis.

The FDA replied Aug. 10 by asking for the records of five of the cases. At the same time, the FDA said it was "actively evaluating" eight other cases linking DES to vaginal cancer reported by physicians at the Massachusetts General Hospital in Boston.

The FDA Nov. 9 proposed changes in labeling guidelines to advise physicians not to prescribe DES for pregnant women.

Dr. John Jennings, an FDA official, said "we have long felt that extreme caution should be exercised in the use of drugs of this sort in pregnancy."

Suit over DES experiment—Three women April 25, 1977 filed a $77 million class action lawsuit against the University of Chicago and Eli Lilly & Co. The plaintiffs charged that during pregnancy they and 1,078 other women had been given DES without their knowledge.

The women had been given the drug while receiving prenatal care at the school's Lying-In Hospital in Chicago in 1951 and 1952. The suit charged that none of the women had been advised that she was participating in a 20-month experiment to test the ability of DES to prevent miscarriages. In the experiment, an equal number of women had been given placebos.

The suit was filed in U.S. District Court in Chicago by attorneys for the Health Research Group, a unit of Ralph Nader's Public Citizen Inc. One of the three plaintiffs was Patsy Mink, a former Democratic congresswoman from Hawaii and currently an assistant secretary of state.

Ironically, the university had concluded as a result of its 1951–52 study that DES was ineffective in preventing miscarriages and discontinued hospital use of the drug.

The university April 26 said a National Institutes of Health-sponsored follow-up survey of 1,250 offspring of the DES mothers had found no evidence of vaginal or cervical cancer in their daughters nor any indication of genital deformity or sterility in their sons.

The university said it had begun contacting the women involved in the DES experiment in 1971 after the Food and Drug Administration banned its prescription for pregnant women.

Mink received a form letter of notification, dated Jan. 29, 1976, in Honolulu March 5, 1976. The letter urged her to have her daughter examined by a physician. It was later found that the 23-year-old woman was afflicted with adenosis, an often pre-cancerous condition also linked to DES offspring.

Lilly, the drug manufacturer, April 27 said its "only involvement" in the university study "was in furnishing the DES and placebos that were used."

Suit dismissed—Wayne County (Mich.) Circuit Court Judge Thomas Roumell May 16, 1977 rejected a $625 million damage suit filed by 144 women and 40 of their husbands. The suit charged that the women had contracted cancer because their mothers had taken DES during pregnancy.

Roumell dismissed the lawsuit because of each woman's inability to identify either a specific DES brand name or manufacturer responsible for her particular illness. The judge ruled in Detroit that the women could not jointly sue the 16 pharmaceutical firms named solely because they all had produced the carcinogenic hormone.

Since DES had not been patented by those who first had manufactured it, the product had been sold under its generic (chemical) name, not under brand names. As a result, lawyers for the women could not pin responsibility for a specific case of DES-related illness on a specific source of the drug. The lawsuit, filed in 1974, had contended that the drug manufacturers were jointly liable for any cancer or other medical problems the women had developed as a result of their mothers having taken DES.

Attorneys for the women had argued for industry-wide liability. They maintained that the drug firms had promoted and sold DES in a negligent manner, aware that it contained a cancer-causing agent called stilbene.

Michigan, with some 85,000 DES daughters, had been a test market for the drug, which had been prescribed to prevent miscarriages. All the female plaintiffs had undergone surgery for removal of cancerous or precancerous lesions.

New study downgrades DES risk. Dr. Arthur L. Herbst, who in 1971 had been the first scientist to warn of the possible association between women who took DES during pregnancy and the incidence of cancer in their daughters years later, reported that the role of DES in the development of vaginal or cervical cancer was less than previously believed. Herbst wrote in the May 1977 issue of the American Journal of Obstetrics & Gynecology "this disease [cancer] is extremely rare among the DES-exposed group and, in fact, is more rare than had been assumed previously."

Herbst, currently chairman of the University of Chicago Medical School's department of obstetrics and gynecology, estimated that the odds of DES offspring developing vaginal or cervical cancer ranged from about one in 10,000 to about one in 1,000. The risk estimate varied so widely because scientists had no valid statistics on how many pregnant women had taken DES between 1947 and 1964, the period when it was prescribed to prevent miscarriages.

Following Herbst's initial report of the hormone-cancer link, the Food and Drug Administration (FDA) had banned the use of DES by pregnant women. It remained available for treatment of prostate cancer, as an estrogen replacement in post-menopausal women and as a "morning after" contraceptive.

Herbst's findings were supported by a Boston pathologist March 6, 1979.

Dr. Stanley J. Robboy of Massachusetts General Hospital, reporting on a two-year study conducted at four medical centers, said that only four cancers of the genital tract were found among a total of 3,339 daughters of women who took DES. In one group of 1,275 daughters who were studied thoroughly, no cancers were found.

Dr. Robboy said, "The results are very encouraging." His study was financed by the Department of Health, Education and Welfare and published in the March issue of Obstetrics and Gynecology.

Reports link estrogen hormones, uterine cancer. Two studies published in the Dec. 4, 1975 issue of the weekly New England Journal of Medicine strongly suggested a causal relationship between the increase in cases of endometrial (uterine) cancer and the increased use of estrogen hormones over the last decade.

Estrogen hormones were taken by millions of American women to alleviate the symptoms and aftereffects of menopause. It was estimated that 25 million prescriptions were being written annually for the so-called replacement estrogens, which supposedly supplied the female sex hormone that the ovaries ceased producing at menopause. Since the 1960s, the hormone had been widely recommended to women as a means to stay feminine and ward off the effects of old age.

The two studies, conducted separately at the University of Washington in Seattle and at the Kaiser Permanente Medical Care Program, a large prepaid medical-care plan in Los Angeles, indicated that users of the hormone faced a five-fold to 14-fold increased risk of developing uterine cancer compared with women who had never taken the drug.

In the Seattle study, researchers found that of 317 women who had endometrial cancer, 152 had been treated with estrogen hormones. Of a like number of women without endometrial cancer (but with other forms of cancer) 54 had used estrogens.

In the Los Angeles study, 57% of those with endometrial cancer had used estrogens, while only 15% of the "control" patients had used them.

Further investigations that were reported in the Washington Post June 3, 1976 and that week in the New England Journal of Medicine appeared to confirm research linking the use of estrogen with uterine cancer.

One investigation, conducted by researchers at the University of Washington in Seattle, found that cancer of the uterus increased as much as 150% between 1969 and 1973 among women taking estrogen during and after menopause. Dr. Noel S. Weiss, who led the medical team, summarized his findings by declaring: "The important point is that it is unlikely the disease is due to some characteristic of the women rather than the medicine...."

Dr. Thomas M. Mack of the University of Southern California, who directed the other study, concluded that there was "a high level of statistical significance" that estrogen caused cancer of the uterus.

A new study reported Aug. 16 in The Washington Post challenged the long-standing contention that taking the hormone estrogen after menopause protected women against breast cancer. Moreover, the study, published Aug. 19 in The New England Journal of Medicine, warned that there was "a definite possibility" of a cause and effect link between the drug and breast cancer.

After studying 1,891 women for an

average of 12 years after they had started estrogen-replacement therapy, researchers found that 15 years after the onset of treatment, the probability of a woman developing breast cancer doubled. The number of women in the study who normally would be expected to develop breast cancer was 39.1—but 49 women, or 25% more than expected, actually developed breast cancer.

Additional evidence of a link between the use of estrogen and development of uterine cancer was provided by a study conducted at Johns Hopkins University and reported Jan. 4, 1979 in the New England Journal of Medicine.

It was the largest study ever conducted of women taking estrogen during menopause. The research with 1,339 women produced data that prompted the scientists to conclude that those who took estrogen pills were six times more likely to have cancer of the uterine lining than those not taking them.

For women who used the pills for more than five years the risk was found to be 15 times greater.

The findings contradicted a November 1978 study by Yale University doctors that also appeared in the New England Journal of Medicine. That report concluded that the suspected link between estrogen and cancer could be discounted because of erroneous research methods. The Yale doctors claimed that uterine cancer was more likely to be discovered in women taking estrogen because they were under a doctor's care.

Hot flashes were said to be the only symptom of menopause against which estrogen had proved to be effective.

Dr. Robert W. Kistner, professor of obstetrics and gynecology at Harvard Medical School, who had spoken out against critics of oral conception and synthetic estrogens, Jan. 10, 1976 had retracted his earlier statements.

Kistner acknowledged in an interview with the Washington Post that his statements regarding the safety of birth control pills and the use of estrogens in the treatment of menopause-related afflictions "cannot be substantiated." Kistner also said that he had given up research on hormonal agents seven or eight years ago and that he did not want to be known as an authority on the subject any more.

Birth-curb pill suspected—Syntex Laboratories had announced Jan. 19, 1970 that it was suspending tests of its "mini-pill" oral contraceptive pending further study of experiments that produced signs of breast cancer in dogs treated with the drug. The mini-pill was so dubbed because it contained only half a milligram of a progestin called chlormadinone acetate.

A spokesman for Syntex said that five dogs treated with the contraceptive developed nodules (lumps containing bacteria) in the breast tissue. One of the nodules, the spokesman said, was found to be cancerous.

The mini-pill was being taken experimentally by thousands of women in the U.S. and was marketed in France, Mexico and Great Britain. The Syntex spokesman said there had been no reports from any of the pills' users that unusual changes in breast tissue had occurred.

All birth-control pills then on the market had synthetic estrogen and progestogen, another synthetic hormone.

Several leading U.S. physicians estimated that nearly half of the 8.5 million American women using birth control pills took pills composed of more than 50 micrograms of estrogen, either in combination or in sequence with progestogen.

Senate hearings on 'the pill'—At Senate subcommittee hearings, which opened Jan. 14, 1970, prominent physicians disagreed on the potentially dangerous side effects of birth control pills. Sen. Gaylord Nelson (D, Wis.), chairman of the Monopoly Subcommittee of the Senate Select Committee on Small Business, said he had called the hearings to question whether the pills' manufacturers had deliberately under-emphasized the risks involved in using birth control pills.

Dr. Hugh J. Davis, a Johns Hopkins specialist in birth control devices, told the senators Jan. 14 that he feared that birth control pills may cause breast cancer that would remain undetected for years. Dr. Davis questioned whether it was wise to have "millions of Americans on the pill for 20 years and then [we] discover it was all a great mistake?"

Dr. Roy Hertz, of the Population Council and Rockefeller University, agreed with Davis. Hertz testified Jan. 15 that only two facts about birth control pills had been substantiated: the pill's high degree of effectiveness in preventing pregnancy and the pill's ability to cause blood clotting problems. Hertz said all doctors prescribing birth control pills should treat each patient as though she were part of a research program. He advocated such safety measures, he said, because too many important questions about the pill's long-range side effects remained unanswered. Hertz also cited examples of laboratory experiments in which animals treated with synthetic hormones similar to those found in the pills developed certain strains of cancer.

Dr. Robert W. Kistner disagreed. He said animals treated with birth-control hormones in laboratory experiments had produced a protective effect against cancer-producing agents. Among the patients at the Boston Hospital for Women, Kistner said, there had been no appreciable increase in the incidence of pre-cancerous conditions in the female cervix between 1964 and 1969 despite an increase in the number of women using birth control pills. (But five years later Kistner retracted this opinion.)

2 pill brands discontinued—Two large pharmaceutical houses Oct. 23, 1970 voluntarily discontinued the production of two brands of birth control pills whose chemical ingredients might have contributed to tissue changes in dogs. The action taken by Eli Lilly & Co. and the Upjohn Co. was made public by the Food and Drug Administration (FDA).

FDA Commissioner Dr. Charles C. Edwards Oct. 23 called the halt in production of the two brands of oral contraceptives "the only prudent course." At the same time Edwards said that there was no cause for alarm among women taking the pills.

The Eli Lilly product was marketed under the name C-Quens. Upjohn used the trade name Provest.

Edwards said that women using either of the two pills should continue to do so until their physicians told them otherwise.

The FDA had required continuing studies of the active chemicals in birth control pills and it was in one such study that dogs developed noncancerous nodules in their breasts when treated with large doses of two chemicals. One of those chemicals was an active ingredient in Provest. The other chemical was part of the makeup of C-Quens. The chemical in Provest was identified as medroxyprogesterone acetate, while the chemical in C-Quens was chlormadinone acetate.

DES 'morning-after' pill—A physician at the University of Michigan Health Service Oct. 25, 1971 made public findings that a "morning-after" birth control pill had safely prevented pregnancy in all 1,000 women of child-bearing age involved in a university study.

Dr. Lucile K. Kuchera described the study and her results in an article published in the Journal of the American Medical Association.

The pill in Kuchera's experiment used DES (diethylstilbestrol).

In Kuchera's study, no pregnancies occurred among the 1,000 women, most of them co-eds, although almost all had had sexual intercourse without using contraception at a time when they would be most fertile.

The women in the study were given the DES-pills twice a day for five days, beginning within 72 hours of intercourse. The study was begun in 1967.

The Food & Drug Administration said Sept. 20, 1973 that it would require doctors to warn patients of possible side effects of DES when it was prescribed as a "morning-after" pill. In giving its approval to the use of DES as a contraceptive, the FDA emphasized that it did not consider the drug safe for use over the long-term. The FDA had announced Feb. 21 that it would approve the use of DES as a "morning-after" pill in emergency situations such as rape and incest.

For over 30 years DES had been approved for use in certain gynecological disorders. But it had been associated with cancer of the vagina and cervix in children of some women who were treated with it during pregnancy.

The decision to allow limited use of

DES was criticized by Dr. Peter Greenwald, director of the Cancer Control Bureau in the New York State Health Department. Testifying Feb. 22 before a Senate labor and public welfare subcommittee, he said doctors would interpret the action on DES as a go-ahead and prescribe it whenever they wanted, despite the risks.

Depo-Provera used in Tenn.—A Tennessee health official admitted Feb. 21, 1973 that his office allowed the distribution of Depo-Provera as a contraceptive for clinic patients and the mentally retarded. The Food and Drug Administration (FDA) had not approved use of Depo-Provera in the U.S. as a contraceptive because it had produced breast cancer in dogs and because scientists believed use of the drug needed more study.

The FDA had approved the drug for use in the treatment of pre-cancerous inflammation of the uterus and terminal cancer of the uterine lining.

Dr. Robert Hutcheson Jr. of the Tennessee Health Department said studies on Depo-Provera in other countries persuaded state officials to use the drug in special cases where neither interuterine devices nor oral contraceptives would work. Hutcheson said Tennessee health officials had the same information as the FDA, "but they came to a different conclusion."

Hutcheson said all patients were told of possible harmful side effects. However, Anna Burgess, 21, of Cumberland County, Tenn., testified before a Senate health subcommittee hearing Feb. 21 that the State Welfare Department urged her to take Depo-Provera and at no time told her of possible bad effects or that the FDA had banned the drug as a contraceptive.

Upjohn Co., sole maker of Depo-Provera, stopped shipments of the drug to Tennessee when it found it was being used as a contraceptive, it was reported Feb. 21.

The FDA then approved limited use of Depo-Provera as a long-term contraceptive Oct. 10, but it ordered that patients be provided with detailed information of its risks.

British report on pill safety—G. D. Searle & Co. May 22, 1974 released a preliminary report on a large-scale British study of the effects of using oral contraceptive pills. Financed by Searle, the study by the Royal College of General Practitioners was begun in 1968 and involved 46,000 British women.

According to the report, users of the pill faced distinct, though rare, health risks. Thrombophlebitis, blood clots in the legs, was found to be 5–6 times more prevalent among users than nonusers. Users exhibited a rate of high blood pressure twice that of nonusers.

On the positive side, the report indicated that oral contraceptives could reduce menstrual disorders, iron-deficiency anemia, pre-menstrual tension and benign cysts of the breast.

The report said the study had found among users a higher occurrence of lung blood clots, coronary artery disease and cervical cancer, but it said that the incidence of these conditions was too "small to justify any conclusions."

Sequentials withdrawn—At the request of the Food and Drug Administration, three major drug companies had stopped the marketing and distribution of sequential oral contraceptives, it was reported Feb. 25, 1976.

The discontinued birth control pills were Oracon, made by Mead-Johnson Company; Ortho-Novum SQ by Ortho Pharmaceuticals, and Norquen by Syntex Laboratories.

The FDA said it asked the drug companies to withdraw the pills because of new studies strongly suggesting that sequential pills posed an increased risk of cancer of the uterus.

Pill warning for doctors—The Food & Drug Administration said April 8, 1977 that doctors and druggists had to be told that birth control pills could cause birth defects, tumors, blood clots and, in women over 40, heart attacks. The action, directed at manufacturers of the pill, put into effect a December 1976 FDA order.

The warning would be included in "physician labeling," information for doctors and pharmacists that was included with the pill and governed advertising claims drug companies could make.

Needless X-ray use charged. Dr. Karl Z. Morgan, professor of health physics at the Georgia Institute of Technology in Atlanta, told the American Cancer Society's seminar for science writers in St. Augustine, Fla. March 27, 1974 that Americans received harmful overdoses of radiation from diagnostic X-rays. Asserting that most U.S. doctors and dentists "didn't have the remotest concept of the risks associated with exposure to diagnostic X-rays," Morgan charged that 3,000 Americans died each year from cancer resulting from unnecessary exposure to diagnostic X-rays.

Morgan, director of health physics at the Atomic Energy Commission's Oak Ridge (Tenn.) National Laboratory 1943–72, urged that outmoded, high-dose X-ray equipment be replaced with new low-dose apparatus; that radiation technologists be appropriately educated, trained and certified; and that dentists reserve use of X-rays for special needs only.

It was estimated before a House subcommittee July 11, 1978 that mothers X-rayed needlessly during pregnancy would produce 70 children a year that could be expected to develop cancer. Ultra-sound had largely replaced X-rays, but X-rays were still used before six of every 100 deliveries.

Stricter rules issued—The FDA July 29, 1974 published a new set of standards designed to reduce public exposure to unnecessary radiation. Under the new rules, which were effective for medical and dental diagnostic equipment manufactured after July 31, X-ray beams were limited to the smallest size necessary to produce an acceptable picture. The rules also contained provisions to minimize film retakes by requiring improvement in equipment reliability.

Curb on breast X-rays—The National Cancer Institute Aug. 23, 1976 issued new guidelines on the use of X-ray techniques, known as mammography, to detect breast cancer. NCI recommended that routine mammography be discontinued for women aged 35–50 unless they showed specific symptoms of breast cancer or otherwise were classified as "high risk."

The guidelines, which would have no regulatory force, were distributed to the 27 detection centers participating in a nationwide screening project, which was jointly sponsored by NCI and the American Cancer Society. NCI acted after recent studies indicated that the risk from irradiation during mammography might outweigh the benefits of the procedure for women under 50. Doctors estimated that an average woman had a 7% chance of developing breast cancer and that each mammogram increased that chance by 1% for women aged 35–50.

Dr. John Bailar 3rd, editor of the Journal of the National Cancer Institute, concluded in a paper published in January that "the routine use of mammography" in screening symptomless women could "eventually take almost as many lives as it saves."

Defending the X-ray screening, NCI Director Dr. Frank J. Rauscher Jr. said Aug. 22 that one-third of all breast cancers were detected in the 35–50 age group. Of these, he said, one-third could not have been detected without the use of mammography. The figures were based on 259,000 women screened for breast cancer at the 27 detection centers.

The NCI May 10, 1977 announced more stringent guidelines on the use of mammograms in its nationwide breast-cancer detection project. The institute restricted mammograms for women under 50 to those with a history of breast cancer or with such a history in the immediate family.

A cancer institute panel May 3 cited figures showing that despite recommendations to discontinue the procedure, issued in August 1976, 75% of the women in the detection project between ages 35 and 49 were still undergoing mammographies. The new guidelines were endorsed by the American Cancer Society, which jointly sponsored the country's 27 breast cancer screening centers.

Psoriasis Therapy Complication Seen. Experimental treatment of psoriasis with a combination of the drug methoxypsoralen and exposure to long-wave ultraviolet light had produced a nonfatal form of skin cancer in about 2% of the patients treated, researchers reported in The New England Journal of Medicine of April 12, 1979.

An estimated 35,000 persons were thought to have undergone the treatment in 1978. It was said to have been unusually effective in controlling psoriasis, an incurable and often debilitating skin disorder involving a scaly rash.

The investigators of the study said, however, that the higher incidence of skin cancer could have been the result of a variety of factors other than the treatment. About half those developing skin cancers had previously been treated with X-rays, some had received other psoriasis treatment that might be linked to skin tumors and some had a history of skin cancers.

Patients who had not had X-ray treatments or previous skin cancers had a normal incidence of skin tumors following the drug-ultraviolet treatments, they reported.

Blood pressure drug & cancer. The National Cancer Institute said May 1, 1979 that reserpine, a drug used to lower high blood pressure, had caused cancers in laboratory animals. NCI studies indicated that reserpine might increase the risk of human breast cancer by 50% to 100%.

Pending a review of this finding, Food And Drug Administration and National Institutes of Health officials agreed that untreated high blood pressure posed a greater risk to life than the drug's potential cancer risk.

Ban Asked on Sleep Aids, Nose Sprays. Officials of the Environmental Defense Fund asked the Food and Drug Administration May 1, 1979 to ban sales of many nonprescription sleep aids, nose sprays and cold medicines because they contained a chemical that had caused liver cancers in mice.

Included were nationally advertised drugs used by over 10 million Americans, such as Sominex, Compoz, Nytol, COPE, Excedrin P.M., Allerest time release capsules, and Vicks Sinex.

EDF's Leslie Dach urged the FDA to seize "immediately" all products that contained methapyrilene, a chemical cited in three studies by the National Cancer Institute and Oak Ridge National Laboratory as "a potential animal carcinogen."

But FDA spokesman Wayne Pines said the agency had not completed its review of the evidence. "We're awaiting the National Cancer Institute's judgment before we decide what our next step is," he said.

Research on Virus & Cancer

Virus linked to breast cancer. The head of a team of scientists from the U.S. and India reported March 12, 1971 that they had uncovered new evidence indicating that breast cancer in humans may be caused by a virus.

Dr. Dan H. Moore of the Institute for Medical Research in Camden, N.J. said, however, that he did not think his team's findings conclusively linked viruses to human breast cancer.

The researchers made the findings after analyzing the milk of 56 women in Camden, Detroit and Bombay, India whose families had a history of breast cancer. After breaking down the milk, the scientists said they found particles that appear virtually identical to viruses known to cause breast cancers in mice. There was no indication that the mouse virus could cause human breast cancer.

The scientists also reported evidence suggesting that women with breast cancer made antibodies that would act against the viruses known to cause breast cancers in mice.

Human cancer virus isolated. A research team in Texas said July 2, 1971 that it had isolated a cancer virus from cells taken from a cancer patient. Specialists saw the development as a significant new lead in the search for human cancer viruses.

The research work, sponsored under a contract with the National Cancer Institute, was done at the M.D. Anderson Hospital and Tumor Institute in Houston. The medical team included Drs. Elizabeth S. Priori, Leon Dmochowski, Brooks Myers and J. R. Wilbur.

The characteristics of the virus and the circumstances of its discovery by the research team indicated that the virus could be linked to the cause of the disease, a lymph gland cancer. The cancer link however, had not yet been proved by the Texas team.

The team isolated a spherical virus called C-type, one that had been the proven cause of cancer in animals. The team's report linked a C-type virus with one of the forms of cancer most widely suspected of being caused by a virus. The disease was Burkitt's lymphoma, a lymph gland cancer.

The cells containing the virus were extracted from a child suffering from a form of lymphoma. Four months after extracting the cells, the research team discovered that the cells in the laboratory tissue culture were releasing large numbers of virus particles in various stages of development. At least one virus particle was found in every cell studied.

New evidence. Scientists at Columbia University in New York were reported Jan. 14, 1972 to have found chemical links between three types of human cancers and viruses known to cause comparable types of cancer in animals.

Dr. Sol Spiegelman, leader of the Columbia research group, emphasized that his team's findings did not prove the link between viruses and human cancer. He said, however, that the Columbia experiments came as close to that link as one could then get.

The work of Spiegelman's group was sponsored by the special virus cancer program of the National Institute of Health.

The experiments at Columbia involved breast cancer, sarcoma and leukemia, some of the cancer types thought most likely to be caused by viruses.

Details of the work were published in the Jan. 17–24 issue of Science, the weekly journal of the American Association for the Advancement of Science.

Among developments involving cancer-virus research in 1973:

University of Minnesota urologist Dr. Elwin Fraley announced April 3 that a research team he headed had isolated a urinary tract virus capable of causing cancer of the bladder, uterer, and renal pelvis.

Memorial Sloan-Kettering Cancer Center doctors in New York City said Aug. 14 that their research showed that cats infected with feline leukemia virus ran a 900-times greater risk of getting leukemia than cats who showed no sign of the virus. While contagious among cats, the virus did not affect humans, the doctors said.

Herpes viruses linked to cancers. Scientists in Washington and Italy announced they had new data linking cancer in humans with viruses, the Wall Street Journal reported Feb. 12, 1973.

Drs. Ariel C. Hollinshead of George Washington University Medical Center in Washington and Giulio Tarro of the University of Naples in Italy concluded that cells of cancerous tissue of the lips and cervix carried herpes viral genes that were not present in normal cells and that "the findings could support an etiological role of herpes viruses" in cancer.

Herpes simplex type 1 virus, the cause of cold sores on the mouth and lips, had been suspected of having a role in cancer of the lip. Herpes type 2, the cause of sores in the genital areas, had been suspect with regard to cervical cancer since the mid-1960s.

At the American Cancer Society's annual science writers' seminar, which was held in Nogales, Ariz., Dr. Ysolina M. Centifanto of Emory University (Atlanta, Ga.) said April 4 she had data connecting herpes viruses with cervical cancer. She said the viruses were transmitted by men to women during sexual intercourse. The men were suspected of harboring the viruses in their genital tracts. Centifanto said women who had had genital herpes infections showed an incidence of incipient cervical cancer eight times greater than women who had never had herpes infections.

Dr. Albert B. Sabin, developer of the Sabin live polio vaccine, told the National Academy of Sciences in Washington April 24 that common herpes viruses were factors in nine kinds of cancer. Sabin said he had not learned what mechanism turned these common viruses into cancer-causing agents.

Duke University Medical Center researchers reported in the May 6, 1978 issue of Lancet that they had found a link between a virus (specifically, cytomegalovirus, a kind of herpes virus) and colon cancer. The scientists detected genetic material from the virus in cancerous colon tissue of four out of seven patients. The virus genetic material was not found in healthy colon tissue from the same patients, or in colon tissue taken from persons without colon cancer.

U.S.-Soviet exchange. U.S. and Soviet medical officials Nov. 18, 1972 exchanged viruses and laboratory mice as part of mutual efforts to find a cure for cancer. The ceremony took place in Moscow between Dr. Nikolai N. Blokhin, an official of the Soviet Academy of Medical Sciences, and Dr. John B. Moloney of the National Cancer Institute.

The U.S.S.R. June 30 had concluded an agreement on cancer drugs with U.S. scientists who had arrived in Moscow earlier in the month to exchange medical information.

The accord was reached after six days of talks and provided for an exchange of experimental drugs, known as antineoplastic agents, which would then be tested in each other's laboratories to determine their effectiveness in retarding the growth of malignant tumors.

The Washington Post reported Jan. 10, 1973 that under a medical agreement, Soviet scientists had provided their U.S. counterparts with six viruses believed to cause cancer in humans.

John B. Maloney of the National Cancer Institute said he had "no idea" the Soviet Union possessed the viruses, which he was "very pleased" to receive. The U.S. had previously sent for testing in Moscow some 32 cancer viruses, including one believed to cause the disease in humans.

Human cancer virus isolated? Scientists at the National Cancer Institute announced Jan. 8, 1975 that they had isolated a virus in a human that could be the first human cancer virus isolated in an uncontaminated state. The virus appeared to be distinct from, but related to, those known to cause myelogenous leukemia—a type of cancer involving the blood—in such close relatives of man as the gibbon ape and the woolly monkey. The newly found virus was obtained from a 61-year-old woman suffering from acute myelogenous leukemia.

The virus could be useful in identifying the cause and treatment of cancer, according to scientists. Scientists stressed that the research in no way suggested that human cancers could be transmitted from person to person.

Radiation & Cancer

Energy, the Atom & Cancer

The connection between radiation and cancer began to emerge at about the end of the 19th Century. As early as 1894, German scientists suggested that excessive sunlight (and its ultraviolet radiation) could produce skin cancer. In 1928 a British scientist exposed experimental animals to intense sunlight and produced skin cancer. The ability of radioactivity to cause cancer became known about this time as a result of work with X-rays and radium. In France, an experimenter induced skin cancer in a rat by means of radium as early as 1910. The development of nuclear weapons beginning in the 1940s provided additional evidence that radioactivity could cause cancer.

The cancer-radioactivity connection did much to dampen early optimism about atomic fuels providing abundant energy for an increasingly energy-hungry world. Controversy grew between those who insisted that the atom could be tamed without excessive danger to humanity and those who held that radiation's cancer-producing capacity (and other atomic dangers) made nuclear development unjustifiable.

Cancer & energy. As the energy crisis became pronounced, growing concern was expressed during 1970 about pollution and increases in cancer:

■Rep. Chet Holifield (D, Calif.), chairman of the Joint Committee on Atomic Energy, Jan. 12 released 1,108 pages of testimony taken during hearings that began Oct. 28, 1969 on the environmental effects of producing electrical power. Commenting on testimony pointing to increasing dangers of water and air pollution from conventional means of producing electrical power, Holifield contended that nuclear reactors could make "a meaningful contribution towards the reduction of pollution now attributed to the electric power industry."

■Robert B. Miller, an attorney for the American Civil Liberties Union, charged in a federal district court in Denver Jan. 12 that safety standards of the AEC (the U.S. Atomic Energy Commission) "grossly underestimate" potential damage from radiation. Miller made the charge at the reopening of a suit to prevent natural gas from being freed from an explosion conducted Sept. 10, 1969 – Project Rulison—in Colorado.

■Former Interior Secretary Stewart L. Udall, during a Jan. 14 panel discussion at the New School for Social Research in New York City, linked pollution problems with population and family planning issues. Citing the increasing need for power plants to serve an expanding population, Udall said "in the interest of national survival we cannot permit this haphazard growth that has been destroying our environment."

■Controversy over the effect of radiation on the environment marked a three-day symposium on engineering with nuclear explosives Jan. 14–17. Dr. Theos J. Thompson, a member of the AEC, said at the opening of the sessions, sponsored by the American Nuclear Society in cooperation with the AEC, that concern by environmentalists about radiation hazards was reaching almost ridiculous levels. He added that such persons did not evaluate the benefits of programs to develop peaceful uses of atomic energy, but had concentrated on very low level effects "whose extreme extrapolation might be detrimental."

Dr. Edward L. Teller, a leading developer of the hydrogen bomb, said Jan. 15 that radiation from peaceful uses of atomic energy "can be easily guarded against." Teller said of the AEC's programs that "no big-scale enterprise has ever been carried out with more assurance [of public safety] than the atomic energy enterprise."

■In response to criticism, the AEC denied Feb. 19 that plutonium released at its Rocky Flats, Colo. atomic bomb plant constituted a health hazard. The statement was in answer to a report sent to AEC Chairman Glenn T. Seaborg Jan. 13 by the Colorado Committee for Environmental Information. The report had said that soil samples taken near the site, 16 miles from Denver, indicated an amount of plutonium that could be stirred up by a strong wind and carried off to be inhaled by people in the area.

In response to the AEC's contention that the quantities of plutonium were "miniscule," Dr. E. A. Martell, a member of the information committee, said that "each plutonium particle in the lung produces millions of times more radiation to the tissue around it than a dust particle carrying natural radioactivity."

The Rocky Flats facility, operated by the Dow Chemical Co., had suffered $45 million in damage May 11, 1969 from a fire caused by spontaneous ignition of plutonium. The information committee had disputed the AEC's contention that no radioactivity was vented during the fire.

New radiation rules proposed—Atomic Energy Commissioner James T. Ramey said March 27 that the AEC was proposing regulations to require industry to take advantage of improvements in technology to minimize the amount of radiation released by new nuclear plants. (Current regulations required only that emissions of radiation be within AEC safety limits.)

Ramey said the proposed rules would not reduce the current maximum permissable limits of radioactivity emitted from nuclear power plants. He denied there was any connection between the proposed changes and a recent case in Minnesota in which the state sought limits on radioactive discharges that would be more rigorous than the AEC's. (In the controversial Minnesota case, the Northern States Power Company, located about 30 miles north of Minneapolis, was granted a permit by the Minnesota pollution control agency for a "stack release" from its water reactor that would limit the firm to about 2% of the radioactivity permitted by AEC standards. The power company had brought suit to challenge Minnesota's authority to set standards more rigid than the AEC's. Four states had petitioned the Federal Government for permission to file amicus curiae briefs supporting Minnesota's position; seven had asked to be added to Minnesota's brief.)

Uranium workers' exposure—A six-month delay in lowering radiation exposure limits for uranium miners was protested Dec. 24 by Wilbur J. Cohen, former secretary of health, education and welfare, union officials, a student environmentalist organization and others. The group sent President Nixon a telegram calling the delay "a serious threat to the health of American workers."

Under an order issued during the Johnson Administration, permissible radiation exposure levels for workers were to be cut by two-thirds beginning Jan. 1, 1971. During the interim between issuing the order and its effective date, a study was to be conducted by the Federal Radiation Council on the impact of the order on the uranium mining industry. After the council was dissolved, the staff work for the study was absorbed by the new Environmental Protection Agency, but the day before the dissolution a request was made by HEW Secretary Elliot L. Richardson for a six-month extension for completion of the study. This was granted by the President.

An AEC-financed study had concluded three months previously that the improved protection for workers would result in an increase of only a few cents a pound in the cost of producing the basic uranium extract.

Cohen, dean of the College of Education of the University of Michigan, was joined in his protest by Esther Peterson, former assistant secretary of labor; Leo Goodman, atomic energy adviser to the United Automobile Workers; Anthony Mazzocchi, Washington representative of the AFL-CIO Oil, Chemical and Atomic Workers International Union; Denis Hayes, national coordinator of Environmental Action, the student group; John Gofman of the AEC's Lawrence Radiation Laboratory; and Dr. Irving Selikof, professor of environmental medicine at the Mount Sinai School of Medicine in New York.

Radiation levels reported safe. A study released Jan. 25, 1971 by the National Council on Radiation Protection (NCRP) in Washington said current precautions against radiation exposure in the U.S. were safe and no tighter standards were required. The council was a nonprofit corporation chartered by Congress. It received information on radiation projects of government agencies, including the Atomic Energy Commission and the Public Health Services.

The council report, based on a 10-year study, said its "review of the current knowledge of biological effects of radiation exposure provides no basis for any drastic reductions in the recommended exposure levels despite the current urgings of a few critics."

The NCRP took issue with recent assertions by Drs. John F. Gofman and Arthur R. Tamplin of the AEC's Radiation Laboratory in California. According to their own estimates of radiation dangers, the two scientists concluded that 32,000 excess cancer deaths would probably occur annually under the average permissible radiation exposure (170 millirems) of the American population. Gofman urged that the radiation exposure limits be reduced to one-tenth their present levels.

The NCRP contended that exposure to the total permissible maximum would result in no more than 3,000 additional cancer deaths a year. It said that although average exposures were far lower than the recommended limit, no exposure could be regarded as safe.

The council recommended for the first time that a maximum permissible radiation dose of 0.5 rem (measurement of radiation dosage) be set specifically for pregnant women to protect the fetus.

Commission plan—The AEC proposed June 7, 1971 that nuclear power plants limit their radiation exposure to 1%, or less, of the amount of radiation permitted under current U.S. guidelines for power reactors. AEC spokesmen said only the Humboldt Bay reactor near Eureka, Calif., and the Dresden reactor no. 1 and possibly the Dresden reactor no. 2, both near Chicago, failed to meet the new guidelines.

U.S. plans breeder reactor. Atomic Energy Commission (AEC) Chairman James R. Schlesinger announced Jan. 14, 1972 that the Tennessee Valley Authority (TVA) and the Commonwealth Edison Co. of Chicago would construct a breeder nuclear power plant in Tennessee, the first of a type that was expected to become the mainstay of future power needs.

Schlesinger said breeder reactors, which would create more fuel than they consume, would reduce thermal pollution of the environment, a problem with current nuclear reactors, because of a more efficient heat exchange system.

"We are reaching the point that supplies of fossil fuel—coal, gas and oil—are recognized to be limited," he said. "Furthermore, the availability of low-grade uranium is not too substantial, with estimates being that at its present rate of use in non-breeding reactors it will be exhausted in several decades."

Possible drawbacks to the breeder reactors were the extreme combustibility of liquid sodium used in the process, and the dangerously long radioactive life of plutonium, the by-product fuel.

U.S. District Court Judge George L. Hart Jr. in Washington March 24 dismissed a suit of the Scientists' Institute for Public Information to force the AEC to issue a general environmental reactor program.

The institute attorney, J. Gus Speth, had said that the type of reactor planned by the government would entail greater risk of explosion, thermal pollution and plutonium emission, and produce more radioactive wastes, than other types, and argued that all the problems should be discussed in public before the program's momentum and budget commitments made it inevitable.

Speth said annual federal expenditures of $100 million and the AEC plan to give the breeder reactor top priority together constituted a major federal act and a legislative proposal, thereby invoking the impact statement requirement.

Judge Hart ruled that the breeder program would have no tangible impact for some time, and that "there is no certainty any kind of system will ever be economically feasible."

Hart's decision, however, was overturned some 15 months later. A three-judge federal appeals panel in Washington ruled June 12, 1973 that the AEC must prepare a formal environmental impact statement for the entire program of breeder reactors.

Writing for the appeals panel, Judge J. Skelly Wright said the program presented "unique and unprecedented environmental hazards." The institute had argued that since such reactors "breed" plutonium—an extremely toxic radiological metal—and that construction of over 1,000 such plants had been projected, the potential harm of such systems should be studied before construction started.

Although the AEC had issued an impact statement for a demonstration reactor near Oak Ridge, Tenn., Judge Wright said the commission had taken an "unnecessarily crabbed approach to NEPA in assuming that the impact statement was designed only for particular facilities rather than for analysis of broad agency programs."

Wright noted that the proposed plants were expected to generate some 600,000 cubic feet of high-level radioactive wastes by the year 2000 and said the problems "attendant upon processing, transporting and storing these wastes, and the other environmental issues raised by the widespread deployment [of such plants] warrant the most searching scrutiny under NEPA."

Reactor safety disputed. Concern within the AEC that standard nuclear power plant safety equipment might be inadequate surfaced during hearings begun by the agency Feb. 2, 1972 in response to criticism by environmental and scientist groups.

Philip L. Rittenhouse of the AEC's Oak Ridge (Tenn.) National Laboratory testified March 10 that he and 28 other nuclear safety experts, many of them AEC employes, questioned the efficacy of the emergency core cooling system. The system was designed to flood nuclear reactors with cool water if mechanical failure caused reactor temperatures to rise dangerously. A cooling failure could theoretically cause an atomic explosion. The AEC had ordered modifications in eight existing plants in 1971 as part of an "interim core cooling policy," after laboratory models of the cooling system had failed to function properly, despite computer predictions of success.

A coalition of 60 environmental groups, the National Intervenors, had asked the AEC Feb. 1 to suspend all nuclear power plant licensing pending full scale tests of the cooling system, scheduled for 1975.

A-plant debate. At a news conference held in Washington Jan. 3, 1973, Ralph Nader and spokesmen for the Union of Concerned Scientists asked the Atomic Energy Commission (AEC) for a moratorium on all construction of new atomic power plants "until all safety-related issues are resolved." Nader promised to continue his compaign to delay massive use of atomic power, on economic and safety grounds in Congress, the courts and among electric company stockholders.

Nader and the scientists' group said the danger of "catastrophic nuclear power plant accidents is a public safety problem of the utmost urgency," and called for output reductions of up to 50% at the 29 operating nuclear reactor power plants. Although "no nuclear explosion could occur," they said, a failure in the emergency core cooling system could cause release of radioactive materials with deaths possible nearly 100 miles from the plant. Nader also said that disposal of radioactive wastes presented safety problems.

Nader charged the AEC with secrecy on the issue and with failure to publicize what he said was a belief held by a majority of AEC scientists that safety problems may exist.

In reply, William R. Gould, chairman of the Atomic Industrial Forum, said in New York that "throughout the civilized world" there was a "massive" shift to nuclear energy as a power source "because of its advantages in terms of fuel supply, economics, environmental affects and public health and safety." He said he was confident that "the extraordinary safety record of nearly 100 operating power reactors worldwide" and "the extremely conservative engineering approach" of U.S. plants would be confirmed at February hearings of the Congressional Joint Atomic Energy Committee.

Outgoing AEC Chairman James R. Schlesinger charged at a Jan. 23 hearing of the joint committee that delays in license approvals for nuclear power plants had at times been prolonged by lawyers looking for "a lucrative substitute for ambulance chasing."

Schlesinger said the AEC was the only federal agency required by law to conduct adjudicatory hearings before licensing plants, and said the hearings had delayed plants for years, although they often covered issues resolved long before in earlier cases.

Nader and Friends of the Earth, an environmentalist group, petitioned a federal district court in Washington May 31 to close 20 nuclear plants. They charged the AEC with a "gross breach" of duty by failing to assure that power plant cooling systems would not fail and cause the release of radioactive materials.

David Brower, president of Friends of the Earth, said "overwhelming scientific evidence" had shown that "the lives of millions of people" were threatened by operation of the plants because of "crude and untested" safety systems. The suit quoted several AEC officials as expressing doubt as to the reliability of back-up cooling systems.

In a statement on the suit, the AEC said it saw no basis for suspending operation of the units, which were at 16 power plants in 12 states. The AEC conceded there were differences in opinion within the commission on the safety systems but noted that a review was already under way to determine whether present core-cooling regulations were adequate.

U.S. District Court Judge John H. Pratt June 28 dismissed the Nader-Friends of the Earth suit on the grounds that the plaintiffs had not exhausted AEC procedures for challenging plant safety and that the AEC was making a proper investigation.

The AEC Aug. 30 rejected a new petition from Nader and Friends of the Earth to close the 20 power plants.

In denying the petition, the AEC stood by its earlier position that existing interim regulations covering core-cooling systems provided "reasonable assurance" of protection of public health and safety.

Cutbacks ordered in power plants—The AEC Aug. 24 ordered 10 nuclear power

Radiation & Cancer

The cancer-producing effects of the ultraviolet rays of sunlight appear to be limited to the skin. It has been observed that the incidence of skin cancer is highest in the southern and western parts of the United States and lowest in the north, and is related to the amount of sunshine in the area. Furthermore, skin cancer occurs more frequently among people who work outdoors, such as sailors and farmers, than among people who can guard themselves against excessive exposure to the sun.

The color of the skin is another factor. Cancer of the skin is most common among fair-complexioned people, and much less frequent among black people and others with dark skin.

Related to the cancer-causing effects of sunlight was the discovery of the cancer-producing effects of ionizing radiation from **radium** and X-rays. This discovery was actually made on human beings. Pioneer radiologists developed dryness, ulcers, and, eventually, cancer of their hands. In 1910, a French worker produced skin cancer in a rat following application of radium to the skin.

Ionizing radiation can cause several forms of cancer in man and in animals. Radiologists and others exposed to increased doses of radiation are more likely to develop leukemia than are people who are not so exposed. The people of Hiroshima and Nagasaki who survived exposure to atomic bombs have been carefully studied by scientists. Information obtained in the course of their investigations leaves no doubt that a single radiation exposure at high doses can produce leukemia in man.

Radium salts, which are deposited in bone, give rise to cancers of the bone. A historical tragedy was the death from bone cancer of factory women who pointed with their lips the brushes they used in painting watch dials with radium.

Man-made sources of ionizing radiation undoubtedly represent one of the more serious potential cancer-producing hazards.

—From "The Cancer Story" (National Cancer Institute)

plants in seven states to cut back power levels 5%–25% pending studies of possible safety hazards.

The AEC said the precaution was taken because of the discovery of shrinkage in uranium oxide pellets in reactor fuel rods. With the shrinkage, the heat of the atomic process was not efficiently transferred to cooling water, narrowing the safety margin in case of cooling system failure. The shrinkage could also cause collapse of fuel rods.

The cutbacks would be in effect until the commission could evaluate new data from General Electric Co., manufacturer of the reactors.

Plant rules tightened—The AEC voted unanimously Dec. 28 to impose stricter safety standards on heating of nuclear fuel and operation of emergency cooling systems in nuclear power plants.

The new rules set the maximum temperature for operation of uranium fuel piles at 2,200 degrees Farenheit, a reduction of 100 degrees from the old standards.

Another rule required that fuel bundles be redesigned to insure that no more than 17% of the reactor-core shielding would oxidize if it came in contact with cooling water.

The commission gave the industry six months to comply with standards.

The Union of Concerned Scientists, an intervenor in the AEC proceeding, said Dec. 28 that the ruling was "cosmetic" and represented a "continuation of the AEC's cover-up of critical safety problems."

EPA radiation authority curbed. Charging that the Environmental Protection Agency (EPA) had "construed too broadly" its responsibilities to set environmental standards on radioactive materials, the White House ordered the EPA to drop its plans to set radiation rules for individual nuclear power plants, the New York Times reported Dec. 12, 1973.

According to the directive, the authority to set such standards would rest solely with the AEC, considered by critics of the nuclear power industry to have a more lenient approach to radiation protection than the EPA.

The order was in a memorandum, dated Dec. 7, sent "on behalf of the President" by Roy L. Ash, director of the Office of Management and Budget, to EPA Administrator Russell E. Train and AEC Chairman Dixy Lee Ray. The memo said its purpose was to prevent "confusion" in the area of nuclear power regulation, "particularly since nuclear power is expected to supply a growing share of the nation's energy requirements."

Ash said the AEC should proceed with its own plans to issue rules and the EPA should discontinue similar preparations to issue standards "now or in the future." The EPA would retain responsibility "for setting standards for the total amount of radiation in the general environment from all facilities combined in the uranium fuel cycle"—flexible standards which "would have to reflect the AEC's findings as to the practicability of emission controls."

The Times quoted Charles L. Elkins of the EPA's office of hazardous materials control as saying that AEC standards were "not adequate."

EPA sets tighter radiation standards—The Environmental Protection Agency May 23, 1975 proposed new standards to protect the public from radiation released by the nuclear power industry. The current federal radiation limits for maximum annual dosage to individuals were 500 millirems to the whole body or any internal organ except the thyroid and 1,500 millirems to the thyroid. The proposed new limits would be 25 millirems to the whole body and 75 millirems to the thyroid.

The tighter standards reflected an assessment of the impact of environmental radioactivity for this and future generations.

Regulations making the new standards legally enforcable were issued by the EPA Jan. 6, 1977.

The new standard also called for reduction of allowable emissions of krypton-85 to one-tenth of current levels by 1983.

EPA Administrator Russell E. Train described the new standards as "an important precedent in radiation protection because they consider the long-term potential buildup of radiation in the environment."

The EPA said most nuclear power plants already conformed to the new standards but that milling and other fuel-supply and reprocessing operations needed to be upgraded to meet the new restrictions.

Columbia reactor decision upheld. A three-judge panel of the U.S. Court of Appeals July 5, 1973 refused to review the AEC's decision to grant Columbia University a license to operate a small nuclear reactor on its New York City campus. Community groups opposing the research reactor had asked the court to review a May 1972 opinion by the AEC's Atomic Safety and Licensing Appeals Board that the reactor would not be "inimical to the health and safety of the public." (The Supreme Court decided June 11, 1974 to let the decision stand.)

Nuclear Hazards to Health

A-power plant 'events.' The Atomic Energy Commission (AEC) reported May 28, 1974 that 861 "abnormal events" had taken place at the nation's 42 nuclear power plants during the year 1973. None of the incidents resulted directly in health hazards, the agency said, but 371 were potentially hazardous. Twelve of the incidents involved release of radioactivity at rates above permissible limits beyond plant site boundaries, although the total amount released was said to be within safety limits.

The report said the incidents included loss of power supply, failures of electronic monitoring equipment and cooling system leaks. Each of the 42 plants recorded at least one "event."

Plutonium leak. The AEC said May 14, 1974 that it had detected leakage of a highly-toxic plutonium isotope from its plant in Miamisburg, Ohio, a suburb of Dayton. The plant produced nuclear power supplies for satellites and other spacecraft.

Based on "preliminary samples," the AEC said, the leakage presented no health problems because it had been found deep in mud in the Erie Canal near the plant, not in air or vegetation. Plutonium-238 was said to be one of the most deadly substances known if inhaled directly into the lungs, but relatively harmless otherwise.

Reactor hazards found slight. According to a study released by the Atomic Energy Commission Aug. 20, 1974, the risks from nuclear power plant accidents were smaller than from other man-made or natural disasters. The study concluded that, given the 100 conventional water-cooled plants expected to be in operation by 1980 (51 were currently operating), the chance of an accident involving 10 or more fatalities was one in 2,500 a year; an accident involving 1,000 or more deaths carried a risk of one in one million a year.

AEC officials emphasized that the study dealt only with the safety of the commercial reactors themselves, and not with risks involved in mining, manufacturing or transporting nuclear materials. The study also failed to include the liquid-metal-fast breeder reactors currently under development.

The report stated that of the approximately 15 million persons expected to be living in the vicinity of the first 100 reactors, one might be killed and two injured in every 25 years. The study noted that power plant reactors could not explode like nuclear weapons because of the fuel used.

AEC Chairman Dixy Lee Ray said Aug. 20 that there was "no such thing as zero risk," but in terms of the study the nuclear industry "comes off very well." She said the risks cited in the study were acceptable and urged that plant construction be continued. Ray said the study had been commissioned by the AEC, but the agency did not "influence" its findings.

Reactions by critics of the nuclear industry were less favorable. Daniel Ford of the Union of Concerned Scientists contended that the study was, "for all practical purposes," an "in-house" effort by the AEC, which had consistently advocated increased nuclear production. Consumer advocate Ralph Nader labeled the report "fiction," expressing doubt that such statistical projections were valid or possible.

The study was criticized in a document released Nov. 23 by the Union of Concerned Scientists (UCS) and the Sierra Club, a conservationist group, as speculative and unreliable.

Speaking for the two groups, Dr. Henry Kendall, a physicist, said in Washington that the AEC's safety claims "are a conceit based far more on their enthusiasm for the nuclear power program than on solid and convincing scientific proof." The UCS and Sierra statement said the AEC study, prepared by Dr. Norman C. Rasmussen, contained a number of flaws. The safety analysis used by Rasmussen to estimate the probability of an accident, they said, had been developed and then abandoned by the aerospace industry and the federal government because it had been found to drastically underestimate existing hazards.

The AEC report was also criticized for the low number of projected casualties based in part on the successful evacuation of persons living near an atomic plant. A major accident at a nuclear plant could kill or seriously injure 126,800 people, 16 times the casualties estimated by the AEC report, the scientists said. They emphasized that there were no "adequate plans or means to evacuate to a distance of 20 miles" in the event of a plant mishap. It could not be assumed, as the Rasmussen report contended, that an evacuation could be achieved while only 5% of the population was in automobiles and 90% were indoors.

The report said the AEC study also failed to consider the fact that plutonium, the more lethal fuel which industry hoped soon to use in its reactors, posed a far greater danger than that considered in the commission's own reactor safety study.

AEC member Saul Levine defended the Rasmussen report Nov. 24, saying that the scientists' criticism of the study's form of analysis would have been correct for the 1960s, but "we have advanced that methodology considerably ... our members are in touch with reality." The AEC, he said, "is confident that the techniques used in the Rasmussen report are the best available."

The Environmental Protection Agency Dec. 4 lauded the methods used in the AEC study but said the projected casualties could be "about ten times higher than those estimated" by the AEC.

The EPA statement was contained in an AEC-requested analysis of the commission's 14-volume study completed in the summer. It said the commission's study was "an innovative forward step in risk assessment of nuclear power reactors."

A second report issued by the EPA expressed concern about the possible effects the plutonium-fueled reactors proposed by the AEC would have on the environment. Before this new fuel was used on a full scale, the problem posed by plutonium disposal should be resolved and a new accident survey should be completed, the EPA said.

Few penalties for violations. Reporting on a study of AEC records, the New York Times said Aug. 25, 1974 that the commission had imposed penalties on only a small fraction of nuclear installations at which violations had been found, despite the fact that many of the violations could have created significant radiation hazards.

According to records for the year ended June 30, the AEC found 3,333 violations in 1,288 of the 3,047 installations inspected. The commission imposed punishment in eight cases: license revocations involving two companies and civil penalties totaling $37,000 against six others.

Under the AEC's three-level classification of the seriousness of violations, 98 were in the top category (violations which had caused or were likely to cause radiation exposures in excess of permissible limits). In category two—defined as violations that, if not corrected, might lead to exposures above permissible limits—there were 2,132 violations. Category three—infractions involving documentation and procedural matters—included 1,103 violations.

The report also noted that a composite ratio of violations and penalties over the past five years was similar to that of the most recent fiscal year: 10,320 inspections; 3,704 installations with one or more violations; and 22 cases involving imposition of penalties.

Cracks found in nuclear-plant reactors. Electric utilities operating 21 water-cooled nuclear reactors were under Atomic Energy Commission (AEC) orders to close down the facilities for a special inspection of cooling systems, it was reported Sept. 22, 1974. The inspection was ordered after cracks were found in pipes of three reactors within 10 days.

According to the AEC, leakage of radioactive water had occurred in only one case, and there was no release of radioactivity into the environment. The AEC also said the reactor's overall cooling system was not impaired.

The Nuclear Regulatory Commission (NRC), a successor to the AEC, ordered 23 reactors shut down Jan. 29, 1975. It acted after finding cracks in the emergency cooling system of an atomic reactor operated by the Commonwealth Edison Co., near Morris, Ill. The leak did not result in the release of any radioactivity to the environment, the NRC said.

The affected 23 reactors produced 14,283 megawatts of electricity, less than half of the 35,000 megawatts generated by the 52 reactors licensed to operate in the U.S.

The Baltimore Gas & Electric Co.'s nuclear power plant in Calvert Cliffs, Md. had announced Jan. 25 it would close Feb. 1 because of unacceptable radiation leaks from the door to the reactor container. The NRC had reported Jan. 24 that the emissions were from three to 10 times above federal standards.

The NRC announced March 7 that 21 of the reactors had passed inspection but that an additional crack had been found at the Morris plant and that one inspection, also at Morris, had been deferred.

At a Congressional hearing Feb. 5, agency officials admitted the cause of the cracks was unknown but considered the shutdown of the plants for the inspection "appropriately prudent."

Another witness, Daniel Ford, executive director of the Union of Concerned Scientists, a public interest environmental group, disagreed. He questioned the fitness of the regulatory licensing procedures, in view of the emergency shutdowns, as well as the safety and reliability of reactors themselves.

Documents made public by the Nuclear Regulatory Commission at Ford's request disclosed concern within the agency about the safety issue. The New York Times published March 9 a report on a policy study by the NRC's Edwin G. Triner concluding that utilities owning most of the nuclear reactors were not sufficiently concerned about safety and performance. A N.Y. Times report published April 6, also based on the newly released material, revealed that several NRC scientists and technicians viewed the test for the cracks in the reactors as unreliable.

AEC denies safety data suppressed. U.S. Atomic Energy Commission Chairman Dixy Lee Ray denied Nov. 15, 1974 that the AEC had suppressed data on the safety of nuclear plants. She conceded that "while there may be some validity for such accusations in the past, the situation has changed today."

Ray's statement was in apparent response to a New York Times report Nov. 10 citing AEC documents showing that since 1964 the commission had sought to conceal studies by its own scientists that found nuclear reactors were more dangerous than officially admitted or raised doubts about safety reactor devices.

Ray cited a number of examples to demonstrate the AEC's openness with the public: the release earlier in 1974 of 25,000 pages of documents developed during the deliberations of the Advisory Committee on Reactor Safety. The chairman also pointed out that in 1973 the AEC had made public "an uncompleted 1965 study" that sought to update a 1957 report on the consequences of a possible major accident at a large nuclear power plant. Such a mishap could kill up to 45,000 persons, and "the possible size of such a disaster might be equal to that of the state of Pennsylvania," the report said.

The cases cited by Ray were questioned by Daniel Ford, an official of the Union of Concerned Scientists, that had been critical of many AEC policies. Ford said the Advisory Committee released the documents only after being faced with a suit under the Freedom of Information Act, and that many of its pages had been heavily edited. As for the 1973 report, AEC memorandums had shown that the 1965 study had been deliberately withheld from publication by the commission for seven years after its completion and that this study also was finally released under the threat of a Freedom of Information Act suit, Ford said.

The New York Times report said some of the AEC's suppressed documents had been leaked to the Union of Concerned Scientists by commission officials.

Hazards at Oklahoma plant. A report released Jan. 7, 1975 by the AEC upheld charges by the Oil, Chemical and Atomic Workers Union of health hazards and other dangers at the plutonium processing plant of the Kerr-McGee Corp. in Crescent, Okla.

The report, based on the findings of AEC investigators, substantiated 20 of the 39 union claims of danger to the health of the firm's workers and said some X-ray negatives of fuel rods being manufactured for a plutonium-powered reactor had been falsified and that some data concerning the rods had not been used properly.

Among the health hazards cited were the sending of a worker into a dangerous area without informing him that a respirator was required to protect him from possible radiation, failure to make certain that the respirators were working and "errors" that resulted in contamination. Since Kerr-McGee started its plutonium operations in 1970, 17 safety lapses in which 73 employes had been contaminated were reported, according to AEC records.

Action Vs. Radiation Dangers

A-plant near populated area barred. The U.S. Seventh Circuit Court of Appeals in Chicago April 1, 1975 barred construction of a 660-megawatt nuclear plant near Portage, Ind. on the southern shore of Lake Michigan. The court ordered the site to be filled in by Northern Indiana Public Service Co., which had been granted a license for the plant by the Atomic Energy Commission.

The court said the AEC had violated its own rules in licensing a plant within two miles of a densely populated area, defined as 25,000 or more people. The population of Portage was projected to exceed that by the time the plant was scheduled for operation, and the court noted that a state park abutting the site had up to 87,000 visitors a weekend.

The court was critical of the AEC for "clustering" nuclear plants on the Lake Michigan shore within relatively short distances of Chicago; eight were within 75 miles of downtown Chicago; six more planned, in addition to the Portage site.

The court acted on a suit to halt construction by a unit of the Izaak Walton League and a business civic group.

Breeder safety study proposed. The Environmental Protection Agency (EPA) April 27, 1975 recommended further study be made of the safety and radioactive-waste disposal problems of a plutonium-breeding reactor. While it was not "necessarily advocating a delay" in development of such a reactor, it said, "sufficient evidence exists to warrant re-examination" of the timing of the breeder program. The suggestion in the report was for a delay of from four to 12 years.

The EPA was critical of some AEC projections—of the probable growth rate of electric power demand, which the EPA found overstated; of the chance of a major accident being one in 10 million, which the EPA called premature; and of the time and effort needed for adequate resolution of environmental and safety problems, which the EPA deemed "highly optimistic."

'Short-term' vs. 'long-term' concern. A study commissioned by the American Physical Society reported April 28, 1975 finding no reason for "substantial short-term concern" about the safety of U.S. nuclear reactors. But it recommended "a continuing effort to improve reactor safety as well as to understand and mitigate the consequences of possible accidents."

The study, by 12 independent physicists, found the safety record so far "excellent," with "no major release of radioactivity." But the group did express concern about the long-term, when an increasing number of reactors would be operating and the likelihood of an accident, although "improbable," became correspondingly greater.

The physicists agreed with the old AEC estimate that the chance of a major accident in an atomic power plant was one in 10 million. But they disagreed with the AEC's estimate that an accident could cause about 310 deaths from cancer. There would be "substantial long-term consequences" from an accident in which radiation was released over a populated area, the panel thought. The AEC estimate was said to be off by as much as a factor of 50 because the cloud of radiation could move 500 miles and endanger people in a 10,000-20,000 square-mile area.

Scientists question A-plant program. A petition calling for a "drastic reduction" in the program for construction of nuclear power plants because of safety hazards was sent to the White House and Congress Aug. 6, 1975 by 2,300 scientists.

The petition urged a major research effort on reactor safety, plutonium safeguards and nuclear waste disposal. The "record to date," it said, "evidences many malfunctions of major equipment, operator errors and design defects as well as a continuing weakness in the quality control practices with which nuclear plants are constructed."

On the radioactive waste disposal problem, it said no "technically or economically feasible methods have yet been proven." Nuclear wastes, it added, could prove "a grim legacy . . . to future generations."

The petition was sponsored by the Union of Concerned Scientists, which circulated it to scientists through mailing lists. The endorsement response was said to have been about 20%.

Fund bill curbs plutonium transport. President Ford Aug. 9, 1975 signed a bill authorizing $222.9 million in funds for the Nuclear Regulatory Commission for fiscal 1976 (July 1, 1975–June 30, 1976). The measure also authorized funding of $52.8 million for the July 1, 1976–Sept. 30, 1976 transition quarter prior to the beginning of fiscal 1977 on Oct. 1, 1976.

The authorization bill, approved by both houses of Congress by voice vote July 31, contained a provision banning the air transport of plutonium until a rupture-proof container could be developed to make the material secure even in the event of an airplane crash.

Atomic engineers resign over safety. Three high-level nuclear engineers for General Electric Co.'s San Jose, Calif. division resigned Feb. 3, 1976 to join a drive against nuclear power, a California initiative scheduled for a statewide ballot in June. It would prohibit construction of new nuclear generating plants and require the phasing out of existing plants unable to meet strict conditions.

The three resigning engineers cited the safety problems as the overriding reason for their move. Aligned with this was their concern that safety problems were not fully reported by nuclear companies to the federal government, which had the regulatory responsibility.

Those resigning, who had from 16 years to 22 years of experience with GE, were Dale G. Bridenbaugh, 44, manager of performance evaluation and improvement at GE's nuclear energy division in San Jose; Richard B. Hubbard, 38, manager of quality assurance; and Gregory C. Minor, 38, manager of advanced control and instrumentation.

A statement from GE Feb. 3 pointed out that the company employed several thousand nuclear engineers and it "emphatically" disagreed with the viewpoint of the three resigning. "The overwhelming majority of the scientific and engineering community, including GE scientists and engineers," it said, "believes the benefits of nuclear power far outweigh the risk."

The engineers said in a paper prepared for the Joint Congressional Committee on Atomic Energy:

> The NRC/AEC in recent years has begun to accumulate radiation exposure data for in-plant operating and maintenance personnel. These data, which correlate radiation history with plant operating time, were documented in WASH 1311 "A Compilation of Occupational Exposure From Light Water Cooled Nuclear Power Plants 1969–1973". This four-year study indicates a substantial increase in personnel radiation exposure required to operate and maintain nuclear plants, indicating a substantial build up of radiation levels in the plants. The major use of these statistics to date has been in commercial presentations by the reactor vendors in order "to prove" that theirs is a superior system for minimum personnel radiation exposure.
>
> The data are limited, but a distinct trend has emerged. In 1969, the average nuclear plant required a total of 188-man rem per year exposure to perform all necessary operation and maintenance functions. By 1973, the average had increased to 544-man rem per year (404 cumulative average). Almost all of the increase in exposure occurred during the maintenance activities experienced at the plants. It seems certain that as plants get old, requiring more maintenance, exposures will increase to a much higher level. Experience in some foreign plants has been even more disturbing. The Tarapur plant in India reportedly has required the mass utilization of more than 1,000 support personnel to operate and maintain that plant.
>
> If a concerted effort is made to back-fit operating plants with necessary safety improvements, personnel exposure will increase to an even higher level. This presents the utility and the country with a real personnel health dilemma. It is absolutely essential that plant safety levels be improved to ensure that the "incredible" accident does not occur, yet performing the modifications will require the exposure of technicians and mechanics to a relatively higher level of radiation, particularly those with special skills such as nondestructive testing and welding. The plant management staff is faced with the moral dilemma of making decisions affecting employees' health and welfare as counterbalanced by improved safety to the public. The labor unions have a similar dilemma in deciding whether or not to work under those conditions.
>
> Individual exposures of many skilled personnel will average close to the maximum of five rem per year. Yet, no design standards have been enforced to make the plant designs compatible with minimum personnel exposure.
>
> Material selection is made with little thought given to its effect (for example, stellite valve seats are commonly used—a high source of Cobalt 60).
>
> Scientists have recently indicated uncertainty in levels of biologically allowable radiation. The Environmental Protection Agency (EPA) has recently been petitioned by the NRDC to reduce the current occupational maximum of five rem per year to a maximum of 0.5 rem per year. The uncertainty involved in exposure limits and management provides a large uncertainty in the continued viability of the nuclear power program. Certainly there is a question as to whether or not such exposures should be allowed. With more and more plants going on line, and radiation levels increasing, this situation will become even more critical in the near future. A serious effort must be launched to minimize, to the extent possible, the impact of in-plant radiation exposure.

In New York state, the federal safety engineer for three nuclear reactors at Indian Point on the Hudson River, 30 miles north of New York City, announced his resignation, citing the safety factor, at a news conference Feb. 9. The engineer, Robert D. Pollard, project manager for the federal Nuclear Regulatory Commission (NRC), planned to become Washington representative of the Union of Concerned Scientists, a research group on energy and nuclear power.

Pollard, 36, chief safety engineer for nuclear reactors in North and South Carolina and Texas as well as at Indian Point, said he could not "in conscience remain silent about the perils associated with the United States nuclear-power program." The Indian Point plants, he said, "have been badly designed and constructed and are susceptible to accidents." He recommended closing down Indian Point Plant No. 2 "at once—it's almost an accident waiting to happen."

Consolidated Edison Co., which owned and operated Indian Point Plant No. 2 and one other plant at Indian Point, rejected Pollard's criticism. Spokesmen for the federal Nuclear Regulatory Commission and the State Power Authority, which recently bought the third Indian Point nuclear reactor from Con Ed, also denied that the plants were unsafe.

NRC chairman William A. Anders and Con Ed chairman Charles F. Luce defended the safety of the plants Feb. 10. Anders described Pollard's safety concerns as nothing more than "generic problems."

Report OKs offshore A-plant. A staff report of the Nuclear Regulatory Commission April 9, 1976 found no significant environmental risk in plans for a "floating" atomic power plant—the world's first such installation—off the New Jersey Coast.

A preliminary environmental-impact statement drafted by the staff said that the risk of radioactivity leak through the air or water was "very low."

The Public Service Electric and Gas Co. projected a $2 billion plant 2.8 miles out in the Atlantic north of Atlantic City. Two reactors, in separate buildings, would be moored in 60 feet of water and would be protected by a breakwater. Electricity transmission lines would be carried inside pipes along both the ocean floor and underground through the wetlands to a switching station about seven miles inland.

Court scores licensings. The U.S. Court of Appeals for the District of Columbia ruled July 1, 1976 that the Nuclear Regulatory Commission had been remiss in its licensing of two nuclear plants because of failure to give adequate consideration to the energy-conservation issue or to nuclear-waste disposal.

In writing the unanimous opinions of two three-member appellate panels, U.S. Circuit Chief Judge David L. Bazelon noted the "apprehensive" public concern about nuclear power.

The two cases involved a nuclear power plant in Vernon, Vt., where the waste-disposal procedure was questioned by an environmental group, and another in Midland, Mich., where environmentalists objected that the alternative of conserving energy, instead of constructing a nuclear plant, had not been considered.

Bazelon held that energy conservation "will have an important . . . role in overall energy policy in coming decades" and that the commission could not dismiss it "without inquiry or explanation" in its licensing process.

Licensing moratorium—In compliance with the court ruling, the NRC Aug. 13 announced a moratorium on the licensing of new nuclear power plants until completion of a study of the environmental hazards of fuel reprocessing and disposal of radioactive wastes. A moratorium also was called against any full-power operation of new A-plants.

Ending the moratorium, the NRC announced Nov. 5 that it would resume new-plant licensing on a conditional basis.

The commission had issued a staff environmental study Oct. 13 and had proposed at the same time an interim rule to incorporate the environmental impact into its licensing procedures. Licenses issued before adoption of the final rule would be on a conditional basis.

Breeder reactor, plutonium use scored. A panel of 21 scientists and economists March 21, 1977 urged major changes in the nuclear energy policy of the U.S., including an end to the crash program to develop a commercial fast-breeder reactor and an indefinite postponement of plans to reprocess plutonium for use as a reactor fuel.

The panel, organized by the Mitre Corp. with a grant from the Ford Foundation, endorsed the continued use of current generation uranium-fueled nuclear power plants, but urged more emphasis on solving safety and radioactive-waste problems. The panelists said adequate electricity for the short term could be generated by a combination of nuclear and coal-fired plants.

The panelists, agreeing with critics of the breeder reactor and plutonium reprocessing, objected primarily to the danger of the worldwide spread of nuclear weapons as a result of the availability of plutonium. They said federal research on the breeder should be continued, but in such a way that commercial use of the breeder would be delayed.

The report was based on two key assumptions: that conventional nuclear reactors, which currently generated about 10% of the electricity in the U.S., would be about as expensive and dangerous to operate as coal-fired plants; and that the current official estimates of uranium reserves and resources substantially underestimated the amount of uranium that would be available during the next two or three decades.

The Ford Foundation said the panelists, who had worked on the study for almost two years, had been chosen because of their middle-of-the-road views on nuclear energy. Among them were John Sawhill, former head of the Federal Energy Administration, and two members of the Carter Administration: Defense Secretary Harold Brown, who was president of the California Institute of Technology when the work on the report was done, and Joseph S. Nye Jr., deputy to the undersecretary of security assistance in the State Department.

Cancer Dangers Stressed

Warning on cancer deaths. Rep. Clifford Allen (D, Tenn.) warned in a statement in the Congressional Record Nov. 29, 1977 that a single year's operation of a nuclear plant could cause hundreds of cancer deaths in future generations. He said:

What price will the people of America have to pay for the electricity generated by nuclear reactors—not just in money that will run into the hundreds of billions of dollars invested, the interest thereon, and for skyrocketing prices for nuclear fuel that is now controlled by international cartels—but in deaths due to cancer and genetic effects resulting from radon and the many other poisonous emissions from the uranium required to fuel the increasing number of nuclear generators constructed, and continuing to be built, throughout the United States?

On Tuesday last, there came to my attention, as your Congressman, certain unnerving and startling evidence of gross errors made by members of the Atomic Safety and Licensing Board in the amount of dangerous and poisonous emissions from nuclear reactors—errors of such enormous magnitude as to stagger the imagination.

This was revealed in a report, and projection of deaths, made by one of the top and most respected nuclear scientists in the Nation, in just the past 2 months.

I refer to Dr. Walter H. Jordan, for many years the Assistant Director of the Oak Ridge National Laboratory, and who is generally regarded by his professional colleagues as one of the foremost authorities in this field.

In an official report, dated September 21, 1977, which is now on file with the Nuclear Regulatory Commission, Dr. Jordan made the flat and unequivocal statement that the amount of radioactive materials emitted into the atmosphere and environment, "released as gas, liquid, or solid as a consequence of operating a reference powerplant for 1 year," to wit: Rn-222, has been grossly underestimated and in error in all of the supposedly scientific calculations relied on, and assumed to be correct by the Atomic Safety and Licensing Board of the Nuclear Regulatory Commission.

The emission of Rn-222, for example, which had previously been figured and stated 74.5 curies, Dr. Jordan said, "would be 100,000 times greater!" The exclamation mark was added by Dr. Jordan, in finding such an enormous error and unbelievable understatement of such emissions by the Nuclear Regulatory Commission, in passing on the safety of uranium-fueled reactors.

Dr. Jordan concludes with this unnerving statement:

> Since the radon continues to seep from the tailings pile for a very long time, the total dose to people over all future generations could become very large. Deaths in future generations due to cancer and genetic effects resulting from the radon from the uranium required to fuel a single reactor for one year can run into hundreds. (See Pohl, Search, Vol. 7 No. 8, Aug. 1976.) It is very difficult to argue that deaths to future generations are unimportant. But it can be shown that the number is insignificant compared to those due to the radon contribution in natural background.

Low-Level Radiation Effects Probed. The health impact of low levels of radiation became a subject of controversy and of congressional hearings in the first months of 1978. Levels of radiation that previously had been thought to pose no dangers were linked to increased cancer rates, according to some studies.

Public attention focused chiefly on reports of cancer in two groups: persons who had been exposed to radiation while witnessing U.S. atomic bomb tests and workers at nuclear facilities. There was a study showing a small, but statistically significant, increase in the rate for certain cancers at the Hanford facility in Richland, Wash., and another study showing much more pronounced increases in cancers among workers exposed to radiation at the Portsmouth Naval Shipyard in Maine.

Hanford, Portsmouth Studies—Alice Stewart, an epidemiologist at the University of Birmingham, England, said Feb. 17 that her study of workers at the Hanford Atomic Reservation revealed that they died of cancer at a rate 5% greater than the general population.

Stewart presented her results to a meeting at the annual convention of the American Association of the Advancement of Science. She had conducted her study with George Kneale (also of the University of Birmingham) and Thomas Mancuso, of the University of Pittsburgh.

The three researchers had published a paper in late 1977 that reported essentially the same conclusion. The paper had come under criticism, and Stewart's talk Feb. 17 was devoted basically to showing that further study had confirmed the original findings.

The study, Stewart said, indicated that the amount of radiation needed to double the incidence of cancer within a population—the so-called "doubling dose"—was quite low. For bone-marrow cancers, the doubling dose was 3.6 rads (an acronym for radiation-absorbed dose). For lung cancer, the doubling dose was 13 rads and for cancers of the pancreas, stomach and large intestine it was 19 rads.

For all cancers in general, the doubling dose determined by Stewart and her colleagues was 33 rads for men and 9 rads for women. Stewart said the figure for women was based on a small sample, but there had been a number of studies indicating women were much more vulnerable to radiation than men.

Stewart said the study indicated that the level of what was considered an acceptable lifetime exposure to radiation should be lowered dramatically—to one-tenth or one-twentieth of its current value.

Stewart's conclusions did not go unquestioned. Seymour Jablon, director of the Medical Follow-up Agency of the National Research Council, suggested Feb. 17 that, while there was "no question" that "something peculiar is going on among Hanford workers," radiation might not be to blame. One of the cancers Stewart had focused on, Jablon said, might be induced by certain chemicals. Jablon also cited the lack of increase in the leukemia rate, which was a cancer often associated with radiation.

Another study of the Hanford workers, presented at an earlier AAAS session and reported in the Feb. 25 Science News, took issue with the Stewart findings. The study, by Ethel Gilbert, an epidemiologist for Battelle Pacific Northwest-Laboratories, said that "neither death from all causes nor death from all cancer types shows a positive correlation with external radiation exposures."

Gilbert found a slight increase over the expected incidence of certain cancers—the same cancers that Stewart had focused upon—but said that, while they "warrant attention, one must consider the possibility that they may be due to other occupational exposures or pre-Hanford radiation exposures."

The differences between the Gilbert and Stewart studies primarily reflected different statistical approaches.

Radiation at the Portsmouth Shipyard became an issue Feb. 19 when the Boston Globe reported that a study had found deaths there from cancer occurred at twice the national rate. The study, conducted by Thomas Najarian, a blood specialist at the Veterans Administration hospital in Boston, found deaths from cancer of the lymph gland were 125% higher than the national rate and deaths from leukemia were 450% higher than the national rate.

The willingness of the Energy Department and the Navy to let the cancer/radiation link be fully investigated also became an issue. Najarian Feb. 28 told the House health and environment subcommittee that those two agencies had tried to block the Portsmouth study.

Two senators—Thomas J. McIntyre (D, N.H.) and John Durkin (D, N.H.)—also testified before the subcommittee Feb. 28, giving some support to Najarian's claim. McIntyre said an aide to Adm. Hyman Rickover had said there was "no problem" at Portsmouth and the Navy "did not want a follow-up study." (Rickover was director of the Division of Naval Reactors.)

Durkin said that Energy Department officials had taken actions that "suggested a desire to suppress" the cancer research.

Rickover told the panel the same day that the Navy was unwilling to accept Najarian's findings without further study. He said the Navy had been cooperating with the Energy Department since December 1977 on plans to study shipyard workers exposed to radiation.

Rep. Melvin Price (D, Ill.) asked the Navy to investigate, and he had the Navy's reply printed in the Congressional Record Feb. 27. It said:

On 19 February 1978 the Boston Globe published an article stating that nuclear workers at Portsmouth Naval Shipyard were running an increased risk of cancer due to exposure to low levels of radiation. The Globe published some statistics of death due to cancer based on a two month review of a number of shipyard workers.

The Navy is concerned about the health of shipyard employees working with radiation as evidenced by the strict radiological control program in effect. The Navy believes that the Boston Globe, on the basis of a brief review of some shipyard employees, has reached conclusions which do not accurately reflect the actual health conditions for employees engaged in radiation work. To properly assess a matter as complex as low-level radiation induced health effects will require a far more detailed and expert analysis than that performed by the Globe. On the basis of Navy experience to date and a considerable body of expert scientific evidence, the Navy considers the risk to shipyard workers performing radioactive work is less than risks normally encountered in industrial activities.

Since the start of the Naval nuclear propulsion program, the Navy established a radiation health program of high standards to maintain personnel radiation exposure as low as reasonably achievable. This program includes keeping detailed medical records including radiation exposure histories on each worker. Prior to starting nuclear work at any shipyard, a separate organization of specially trained shipyard personnel was established to implement the radiation health program. This program of strict radiological controls has continued to the present. As a part of this program comprehensive medical examinations are given to all employees who receive radiation exposure and the results of these medical examinations are reviewed by doctors with knowledge of radiation medical effects. With any indication of a radiological problem, whether identified by medical doctors, trained radiological control personnel, or concerned employees, a thorough investigation is conducted.

The radiological safety standards and procedures used by the Navy for radiation workers have not been developed independently by the Navy, but are based on the recommendations and requirements of the U.S. Environmental Protection Agency (which has incorporated the functions of the U.S. Federal Radiation Council), the U.S. National Council on Radiation Protection and Measurements which was chartered by Congress to recommend radiation safety standards for use in the United States, the U.S. Nuclear Regulatory Commission, and the International Commission on Radiological Protection. They are also based on standards which have been reviewed and accepted by the U.S. Department of Labor.

Thus, they compare with standards used throughout the United States and the rest of the world for work of this nature. The estimates of effects of radiation on humans on which radiation limits are based have also been reviewed by the U.S. National Academy of Sciences in 1972, the United Nations Scientific Committee on the Effects of Atomic Radiation in 1977 and the International Commission on Radiological Protection in 1977. These reviews have shown no need to reduce the radiation exposure limits that have been in use.

Although the Navy's program is based on Federal occupational radiation exposure limits of 3 rem per quarter year and no more than a total of 5 rem per year, the Navy's own radiological control procedures maintain shipyard personnel radiation exposure below these limits. As exposure reduction controls and techniques improved, total personnel exposure was reduced even further. As the number of nuclear ships nearly doubled, the amount of radioactive work to keep these ships in operation increased. In spite of this, the trend in total radiation exposure throughout the Naval nuclear propulsion program has been down for the past decade.

The radiological controls used in shipyards are extremenly strict. Personnel are held individually accountable for compliance. Each employee is informed of his radiation exposure and is required to keep his own exposure to a minimum.

Shipyard radiological practices are controlled by a group of specially trained shipyard personnel, and a separate independent shipyard organization also checks all aspects of radiological control. Further, the Naval Sea System Command conducts periodic in-depth inspections which fully evaluate the effectiveness of the shipyard's radiological program.

The Navy has applied the Federal radiation exposure limits so rigorously that no one in the Naval nuclear propulsion program has exceeded these limits in this decade. For this reason and because radiation exposures in the Naval nuclear propulsion program have not been greater than for many others in the nuclear industry, the Navy has not conducted its own epidemiological study. Rather it took cognizance of the work of others, such as the Department of Energy, who were conducting studies of long term effects of low level radiation. The Navy did, however, survey the health of Navy personnel who operate nuclear-powered submarines who were exposed to low levels of radiation. These surveys indicated no problems such as described in the Globe article.

The Globe article stated that the workers may have received higher radiation exposures than measured by dosimetry badges because of breathing radioactive dust or getting radioactivity on their skin and in wounds. The Navy was aware of such possibilities before radioactive work started in nuclear ships. Thus, the shipyards have always monitored radioactivity in the air and on workers' skin. Workers with open wounds are removed from radioactivity work. Airborne radioactivity has been controlled for workers to the same levels permitted for members of the general public; radioactivity on skin is controlled to levels too low to detect. In addition, the Navy has had a rigorous program for measuring personnel for internally deposited radioactivity. This program has shown that no civilian or Naval personnel in the Naval nuclear propulsion program has ever exceeded one tenth of the exposure limits from internally deposited radioactivity.

In November 1977, a study was published of the effects of low level radiation among radiation workers at the Department of Energy's nuclear facility at Hanford, Washington. This study, which was funded by the Department of Energy, indicated a possible increased risk of cancer. While the results of this study have been discounted by many reviewers, the report presented an indication of a potentially higher cancer risk due to low level radiation exposure than had previously been expected. Accordingly, the Navy began working with the Department of Energy to determine the feasibility of conducting a study on Naval shipyard workers. Initial discussions and meetings in early December 1977 led to a formal request for this study on December 30, 1977. After preliminary work was done in January, Department of Energy consultants reviewed the Navy's radiation health program including specific review of a representative shipyard on February 14.

These consultants concluded a mortality study of shipyard workers is feasible, and on 16 February 1978, the Department of Energy agreed to perform such a study on Naval shipyard workers using the Portsmouth Naval Shipyard as a model. Portsmouth Naval Shipyard was selected because it was the first Naval shipyard to overhaul nuclear submarines.

To ensure proper conclusions can be obtained, scientific groups which conduct such a study must include specialists in epidemiology as well as in statistics. The study requires detailed review of medical records on almost all workers. This is necessary since there are many factors which can influence death rates such as smoking, race, age, medical history, and environmental hazards. Thus, such a study requires extensive investigation and a number of years to complete. For example, the mortality study of workers exposed to low-level radiation at Hanford, Washington has been based on about 12 years of review of tens of thousands of medical records.

Every organization which has recommended personnel radiation exposure limits has stated that there is some risk at all levels of exposure to radiation, including that received from cosmic radiation, from building materials, from radioactivity naturally present inside the body, and from medical X-rays. The Federal limits currently used were set so that these risks would be small compared with other risks normally accepted in daily life.

There are recognized risks involved in the things people do every day—both occupationally and in leisure time. The American Cancer Society for example, reports that the risk of death in any one year for smokers to die of smoking-related disease is 1 in 160. The National Safety Council reports that the risk of death in any one year from an automobile accident is 1 in 4000. Navy shipyard statistics reveal an annual risk of slightly less than 1 in 10,000 for death resulting from an industrial accident, which is a rate normally used to describe a relatively safe industry. The risk estimates available to the Navy are contained in reports by the U.S. National Academy of Sciences, the United Nations Scientific Committee on the Effects of Atomic Radiation and the International Commission on Radiological Protection. The consensus of these risk estimates for exposure to low levels of radiation is that the risk of a shipyard worker dying of a disease caused by radiation exposure from his work at the shipyard is less than any of the risks mentioned above.

The Navy does not have the data used by

the Globe in preparation of their article. Even without this information the Navy considers the Globe study has limitations in not having had radiation exposure information available and in the small size of the group sampled. Obtaining correct conclusions in a matter of this complexity requires accurate data, and complete returns from a large percentage of the affected group.

The weight of evidence from numerous other studies and the simplistic approach of the Globe's study lead the Navy to conclude it is not credible that radiation from Naval nuclear propulsion plant work at Portsmouth Naval Shipyard or any other shipyard has doubled the total cancer rate for workers and Naval personnel. In any event the Navy intends to do everything possible to protect its workers and Naval personnel from any harmful effects of their work environment. To this end, and as previously stated, the Navy has requested the Department of Energy to initiate a study of the effects of radiation on shipyard workers. The Navy will also continue to enforce its strict radiological controls in shipyards and in ships.

Federal probe—On Jan. 31, 1979 federal health investigators and civilian experts began studying allegations that workers at the Portsmouth Naval Shipyard suffered leukemia at up to six times the national rate. The probe was ordered by Congress because of Dr. Thomas Najarian's studies and his claim that the cancer rate among 1,700 former workers who died from 1959 to 1977 was double the national average and the leukemia rate was four to six times the national average.

The study eventually could encompass as many as 500,000 workers who had been exposed to low-level nuclear radiation at nine civilian and Navy shipyards since the mid-1950s.

Najarian was reported to have modified his views. Sen. Gordon J. Humphrey (R, N.H.) wrote in the Portsmouth Herald June 29:

Last week, Dr. Najarian came before the Health Subcommittee on which I serve, and told the committee that his earlier results were in error. A more careful reanalysis of his data by Dr. Colton of Dartmouth showed no significant statistical difference in overall cancer rates. Thus, Dr. Najarian's earlier study has been substantially repudiated.

The shipyard has an excellent safety record, and its radiation protection procedures are first-rate. The average lifetime exposure to workers exposed to shipyard radiation is less than these same personnel have from exposure to natural background radiation or to medical sources such as X-rays.

I submit that this risk is small compared to the risks in other industrial activities and is small compared to the risks normally accepted in daily life outside work.

Let me add two items of personal interest. My office building here in Washington is constructed of granite blocks which contain a small amount of uranium. The measured radiation from these blocks combined with the natural background radiation and the radiation I have received from X-rays is about the same as the exposure that shipyard workers receive.

In addition, the radiation I received from cosmic rays as an airline pilot exceeds the levels which most shipyard workers receive.

Hanford cancer issue spurs study demand. Two labor unions asked the Department of Health, Education & Welfare Jan. 30, 1979 to take over job radiation health studies that had been conducted by the Energy Department.

The International Association of Machinists and Aerospace Workers and the United Steelworkers of American wrote to HEW Secretary Joseph A. Califano Jr. urging that HEW take over the studies. The unions cited "alarming" behavior by Energy Department officials.

The United Steelworkers asked HEW to finance the studies of Dr. Thomas Mancuso of the University of Pittsburgh, who had been removed from a radiation project by the Energy Department.

Mancuso, a leading radiation epidemiologist, was granted funds in 1964 to study the effects of radiation exposure on workers at the government's nuclear facilities at Hanford, Wash., and Oak Ridge, Tenn.

According to Energy Department documents turned over to Mancuso under the Freedom of Information Act, the scientist had lost his job in 1974 because he refused to contradict a study showing elevated cancer levels in the Hanford workers. Mancuso had also discovered long-range radiation problems in the Hanford workforce.

After he was dropped from the study, Mancuso released findings in 1976 showing a 6% increase in certain cancers among Hanford workers. Energy Department officials at the time criticized his findings as the "result of an inappropriate use of statistical methodology" but later acknowledged that they raised serious concern about the adequacy of the government's radiation exposure standards.

$10.5 million award for exposure. A federal jury in Oklahoma City May 18, 1979 awarded $10.5 million damages to the estate of Karen Silkwood, a laboratory technician contaminated by radiation in 1974 while an employee at the Kerr-McGee Corp. Cimarron plutonium plant. The exposure was said to have threatened her with a high probability of contracting lung cancer.

Kerr-McGee was ordered to pay the award for its negligence in allowing Silkwood to become contaminated.

The jury's decision was seen as a rejection of federal radiation safety standards and industry safety claims. The verdict was the first in the U.S. dealing with radiation contamination contracted outside of a nuclear facility.

In November 1974, the 28-year-old Silkwood had reported for work at the Cimarron plant for three successive days contaminated with radiation. She had been active in labor organizing efforts at the plant and was investigating allegedly unsafe conditions there.

The source of the radiation was found to be plutonium at Silkwood's apartment. Both sides agreed the substance had come from the plant. Kerr-McGee argued that Silkwood had tried to prove that the Cimarron facility was dangerous by deliberately exposing herself to plutonium.

Silkwood family lawyers contended that Silkwood was horrified by the contamination and they suggested someone had tried to intimidate her through plutonium exposure.

Silkwood was killed in an automobile crash outside Oklahoma City on Nov. 13, 1974. She was on her way to meet a New York Times reporter and a union official in an attempt to document her allegations of inadequate safety regulations and practices at Cimarron. Kerr-McGee, the nation's largest miner and processor of uranium, manufactured nuclear reactor fuel rods at the plant.

The Oil, Chemical and Atomic Workers Union contended that her car was bumped from behind and forced off the road, and that the evidence she carried was stolen. Oklahoma state police claimed that Silkwood was heavily tranquilized at the time of the accident, and had fallen asleep at the wheel. The Federal Bureau of Investigation had conducted its own probe and concluded that there was no foul play.

Silkwood's death was not a direct issue in the trial. Judge Frank Theis ruled in September 1978 that a part of the original suit that alleged conspiracy by Kerr-McGee to violate her rights had been improperly drawn as a class action. His ruling had been appealed.

The major issue in the 1979 trial, which began March 6, was the safety of the operation of the Cimarron plutonium plant. Plutonium was considered so dangerous a substance under Oklahoma law that companies were charged with "strict liability" to control it.

Former Cimarron plant officials testified that safety was a priority and that workers were well trained and warned of the radiation hazards of plutonium. But the Silkwood family lawyers produced former workers who claimed that plutonium leaks were common, that risks of cancer were never mentioned and that plutonium was easily removed from the facility.

(The Cimarron facility ceased production and went on standby status in late 1975, after its contract expired.)

Kerr-McGee attorneys argued that not only was Silkwood responsible for her own contamination, but also presented witnesses who claimed that she was not harmed by her exposure.

Dr. John Gofman, a nuclear physicist testifying for the plaintiffs, had denounced government radiation standards as meaningless and claimed that after her exposure Silkwood had "a 100% probability" of getting lung cancer.

In his instructions to the jury, Judge Theis explained that plutonium was so inherently hazardous that Kerr-McGee could be held liable for damages regardless of whether the company was actually negligent.

Theis also told the jury the only way Kerr-McGee could be relieved of its liability was if the company could prove Silkwood had deliberately removed the plutonium from the plant.

During the trial, Silkwood family lawyers had asked that the amount of their suit, originally $11.5 million, be raised to $71.5 million. Theis told the jurors that he had not ruled on the request because it was unnecessary to do so. He placed no limit on damages that the jury could award.

(Earlier in the proceeding, Theis had barred testimony about Silkwood's character. That testimony would have included allegations of drug involvement, homosexuality, and mental troubles, the Washington Post reported. The Post said testimony also would have indicated that Silkwood had made suicide threats well before her contamination with plutonium.)

The jury awarded the Silkwood estate—which included her three children by a marriage that ended in separation—$505,000 in actual damages and $10 million in punitive damages.

The nuclear power industry had sought to divorce itself from the Silkwood case. Industry spokesmen had contended that the Cimarron plant was not typical of the industry. However, Bill Perkins of the Atomic Industrial Forum acknowledged the verdict would have "a psychological and political impact."

The Three Mile Island Accident

A nuclear power plant incident that began in late March 1979 released some radiation, appeared to threaten an explosion or "meltdown" and provoked speculation that many people in the area might become cancer victims as a result of the highly publicized events.

Threat from Pennsylvania incident. A series of breakdowns in the cooling system of the Three Mile Island nuclear power plant's No. 2 reactor led to a major accident in the early morning hours of March 28. The Three Mile Island facility, owned by the Metropolitan Edison Co. and two other utilities, was located 10 miles south of Harrisburg, Pa. in the Susquehanna River Valley.

By Friday, March 30, the Nuclear Regulatory Commission warned of a possible core meltdown, a catastrophic event that could involve major loss of life, and also raised the threat of an explosion of a hydrogen gas bubble that had formed in the overheated reactor vessel of the crippled plant.

Also, on March 30, Pennsylvania Gov. Richard Thornburgh, concerned by Three Mile Island's continuing emission of radioactive gases, advised pregnant women and preschool children within a five-mile radius of the plant to leave the area. It was feared that people in an even wider area might ultimately become cancer victims as a result of the radioactivity.

Over the weekend, nuclear experts worked to cool down the overheated uranium fuel core and to reduce the size of the potentially dangerous hydrogen bubble. Evacuation plans for citizens living 10 to 20 miles downwind of the facility were prepared for use when or if technicians decided to force the hydrogen gas bubble from the reactor vessel.

On the fifth day after the accident, President Carter was able to visit the site and announce that the reactor was stable and that radiation levels near Three Mile Island were "quite safe."

On April 2, NRC and Met Ed officials announced a dramatic reduction in the size of the potentially dangerous gas bubble and a further cooling of the reactor core. The following day, seven days after the accident, it was announced that the hydrogen gas bubble had been eliminated.

NRC and utility experts said they would continue their efforts to bring the reactor to a "cold shutdown" state.

The accident threatened the future of nuclear power in the United States and called into question the safety systems regulated by the NRC and used by the nuclear power industry.

Three Mile Island No. 2 had only been operating for a short period of time, since December 1978. Three Mile Island No. 1, in operation since 1974, had been closed for routine maintenance when the accident occurred.

Day One: ***The Accident*****—**Early on the morning of March 28, a malfunction in the cooling system at the No. 2 unit of the Three Mile Island facility led to the closing down of the reactor and the release of radiation into the air. The explanation of the sequence of events that led to the accident was later hotly contested by Metropolitan Edison Co. (Met Ed), the NRC, the state of Pennsylvania and companies that had constructed elements of the reactor system.

According to Met Ed, the accident began at 4 a.m. when a key part of the plant's cooling system failed. Vice President for Generation John G. Herbein claimed that a valve had failed in a pump in the primary core cooling system.

(But officials of Babcock and Wilcox, which designed and built the reactor, said there were no valves inside the pumps. That position was supported by an official of Bingham-Willamette Co., which built the pump.)

Met Ed officials March 28 said the flow of water used to take heat away from the nuclear reactor was interrupted, which led to the stopping of the steam turbine and a consequent shut down of the reactor by means of the automatic computer-directed insertion of the control rods between the fuel rods.

The reactor continued to generate heat, and as a result the emergency cooling system automatically began operating. But at some point in the transition from the primary cooling system to the emergency core cooling system, a plant operator turned off the emergency system and, after a period of time, turned it back on. At that point, it was believed, the core was damaged, as some of the pellets of enriched uranium fuel became so heated that they either melted through or ruptured the zirconium-clad tubes that held them.

Somehow, some of the water used to cool the core, whether from the primary or emergency systems, spilled onto the floor of the reactor building. When some of that radioactive water became steam, it was vented into the atmosphere above the plant to relieve pressure.

The radioactive steam was at first thought to be the sole source of radiation outside the plant. Later, however, the NRC reported that the radiation, which had

Measuring Exposure to Radiation

Radiation exposure was measured in a variety of units:

- Roentgens, a measure of the quantity of X-ray (or gamma ray) radiation in the air.
- Rads, (radiation absorbed dose), a measure of the amount of any kind of ionizing radiation absorbed in body tissue.
- Rems, (roentgen equivalent man), a measure of the quantity of any ionizing radiation with the same biological effectiveness as one rad of X-rays.

Since rems indicated the extent of biological damage to the human cell, and not the actual intensity of radiation, they were often used in assessing potential health hazards. A rem was a large quantity of exposure. So experts tended to use millirems in their calculations.

The accepted maximum annual exposure to man-made, nonmedical radiation for the general public was between 200 and 500 millirems. A complex formula for workers exposed to radiation allowed about 5,000 millirems a year. The typical amount of radiation an American got from all sources was 200 millirems a year. The exposure level from a standard diagnostic X-ray was between 45 and 75 millirems.

Although they lacked hard proof, scientists agreed that the addition of almost any amount of radiation, no matter how small, was bad because it could cause future cancers or mutations in a small number of people. As was true with many other suspected carcinogens, different humans had different tolerance levels.

penetrated four-foot thick walls, had been traced directly to the nuclear materials (the damaged core) within the plant.

By 7 p.m. the uranium fuel in the core was still so hot that the plant's managers had to vent more steam into the atmosphere to prevent an explosion in the containment building.

The direct result of the venting was the release over a four-county area of small amounts of radioactive iodine, krypton and xenon. NRC spokesman Carl Abraham described the radiation levels surrounding the plant as "quite low" and not dangerous to humans.

There was no apparent serious radiation exposure for Three Mile Island workers, but a plant spokesman said some of the 60 employees on duty were contaminated but did not require hospitalization.

Estimates of the amount of radiation released were increased during the day, at one point reaching a level of seven millirems. In a statement at 5 p.m., the NRC said its maximum confirmed measurement, at a site a third of a mile from the plant, was three millirems. At the seven millirem level, a human exposed for 24 hours would receive 168 millirems. [See box on radiation exposure]

Day Two: *Radiation Leaks Continue*— Radioactivity continued to leak from the Three Mile Island plant March 29, with low levels of radiation detected in the atmosphere as far as 20 miles away.

By the evening of March 29, Met Ed and NRC officials said the reactor had cooled enough to allow technicians to turn off the emergency core cooling system. The reactor was said to have cooled to less than 200 degrees Fahrenheit (92 degrees Celsius).

Radiation leakage was expected to continue for 24 hours to a week.

Met Ed and NRC officials said the highest levels of radiation outside the plant were about 20 millirems an hour. NRC Chairman Joseph Hendrie, appearing before the House Interior subcommittee on energy and the environment, said the plant was still very radioactive.

Hendrie said one gauge inside the containment building showed radiation readings near the ceiling of as much as 20,000 rems an hour, a highly lethal amount. But Hendrie said that reading was being questioned because another gauge near the floor reported 10 rems an hour.

He also said a single sample of milk taken about five miles from the plant appeared to contain amounts of radioactive iodine. But he added that the levels were so close to the "threshold," or minimum measurable level, that the milk reading was being questioned.

Hendrie said the reports did not suggest there would be any "significant" impact on the health of residents in the area. He said the readings "should" start dropping as the plant's radioactivity waned.

Met Ed officials, at a press conference in Hershey, Pa., reiterated their belief that the continued radioactive releases were well below harmful levels.

Herbein, vice president for generation, claimed, "We didn't injure anybody through this accident, we didn't seriously contaminate anybody and we certainly didn't kill anybody. The radiation off-site was absolutely minuscule."

Herbein said radiation readings indicated the level of exposure ranged from up to 20 millirems an hour at the site and as much as seven millirems in nearby towns.

Asked whether he thought any residents of the Susquehanna River Valley should seek medical attention, Herbein replied: "No, I don't think they should see a doctor. There is nothing like that kind of concern."

At a news conference in Harrisburg, some 11 miles from the Three Mile Island facility, Pennsylvania Gov. Richard Thornburgh said his office had received many calls from pregnant women asking advice about leaving the area. He said that he and his aides saw "no need to consider evacuation at this time."

Several critics of nuclear safety disagreed with that assessment, however. "Every dose of radiation is an overdose," said Nobel Prize-winning biologist George Wald, professor emeritus at Harvard University. "A little radiation does a little harm and more of it does more harm."

Ernest Sternglass, professor of radiology at the University of Pittsburgh, flew to the area and reported that his findings corresponded to a major fallout pattern from a nuclear bomb test.

"The reaction of the community should be to stand up and scream," Sternglass said. "Risk for pregnant women and young children is significantly increased."

"It's not a disaster where people are going to fall down like flies. It's a creeping thing."

According to the New York Times, however, few residents in the general area around Three Mile Island were concerned enough about the radiation levels to leave.

The accident focused attention on another issue: the possibility of a "worst case scenario" in which a complete "meltdown" of the radioactive core at the plant would release lethal radioactivity over a wide area.

This "worst case" catastrophic accident had formed the basis for the plot of a popular film, *The China Syndrome*, which had been released just before the Three Mile Island accident. (The title referred to a meltdown that would cause the uranium core to melt figuratively through the earth all the way to China.)

In his testimony before Congress, NRC Chairman Hendrie said, "I don't think we were anywhere near a fuel meltdown, but we suffered damage to the reactor core, which is significant."

"This is the first time we've had this level of core damage at all in the history of the civilian program," he added.

Met Ed officials angrily denied that the situation at the reactor had ever remotely approached a core meltdown.

Day Three: *Meltdown Threat Seen*—A new burst of high radiation escaped into the air from the Three Mile Island nuclear power station March 30, and Pennsylvania Gov. Thornburgh urged pregnant women and preschool children within a five-mile radius of the plant to leave the area at once.

Meanwhile, the crisis worsened as the NRC said the reactor faced "the ultimate risk of meltdown" and the entire population within five miles of the plant might have to be evacuated.

The new burst of radiation was released, according to the NRC, when an automatic device vented gases from the reactor's cooling water system between 6:40 a.m. and 9 a.m., because of a dangerous buildup of the gases.

Plant officials said they had not expected the gas pressure in the tank to rise, but that once the increase occurred, the decision to vent the gases was deliberate.

But Pennsylvania's director of the bureau of radiological health, Thomas Gerusky, said the emission was "unexpected, unplanned and they [the company officials] could not stop it."

Gerusky said early afternoon readings in the vicinity of the plant registered 14 millirems (compared with a 0.1 millirem reading in a nonaccident situation.)

The NRC said that immediately after the morning leak that 1,200 millirems were detected above the facility.

But nuclear industry officials said that the latest plume of radioactive gas had a maximum radiation level of 350 millirems an hour.

Thornburgh called a news conference to order 23 schools closed and to urge tens of thousands of residents of central Pennsylvania to stay indoors until further notice.

(About 500,000 people, including those in the cities of Harrisburg, York, Lancaster, and Lebanon, lived in a 15-mile radius of the Three Mile Island plant.)

By the evening some 150 pregnant women and children were reported at a shelter in Hershey. Several thousand schoolchildren were also removed from the plant area.

Thornburgh said that although the radiation leakage was no greater than the first day of the accident, he believed "an excess of caution" was best.

Met Ed angered Thornburgh and other Pennsylvania legislators with the venting, which had not been announced, and also by the dumping of 400,000 gallons of slightly radioactive waste water into the Susquehanna River on Thursday night (March 29).

Herbein had defended those actions at a news conference, saying, "I don't know why we need to tell you every step we take. We certainly feel a responsibility for people who live around our plant and we need to get on with our job."

Pennsylvania officials reportedly had put together an evacuation plan to move the residents of small towns within a 10-mile radius of the plant within one hour. The plan called for the evacuation of Harrisburg residents within two hours. The evacuees would be moved upwind in the event of an explosion or meltdown that released radioactivity.

Day Four: *Conflict Over Bubble*—The threat of a major disaster at the Three Mile Island plant had apparently receded March 31, as federal officials noted a cooling and slowdown in abnormal activity within the reactor core.

But at a news conference in Washington, NRC Chairman Joseph Hendrie said evacuation of citizens living 10 to 20 miles downwind of the facility was "certainly a possibility" when or if technicians decided to force a hydrogen gas bubble from the reactor vessel. It was thought that the bubble was blocking cooling water from some of the reactor's uranium fuel rods.

Meanwhile, engineers for the Met Ed claimed to have "bled" the dangerous hydrogen bubble down in size by one third.

But Harold Denton of the NRC, speaking in Harrisburg, sharply challenged that statement. And NRC officials said there had been an increase of oxygen in the giant gas bubble, increasing the danger the highly flammable hydrogen gas would ignite.

Also on March 31, the NRC revealed that there had been an earlier hydrogen explosion on Wednesday, the first day of the accident, which Met Ed had not told the NRC about until Friday. The NRC said the hydrogen blast occurred not long after the start of the accident, at 4 a.m.; the utility said it happened at 2 p.m. Thursday.

Gov. Thornburgh extended his advisory that preschool children and pregnant women stay at least five miles from the plant. The governor's office said it was no longer necessary for people to stay indoors and keep the windows sealed.

It was believed that about 5% of the 20,000 persons who lived within a mile of the Three Mile Island plant had voluntarily left the area. Civil defense officials said at least 1,200 persons had gone to emergency shelters.

As the radiation continued to leak from the plant, officials in nearby states said they were not overly concerned about contamination, but they had stepped up monitoring of air and water, and in some cases, milk. No increase in radiation had been reported.

The NRC began March 31 to "blanket the countryside" with devices to monitor and record accumulated radiation. Until that action, monitoring outside the plant site had consisted of spot checks that determined radiation at a specific time and place.

Day Five: *Carter Visits Plant*—President Carter, who toured Three Mile Island April 1, was told that conditions there were stable. He urged residents of the Susquehanna River Valley area to cooperate if emergency measures became necessary.

Some government officials expressed cautious optimism that the crisis was easing. The reactor core was said to be cooling, though serious danger remained from the hydrogen gas bubble.

After his tour of the plant, Carter promised "a thorough inquiry" into the causes of the accident, and pledged he would be "personally responsible for thoroughly informing the American people about this particular incident and the status of nuclear safety in the future."

Carter** said that radiation levels near the Three Mile Island facility were "quite safe," but cautioned that officials at the plant faced critical decisions in the following days on measures to dissipate the gas bubble.

He added: "The primary and overriding concern for all of us is the health and safety of the people of this area."

"As I have said before, if we make an error, all of us want to err on the side of extra precautions and extra safety."

Civil defense officials said that some 50,000 of the 950,000-plus residents of the four-county area surrounding the plant had left their homes by Sunday morning.

"I'd say it's increasing every couple of hours, based on the calls from residents we're getting here," said Paul Leese, civil defense director for Lancaster County.

Meanwhile, Gov. Edmund G. Brown Jr. of California asked the NRC in a telegram

**In 1952, as a naval officer, Carter was assigned to the Atomic Energy Commission's division of reactor development at Schenectady, N.Y. At Schenectady, he taught mathematics and reactor technology to prospective crew members of the USS *Seawolf,* the nation's second nuclear submarine. At that time, he also took graduate courses in nuclear physics.

for a "precautionary and temporary" closing of the Rancho Seco nuclear power plant, near Sacramento. Since the Rancho Seco plant was built by Babcock and Wilcox, and was almost identical to Three Mile Island, Brown said, he was concerned about the question of a generic defect.

Speaking on the ABC broadcast interview program *Issues and Answers* Rep. Morris K. Udall (D, Ariz.) suggested that "once the dust settles" that the NRC study the safety record and performance of the eight Babcock and Wilcox plants in operation.

Day Six: ***Gas Bubble Shrinks***—Federal and utility nuclear experts said April 2 that the large gas bubble that had formed at the top of the reactor pressure vessel had shown a "dramatic drop" in size.

While NRC officials expressed surprise and relief, Met Ed experts insisted they had expected the bubble to shrink.

"The whole thing has been a planned process since it began last Friday," said John Hilbish, a Met Ed nuclear engineer. "Based on the game plan, this is exactly what we expected to happen."

NRC estimates of the size of the bubble Monday night (April 2) ranged from 47 to 150 cubic feet—down from 850 cubic feet several days earlier. Met Ed officials claimed the bubble had virtually disappeared.

On Friday (March 30) Met Ed technicians began "degasifying" the bubble by spraying the circulating liquid in the reactor's primary cooling system into a portion of the plant called a pressurizer.

The cylindrical pressurizer was designed to allow the operators of the plant to raise or lower pressure in the cooling system. The pressurizer was located outside of the reactor vessel but within the containment building.

When the coolant was sprayed into the pressurizer, hydrogen was removed from the liquid. Then the coolant was recirculated into the reactor vessel where it absorbed more hydrogen from the bubble.

From the pressurizer, the radioactive hydrogen was vented into the containment building. NRC officials said the two recombiners were started to keep down the level of the potentially explosive gas in the building.

The fuel temperatures in the core continued to drop, with officials claiming that only two fuel bundles remained over 400 degrees Fahrenheit (202 degrees Celsius), as compared with Sunday (April 1) when four fuel bundles were over that mark.

The NRC's Harold Denton said he would like to see the reactor temperature brought down to a "cold shutdown temperature—normally thought of in the 170 to 180 degree range."

Denton also said that general radiation levels monitored by instruments at 37 locations around Three Mile Island were continuing to drop. He said the highest radiation reading during the past 24-hour period at a station five miles northeast of the plant was 1.1 millirems an hour.

The containment building, however, continued to retain extremely high radiation levels. An instrument April 2 measured the radiation level near the dome at about 30,000 rems an hour. (Many doctors believed a human exposed to 400 rems would die in a short time.)

The NRC raised the possibility that Three Mile Island was so contaminated that it might never reopen to generate electricity.

"It might be a $1-billion mausoleum," said Sen. Gary Hart (D, Colo.), chairman of the Senate Public Works subcommittee on nuclear regulation. "It might be more expensive to clean up the plant than it was to build it."

Gov. Thornburgh announced that his recommendation that pregnant women and preschool children stay outside the area within a five-mile radius remained in effect until further notice. He also said a liberal leave policy for state employees implemented that day would stay in effect.

Red Cross officials said that about 40% of the estimated 133,000 persons living within a 10-mile radius of the plant had left the area. A spokesman for the Hospital Association of Pennsylvania said that the six general hospitals within a 10-mile radius of the plant were releasing ambulatory patients and restricting admissions to emergency cases. The hospitals had about 50% of normal occupancy.

Day Seven: ***Cooldown Continues***—The Three Mile Island No. 2 reactor continued to cool April 3, and the NRC announced that the hydrogen bubble trapped in the reactor vessel had been eliminated.

Authorities said the danger of a major new accident had lessened significantly.

NRC official Denton said a few small bubbles might still exist in the primary cooling system, but he claimed "they don't present any significant safety problem."

Denton and his aides said the emergency could not be declared over until the high temperatures in the reactor fell further.

At the same time, U.S. officials revealed that "very small amounts" of radioactive iodine had been detected for the first time in samples of milk taken from farms in the area.

Gov. Thornburgh, reacting to that announcement and the fact that small releases of radioactive gases continued to take place, did not lift his advisory that pregnant women and preschool children stay out of the plant area.

Denton said the highest iodine level discovered by the Food and Drug Administration was about 31 picocuries per liter, and the level in most of the samples was 10 to 20 picocuries. The FDA considered 12,000 picocuries per liter dangerous. (During the fallout from a Chinese nuclear test, Denton said, levels of 100 to 300 picocuries a liter were reached.)

As for radiation exposure, federal and state officials projected that the cumulative radiation dose level for local residents would be less than 100 millirems.

The containment building had the highest level of contamination recorded in commercial nuclear operations history. Waste water in sump tanks in an auxiliary building was also so highly radioactive that it could not be inspected. A clean-up of those tanks could not begin for weeks or months, but they presented a greater danger than the reactor or containment building because they were more exposed to the environment.

In another development, The Washington Post reported April 3 that the trouble at Three Mile Island actually began at 3 a.m. Wednesday (March 28) and not at 4 a.m., as claimed by Met Ed.

The Post quoted Glenn A. Seiders, a Met Ed worker, who said he was summoned to the facility shortly after 3 a.m. when control room alarms showed trouble. Seiders said that plant officials realized by 4 a.m. that a serious situation had developed.

Day Eight: ***Errors Detailed***—Federal safety investigators in their first official report told the Nuclear Regulatory Commission April 4 that a series of human, mechanical and design errors had contributed to the Three Mile Island accident.

Darrell Eisenhut, deputy director of the NRC's division of operating reactors, told the five NRC commissioners that Metropolitan Edison Co. had closed three auxiliary cooling pumps for maintenance "at least two weeks" before the accident and had kept them closed until the accident occurred.

Eisenhut told the commissioners that it was a major violation of federal regulations.

Eisenhut listed several other errors that he said had contributed significantly to the incident: electrical magnetic relief valves had failed to close as planned after opening to release a buildup of water pressure in the reactor; plant operators apparently received incorrect readings from the pressure level indicator about the amount of water in the reactor; and on two occasions after the accident began, operators in the control room "prematurely" turned off the emergency core cooling system.

Despite the errors, the special NRC investigating team recommended against requiring the immediate shutdown of the eight Babcock and Wilcox built reactors or of the 61 other similar reactors built by other manufacturers.

The NRC staff said that the reactors could continue operating without "undue risk to the public." But the NRC team did say that all plants designed by Babcock and Wilcox might share some of the design features that apparently contributed to the incident.

In Harrisburg, the NRC's Harold Denton said conditions at the Three Mile Island No. 2 reactor remained "stable."

Radiation monitoring in the countryside around the facility showed "most levels are slightly above background radiation," according to an NRC spokesman.

In Washington, Health, Education and Welfare Secretary Joseph A. Califano Jr. told the Senate Human Resources health subcommittee that those persons within five miles of the plant had received as much as 80 millirems of radiation since March 28. Califano claimed that the number of cancer deaths in Pennsylvania was not expected to rise above normal. But he said that "great uncertainties still remain about the relationship between cancer deaths and low-level radiation."

Califano announced HEW would start long-term health studies of workers near the plant as well as pregnant women, their children when born and a sample of the general population exposed to radiation.

NRC Chairman Joseph M. Hendrie testified that it was not until Saturday (March 31) that his agency installed dosimeters to measure accumulated radiation levels. Until that time, he said, the NRC relied on Met Ed for offsite radiation readings.

Hendrie also said that releases of slightly radioactive water into the Susquehanna River and the venting of steam into the air had been done without prior NRC approval.

Subcommittee Chairman Sen. Edward M. Kennedy (D, Mass.) criticized the NRC for allowing Met Ed to make decisions "which pose potential implications for public health."

Day Nine: ***Carter Forms Panel***—President Carter announced April 5 the formation of an independent commission to investigate the Three Mile Island accident.

At the Three Mile Island plant, engineers had decided to pump radioactive gases that had formed in a storage tank back into the reactor containment building.

There were still "hot spots" in the reactor core, where temperatures were at least 328 degrees Fahrenheit (164 degrees Celsius).

State civil defense officials estimated that some 80,000 people living near the plant went away over the weekend, but by late Thursday (April 5) about 85% of the evacuees had returned.

Day 10: ***NRC OKs Babcock Reactors***—The NRC announced April 6 that eight nuclear reactors built by Babcock and Wilcox, the manufacturer of Three Mile Island No. 2, would be permitted to continue generating electricity at full power.

The decision was announced in a letter from Chairman Joseph M. Hendrie to California Gov. Edmund G. Brown Jr., who had requested a temporary closing of the Rancho Seco reactor near Sacramento.

In his reply to Brown, Hendrie cited a number of steps the NRC had taken at plants with Babcock and Wilcox reactors, including special warning bulletins sent to plants and the assignment of NRC inspectors to assist operators in the event of trouble.

At the plant meanwhile, a radiation buildup caused by faulty pumping equipment briefly delayed efforts to cool down the reactor, the NRC reported.

Engineers fixed the equipment, which was not identified, and resumed pumping radioactive gas from tanks in an auxiliary building back into the containment building.

Officials said a small amount of radiation had been vented from the auxiliary building because of the equipment problem. An NRC spokesman said airborne radiation levels never rose above 0.3 millirems an hour, within the radiation range of the previous 24 hours.

In Washington, the White House April 6 sought to assure consumers that food from the area was safe.

"The President is concerned about reports that some members of the public fear the purity of food from the area surrounding the Three Mile Island nuclear plant," a statement said. "These fears are not grounded in fact. Current readings show nothing to fear from food grown, harvested or produced in that area."

Day 11: ***Radiation Said Down***—Pennsylvania Gov. Richard Thornburgh and the NRC's Denton toured the area near Three Mile Island April 7. They told residents that the reactor was cooling down and that radioactivity was extremely low.

Since there had been some releases of radioactive gases and iodine into the atmosphere, Thornburgh said, his advisory warning—that pregnant women and preschool children remain five miles from the plant—remained in effect.

"We're trying to be as cautious as possible and not increase the psychic costs of the whole incident," Thornburgh said. "I don't want to give advice to people and then have to counter that and ask them to move out again."

In Washington, meanwhile, a panel of scientists concerned about nuclear radiation hazards charged that the government was withholding information about the accident and understating the damage to the environment.

The scientists included Karl Z. Morgan of the School of Nuclear Engineering of Georgia Tech, Dr. Ernest J. Sternglass of the University of Pittsburgh Medical School and Rosalie Bertell of the Ministry for Concern for Public Health in Buffalo, a public interest group.

Sternglass said he was suspicious of the official announcements of radiation emissions. "I don't believe that even the President and his wife were told the actual dose levels," he said. "He may have gotten more than the one millirem he was promised."

Sternglass said that over the course of 10 days there was 400 millirems of gamma radiation, equal, he said, "to the accumulated fallout on the East Coast of 25 years of weapons testing."

Day 12: *Iodine Said Stabilized*—Top NRC official Robert Bernero said April 8 that engineers had applied sodium thyosulfate and hydrazine to radioactive iodine in the Three Mile Island plant over the weekend and were successful in stabilizing it.

"Iodine doesn't dissolve freely," Bernero said. "Iodine is one of the principal contributors to radiation doses. It can get into kids' milk and cause thyroid cancer. Now airborne releases of iodine are less likely."

Iodine had been detected in what was termed small and relatively harmless amounts in milk from the Pennsylvania dairy farmland near the Three Mile Island site.

Bernero also said that engineers had started up their degasification plan to eliminate radioactive gases within the cooling system and start the process of a safe, cold shutdown of the reactor.

The NRC said a small cloud of radiation burst from the plant site Saturday night (April 7) during a continuing operation to depressurize the cooling system.

NRC officials said that latest average maximum reading on radiation levels around the plant was .05 millirems an hour at a spot a mile from the reactor. They called the level insignificant.

Day 13: *NRC Says Crisis Over*—Harold Denton, the federal official in charge of the Three Mile Island nuclear plant, said April 9 that "the crisis is over."

Gov. Thornburgh rescinded his advisory warning pregnant women and preschool children to stay away from the plant, and he also lifted his order closing 23 schools within a five-mile radius of Three Mile Island. He said there was no threat to public health from milk or drinking water in the area.

Engineers continued to remove radioactive gases from the cooling system.

The NRC said low levels of radiation continued to seep from the plant, at the level of 1 to .1 millirems an hour. Denton said he doubted there would be another major release of radiation but said authorities would have enough time to order an evacuation.

Denton also said the maximum possible dosage any person outside the plant could have received since March 28 was less than 100 millirems. The NRC said 12 plant workers had absorbed doses between two and three rems, while three received more than three rems.

Final Shutdown Started. The final cooling process to bring the No. 2 reactor of the Three Mile Island nuclear power plant to cold shutdown began April 13.

Using a steam generator to draw off heat, the Nuclear Regulatory Commission and Metropolitan Edison Co., the plant's operator, managed to cool the reactor core to some 230 degrees Fahrenheit (110 degrees Celsius), down from 280 degrees Fahrenheit (138 degrees Celsius). Some of the damaged fuel rods remained at temperatures over 300 degrees Fahrenheit (149 degrees Celsius).

The engineers and technicians moved cautiously, fearful of creating a potentially explosive hydrogen gas bubble in the reactor vessel or of allowing bursts of radiation to escape.

But on April 14 and 15, as the cooldown continued, bursts of radioactive iodine vented from the plant. The escape of iodine reached a peak April 15, when 95 picocuries of iodine-131 were measured on the east bank of the Susquehanna River, less than a mile from the Three Mile Island facility.

(The standard allowable limit away from the site of a nuclear plant was 100 picocuries to a cubic meter.)

The NRC said April 18 that the danger was gone that another hydrogen bubble could appear in the reactor vessel. But the NRC said radioactive iodine continued to leak at higher than normal levels.

One of 16 air samples taken close to Three Mile Island showed 200 picocuries to a cubic meter. But an NRC spokesman said the amounts were not a health hazard.

NRC Transcripts Released. The House Interior and Insular Affairs Committee April 12 made public transcripts of the Nuclear Regulatory Commission's closed-door meetings during the Three Mile Island nuclear crisis. The committee had forced the NRC to release the transcripts by threatening a subpoena if they were not turned over.

The transcripts, several hundred pages long, covered a fairly continuous NRC meeting that began Friday morning March 30 and ran through Wednesday, April 4.

The transcripts were made from tape recordings whenever at least three of the NRC's five commissioners were present.

The records of the meetings showed that the five commissioners and the NRC's technical staff were at times highly disturbed by receiving incomplete information from the accident site and with being forced to predict and evaluate future events. The officials were unsure of whether to recommend the evacuation of the people living around the Three Mile Island plant.

Two days after the accident, on March 30, NRC Chairman Joseph M. Hendrie, said of the crisis facing both him and Gov. Richard Thornburgh (R, Pa.): "We are operating almost totally in the blind; his information is ambiguous, mine is nonexistant and—I don't know—it's like a couple of blind men staggering around making decisions."

Also on March 30, the NRC director of the division of systems safety, Roger J. Mattson, described the damage to the No. 2 reactor at Three Mile Island:

"My best guess is that the core uncovered, stayed uncovered for a long period of time," he reported. "We saw failure modes the like of which has never been analyzed."

Mattson told the commissioners that there had apparently been a hydrogen explosion at the plant 10 hours after the first signs of trouble.

Hendrie: It sounds to me like we ought to say where we are. I don't like the sound of depressurizing and letting that bubble creep down into the core.

Mattson: Not yet. I don't think we want to depressurize yet. The latest burst didn't hurt many people. I'm not sure why you are not moving people. Got to say it. I have been saying it down here. I don't know what we are protecting at this point. I think we ought to be moving people....

Kennedy*: How far out?

Hendrie: How far out?

Mattson: I would get them downwind, and unfortunately the wind is still meandering, but at these dose levels that is probably not bad because it is (inaudible).

Mattson: I might add, you aren't going to kill any people out to 10 miles. There aren't that many people and these people have been—they have had two days to get ready and prepare. It's too little information, too late unfortunately, and it is the same way every partial core meltdown has gone. People haven't believed the instrumentation as they went along. It took us until midnight last night to convince anybody that those goddamn temperature measurements meant something. By 4 o'clock this morning B and W (Babcock and Wilcox) agreed.

At a meeting on Saturday, March 31, the transcripts showed that the NRC members were seriously concerned about the possible consequences of a hydrogen explosion or a core meltdown.

---

*NRC member Richard T. Kennedy

Hendrie briefed his fellow commissioners at the March 31 meeting on the amount of time there would be to evacuate people if the meltdown sequence began.

NRC Orders Babcock Plants Shut. The Nuclear Regulatory Commission April 27 ordered the temporary shutdown of all operating nuclear power plants constructed by Babcock and Wilcox Co.

The NRC's decision to close the plants came shortly after the operators of the seven facilities involved had offered to close their power stations voluntarily.

After receiving that offer, the NRC decided to issue a shutdown order rather than rely on letters of agreement from the firms.

"We have to let them know who are the regulated and who are the regulators," one NRC member said.

Harold Denton, the NRC's director of nuclear reactor regulation, told the commission that the seven utilities would close the plants to conduct safety analyses, make safety modifications, prepare new emergency procedures and improve training of plant operators.

The changes required for reopening involved improving the plants' backup feedwater cooling systems; putting safeguards on the control systems; improving the reactors' ability to close down automatically; studying detailed analyses of the plants' responses to accidents, and beefing up control room staffs.

Three Mile Island Reaches Shutdown— The NRC said April 27 that the No. 2 reactor at Three Mile Island had come to a shutdown condition.

NRC spokesman Karl Abraham said the last remaining pressure gauge had failed and technicians decided to take advantage of the failure to stop a reactor pump permanently rather than restarting it only to stop it again later.

"The water is circulating naturally without the use of a pump. This is called natural circulation," Abraham said.

The NRC had said that when natural circulation began it would be the equivalent of a cold shutdown of the reactor.

The water in the system, which could not be allowed to boil, remained at about 225 degrees Fahrenheit (107 degrees Celsius), but was not boiling because it was under pressure of 1,000 pounds per square inch. The boiling point of water at that pressure was about 545 degrees Fahrenheit (285 degrees Celsius). Cold water in the cooling system prevented the uranium fuel from melting and causing a release of radiation from the plant.

One cancer death called possible. Health, Education and Welfare Secretary Joseph A. Califano Jr. May 3 said statistical probability indicated that at least one cancer death caused by radiation could be expected among the two million people living within 50 miles of the Three Mile Island nuclear accident site.

Califano said the radiation levels, which were nearly twice as high as originally estimated, could cause as many as 10 additional nonfatal cancers. The HEW secretary also told the Senate Government Affairs subcommitte on energy, nuclear proliferation and federal services that some investigators were estimating up to 10 deaths.

Califano had testified in April that the number of cancer deaths in the Three Mile Island area were not expected to rise.

Gravel says 12 will die—Sen. Mike Gravel (D, Alaska) May 15 rejected "the false claim that no one was killed or injured by the accident." He said in a statement in the Congressional Record:

> While it is true that the amount of radiation released was not enough to cause people to drop dead in the streets from acute radiation poisoning, we must remember that exposure to even tiny amounts (such as the amounts released at TMI) can cause cancer and leukemia, in addition to genetic injury. Whether the victims of radiation poisoning die immediately or 5, 10 or 20 years after their exposure is not of enormous importance—they will still be just as dead.
>
> Based on figures supplied by the Nuclear Regulatory Commission, it can now be established that 12 human beings have been irreversibly condemned to die from cancer or leukemia due to this ac-

cident. The number could be, and in all probability is, considerably higher.

Protests Sparked Abroad. The accident at Three Mile Island, in some measure a fulfillment of the predictions of nuclear critics, served as a rallying cry for demonstrations against nuclear power around the world. In Hanover, West Germany, some 35,000 to 50,000 persons gathered March 31 to protest a planned facility to process and store nuclear waste, shouting "We all live in Pennsylvania!"

In Denmark, which did not have any nuclear power plants, rallies were held to demand that two Swedish nuclear plants located close to the Danish border be closed, the Wall Street Journal reported April 3. A newspaper in Copenhagen described the accident at Three Mile Island as "a blessing in disguise" for pointing up the perils of nuclear power, the New York Times reported April 1.

In the small French town of Chooz, where the government planned to expand a nuclear power station, women locked up the mayor in the city hall for several hours, according to the Wall Street Journal April 3. French Socialist Leader Francois Mitterrand urged that construction of nuclear power plants be halted while a study was conducted to determine whether nuclear power was safe, the Journal reported.

Opposition political leaders and local officials elsewhere also expressed opposition to or reservations about nuclear power. Former Swedish Premier Thorbjorn Falldin called on the government March 31 to close down the Ringhals 2 reactor, which was of the same type as that on Three Mile Island.

In Italy's Montalto di Castro, proposed site of a new nuclear facility, Mayor Alfredo Pallotti sent a telegram to the government April 1 demanding "new guarantees that every precaution would be taken to insure the safety of residents." There were protests in South Africa against the country's first nuclear power station, located on the Atlantic coast north of Capetown, the New York Times reported April 2.

A coalition of environmentalists, union officials and Communist Party members in Japan called on the government and utility companies April 2 to stop operations at the 19 nuclear plants in the country.

Government Reactions Vary—The governments of most Western countries expressed concern about the implications of the accident, but there appeared to be considerable variation in the likely impact of the accident on the nuclear policies of different countries.

In Sweden, the major political parties agreed to hold a referendum on nuclear power before having the government proceed with the authorization of any new nuclear plants, the Wall Street Journal reported April 5.

The French government, on the other hand, revealed April 5 that it had officially approved plans to accelerate the country's shift to reliance on nuclear energy. The government's program called for 50% of France's electricity to be supplied by nuclear power plants by 1985, compared with 13% currently.

French Industry minister Andre Giraud insisted April 1 that an accident of the kind at Three Mile Island could not occur at French nuclear facilities. "Even in the event of a similar leak," he said, "our power stations are built so that they would contain the escaped radioactivity."

However, the French government said April 1 that it had sent a team of scientists to Pennsylvania to investigate the causes of the U.S. accident. The West German government announced the same day that it had also dispatched scientific investigators.

British Prime Minister James Callaghan said April 3 in Parliament that he could "assure the country that the incident which took place in Harrisburg could not take place here because of the different type of reactors. We have been very wise in concentrating on a safer type of reactor."

News media in the Soviet Union reported the accident in terms suggesting that it was the result of U.S. engineering and regulatory incompetence or the lack of concern for safety problems that, according to the Soviets, characterized private industry in capitalist countries.

A Soviet nuclear energy official said April 4 that the U.S.S.R. had "perfected protective systems. . . . Soviet safety norms simply rule out any escape of radiation.

They are set up at several echelons and are fully automated and reliable."

Domestic Protests. The accident at Three Mile Island unleashed a series of protests and demonstrations, as anti-nuclear power forces in the U.S. repeated their claims that atomic energy was dangerous and a threat to the environment.

On another front, several states moved to curtail or reassess their commitment to nuclear power. On April 2, Illinois Gov. James R. Thompson, a Republican, ordered the state Commission on Atomic Energy to conduct a technical review of the state's seven nuclear power reactors. He called it a precautionary move, not the result of any problems at the facilities. (Illinois had more plants in operation than any other state, with seven, and 17 more were planned.)

New York state officials April 5 announced the cancellation of a huge nuclear power plant in Cementon, N.Y., the proposed 1,200-megawatt Greene County facility. The Power Authority of the State of New York said construction costs, licensing delays and the Three Mile Island accident each played a part in the decision. The authority said it would seek federal approval to build a coal-burning facility at the site, 120 miles north of New York City.

On April 6, Columbia University's engineering faculty agreed to a request by the school's president, William J. McGill, not to activate a small nuclear reactor on the University's Morningside Heights campus in Manhattan.

Supporters of nuclear energy won a surprising victory April 7 in Austin, Texas when voters approved continued participation in a 2,500-megawatt nuclear power plant, the South Texas Nuclear Project, under construction at a Gulf Coast site 160 miles southeast of the city. Voters approved, by a 28,430 to 25,037 vote, a $216-million bond issue necessary to cover cost overruns that had doubled the cost of the plant.

"In light of Harrisburg, this is a phenomenal victory," said Neal Spelce, a consultant for the pro-nuclear power Committee for Economic Energy.

Some 65,000 people marched in an anti-nuclear power demonstration in Washington May 6. The protest march, from the White House to the Capitol, was the largest against nuclear power in the U.S. to date.

Speakers at the demonstration included Gov. Edmund G. (Jerry) Brown Jr. (D, Calif.), consumer advocate Ralph Nader, California political activist Tom Hayden and his wife, actress Jane Fonda.

Brown told the crowd that reliance on nuclear energy was a "pathological addiction " that was "storing up for generations to come evils and risks that the human mind can barely grasp."

Repeating his earlier comments on the growing political importance of the issue, Brown told reporters that nuclear energy would be an issue in the 1980 presidential campaign.

In a related development, Sen. Edward M. Kennedy (D, Mass.) May 7 called for a moratorium on construction of nuclear plants and a case-by-case examination of all existing reactors. Kennedy said all safety questions should be answered before there was any new construction.

Danger from Radioactive Wastes

One of the principal dangers of nuclear development is the failure so far to devise a safe way of disposing of wastes, many of which will remain radioactive for thousands of years and therefore constitute a virtually permanent cancer threat.

Facts called suppressed. Sen. Frank Church (D, Ida.) had accused the Atomic Energy Commission March 6, 1970 of not releasing to the public a 1966 report by a panel of the National Academy of Sciences critical of AEC procedures for storing radioactive waste.

The report, made available to the press March 6, said that the four major AEC plants where waste was stored were located in poor geological areas for such uses, that the practice of storing waste in the ground could pose a hazard through build-up, and that there was no uniform standard among the plants for determining the degree of radioactivity of waste materials. The panel had said that it saw no immediate danger in the way the AEC was storing or disposing of nuclear wastes.

John Erlewine, AEC assistant general manager for operations, was reported March 6 to have said that the report was only one of many not published by the AEC. He also said that while the AEC was putting waste into the ground it did not necessarily intend to leave it there and its operations were within the standards laid down by the Federal Radiation Council.

Four federal agencies had told the AEC it was careless in its disposal of radioactive wastes, according to the Washington Post March 13. The paper cited a report prepared for Church by the Bureau of Radiological Health, the Bureau of Sport Fisheries and Wildlife, the U.S. Geological Survey and the Federal Water Pollution Control Administration. The agencies recommended that the AEC keep at least two feet of clay or gravel between atomic burial pits and the exposed basalt formations below (the AEC then required no minimum protective barrier) and that the commission take steps to keep atomic burial sites free of flood waters.

Kansas A-waste plan scored. A geological report submitted to Kansas Gov. Robert B. Docking in December 1970 and published Feb. 16, 1971 criticized the plans of the Atomic Energy Commission (AEC) for burying radioactive wastes in salt mines at Lyons, Kansas. The report said the AEC had "exhibited remarkably little interest" in studying the effects of radiation and heat on the salt, that plans for transporting the radioactive waste across the state were "completely inadequate" and that emergency plans "do not exist at all." The New York Times reported March 17 that the AEC had assured opponents of the project in Kansas that the dumping scheme would be abandoned if safety problems arose.

Wastes used in buildings. James R. Schlesinger, AEC chairman, said Dec. 6, 1971 that the government might pay part of the cost of removing radioactive sands used in home construction in Grand Junction, Colo., accepting "moral responsibility" along with state authorities, uranium mills and building contractors.

The sands, waste products from nearby uranium processing mills, contained radium and other radioactive substances, and had caused detectable radiation levels at 5,300 sites in the community, in some cases exceeding health standards.

Colorado Gov. John A. Love said Dec. 5 that since the federal government was the sole uranium customer, it had sole responsibility to pay the estimated $12 million $20 million removal cost.

Model state law on wastes. The Environmental Protection Agency offered a model state law to control radioactive tailings (wastes) from Western uranium processing mills (reported Feb. 18, 1972).

The law, presented at a state-federal Southwestern water pollution conference in Las Vegas, would hold uranium mills responsible for the tailings, and require contouring and planting of grass. The tailings were a problem in nine Western states—Wyoming, Colorado, Utah, South Dakota, New Mexico, Texas, Arizona, Washington and Oregon, where 15 operating and 20 defunct uranium mills would be joined in the next 10 years by 10 new plants.

The AEC had refused legal responsibility for plants built before the 1969 Environmental Policy Act, but said waste control would be required before any new mills were licensed.

AEC to review waste policies. Atomic Energy Commission (AEC) Chairman

Dixy Lee Ray ordered a re-evaluation of nuclear waste management programs after a controversy developed over leaks from waste storage tanks at the AEC facility at Hanford, Wash., it was reported Aug. 28, 1973. Dr. Ray conceded that radioactive waste management had at times been "sloppy" and "negligent," but she said public health had not been endangered.

The 115,000-gallon Hanford leak had been confirmed June 8. The AEC reported July 31 that an investigation had found questionable waste practices being followed by a private contractor, the Atlantic Richfield Hanford Co. The AEC said the leak had gone undiscovered for six weeks because a company supervisor had not read reports showing waste levels dropping steadily in the holding tank.

The AEC reported, however, that the liquid waste had stabilized at a point underground where there would be no hazard to ground water.

Four environmentalist groups filed suit in federal district court in Spokane Aug. 1 seeking to prevent resumption of the Hanford operation after repair of the leaks. The suit accused the AEC of failing to file the required environmental impact statement for the Hanford operation and of violating radioactive wastes sections of the Atomic Energy Act of 1954.

The plaintiffs alleged that, in addition to accidental leaks of high-level wastes, low and intermediate-level wastes had been deliberately disposed of in the soil, endangering water supplies. The AEC said the high-level wastes had been contained and the other wastes posed no dangers. The suit was dismissed Aug. 17 after the AEC agreed to file an environmental impact statement.

Conference asks waste-disposal data exchange. Representatives of seven leading nuclear energy users—Britain, Canada, France, Japan, Sweden, the U.S. and West Germany—agreed at a conference in Denver, Colo. July 12, 1976 to increase their exchange of information on the disposal of nuclear-waste material.

The conferees agreed that without a safe system for storing radioactive wastes, public apprehension would seriously curtail nuclear-energy programs.

The conferees agreed to set up an international committee of waste-handling experts. Under discussion were plans such as storing the wastes in steel canisters and burying them in deep-lying salt deposits in the U.S. and West Germany and in crystalline rocks in Canada.

A-waste centers called hazard. Ralph Nader released a draft report by a nuclear expert Sept. 7, 1976 concluding that "a major radioactive waste problem already exists" in the U.S. The report was prepared by Mason Willrich for the Energy Research and Development Administration.

The report said that the federal government's past handling of radioactive material had been "marred in a sufficient number of instances to be a cause for concern" and that the system of storing wastes soon "will be unworkable." It said further that the escape of radioactive material into the air and water would "constitute a radiological hazard for hundreds of thousands, perhaps millions of years."

It was estimated that 75 million gallons of high-level radioactive waste and 51 million cubic feet of low-level waste were stored at nine different sites in the U.S. The federal military reactors were said to be producing 7.5 million gallons of liquid high-level waste a year and the commercial reactors were expected to produce a total of 60 million gallons of such waste by the year 2,000.

Federal production of low-level radioactive waste was put at 1.3 million cubic feet a year, the commercial production was estimated at a total of 50 million cubic feet by 2,000.

At the Hanford site, the government's major storage area, 18 leaks had resulted in losses of 430,000 gallons of high-level wastes into the surrounding soil, the Willrich report said.

Radioactive Waste Sites Found. The Energy Department was beginning an aerial search by helicopter for radioactive dump sites in 20 square miles in Denver, it was reported March 5, 1979.

Some sites had been discovered after an Environmental Protection Agency employee, researching old Bureau of Mine records, had found that the Colorado radium industry, which flourished 50 or 60 years ago, had several refineries located in Denver.

Radium was a known cause of cancer and could produce birth and genetic defects. In the early 1900s, however, many doctors and scientists believed radium was a medical cure-all.

The aerial search in Denver was an expansion of a survey in six states to determine if radiation contamination from radium dump sites posed health hazards to people living or working in buildings constructed on those sites.

EPA officials and staff members of the Colorado Department of Health had confirmed 15 sites of excessive radiation emission in Denver. Nearly 100 Denver residents had been found to work in areas where gamma radiation exceeded acceptable limits. The Colorado Department of Health was conducting tests on the individuals involved.

One Denver brick and tile company was asked to tear down or move two buildings to allow the removal of a radium dump.

Although Denver was the immediate focal point of the Energy Department, EPA and local concern, it was believed that radium deposits were located in Chicago, Baltimore, New Jersey, Pennsylvania and New York City.

A-Weapons & Tests

The testing of nuclear weapons is said to increase the incidence of cancer by spreading carcinogenic radiation for great distances from the test sites. Contamination with cancer-causing radiation is also reported to have been great at and near test sites. Almost any plant that produces nuclear weapons, it is charged, also produces cancer, almost as a by-product, both in the plant and its vicinity as well as in areas where radioactive products or wastes may be stored or shipped.

Nevada site contaminated. In a report made public Aug. 20, 1970, the Atomic Energy Commission disclosed that a 250-square-mile area of its Nevada A-testing site was contaminated with poisonous and radioactive plutonium 239.

The report, submitted in July to the White House Council on Environmental Quality, said the contamination had occurred in tests conducted in 1958 to determine whether the crash of a U.S. bomber could trigger a nuclear explosion.

Large parts of the contaminated zone, which constituted one-fifth of the AEC's Nevada test area, were reported Aug. 20 to have been sealed off to the public. An AEC spokesman said, however, that health hazards could result only if the plutonium was stirred up into the atmosphere by a wind to pollute the air.

The report revealed that one out of every 12 underground atomic tests carried out since the 1963 treaty banning atmospheric tests had leaked some radioactivity "off site," but the amount was said to be one-tenth of the public exposure level considered safe by the Federal Radiation Council.

AEC tests to resume. Officials of the Atomic Energy Commission declared May 14, 1971 that underground tests at the test site in Nevada would resume "in early June," following suspension of all tests during investigation of the circumstances that caused a test Dec. 18, 1970 to expel a radioactive cloud.

The AEC report said the venting of radioactivity in the Dec. 18 test, code-named Baneberry, had been caused "primarily by the earth around the explosive device being more saturated with water than had been anticipated." Test resumption was approved "under more stringent and detailed technical analysis and review procedures," including "a closer examination of the geology of test locations."

The tests were resumed June 16.

In a related development, the Swedish government delivered a memorandum April 30 to the U.S. embassy in Stockholm declaring that an increase in radioactivity over Sweden in December 1968 could be attributed to a U.S. underground nuclear test Dec. 8, 1968. The note said the test was in violation of the 1963 treaty limiting the release of test radioactivity across national borders. An AEC spokesman replied April 30 that of some 30 underground tests conducted by the U.S. in 1968 only one had caused a "very small amount of radiation" offsite.

U.S. explodes H-bomb under Amchitka. The most powerful underground nuclear test conducted by the U.S. was executed Nov. 6, 1971 on the Alaskan island of Amchitka in the Aleutians, five hours after the Supreme Court denied a last-minute appeal by environmental and antiwar groups for a temporary injunction.

The test, code-named Cannikin, was conducted in the face of strong opposition from Canada, Japan, some U.S. senators and thousands of U.S. citizens, all of whom feared possible adverse ecological consequences. However, the major earthquake and tidal wave feared by test opponents failed to materialize, and the AEC reported no trace of radioactive leakage.

The five megaton blast (equivalent to a force of 5 million tons of TNT) was detonated at 5 p.m. (EST) in a 54-foot wide chamber at the bottom of a 6,000 foot hole on Amchitka. It caused a ground side roll on Amchitka and on the island of Adak, 190 miles away from the test area.

AEC Chairman James R. Schlesinger said the explosion had recorded 7 on the Richter scale, with the effects "well within the range of projections." (Major earthquakes record magnitudes of 7 or more on the Richter scale).

A petition signed by 12 leading American scientists, including three Nobel Prize winners, had urged Nixon Nov. 5 to delay the test to allow "full public and Congressional debate on the issue" before a final decision was made.

Supreme Court bars delay—Meeting in special session to hear oral arguments for and against the test, the Supreme Court Nov. 6 voted 4–3 against a temporary injunction. A last-minute brief filed Nov. 4 by the Committee for Nuclear Responsibility Inc. and seven other environmental, antiwar and American Indian groups had asked for at least a week's postponement of the test to hear their contention that the AEC had downplayed the test's environmental risks in violation of the 1969 National Environmental Act.

Conference urges A-test ban. A call for a halt to all tests of nuclear weapons, "especially those carried out in the atmosphere," was approved June 12, 1972 by a committee representing all nations attending the World Conference on the Human Environment in Stockholm. The vote was 48–2, with France and China dissenting and 14 nations, including the U.S. and Great Britain, abstaining.

Approval of the recommendation, introduced by Peru and New Zealand, came amid protests in Stockholm and several foreign nations against an imminent French nuclear test in the South Pacific. Nevertheless, a French spokesman said June 12 that his country would not consider itself bound by the conference vote, since it was simply a recommendation with which France disagreed.

Colorado A-blast tests for natural gas. Three 30-kiloton (equal to 90,000 tons of TNT) nuclear devices stacked in a steel well casing were detonated simultaneously May 17, 1973 more than a mile below the Piceance Creek basin in Rio Blanco County, in northwest Colorado.

The blast, in the AEC's Plowshare Program for developing peaceful uses of atomic energy, was aimed at breaking up sandstone formations in an effort to release natural gas trapped deep underground. It was the third such experiment in Plowshare's gas stimulation program.

AEC officials said initial checks after

the blast indicated there had been no above-ground radiation leakage.

The experiment, called Project Rio Blanco, was jointly sponsored by the AEC and the CER Geonuclear Corp., a private Las Vegas concern.

Environmentalists had attempted to halt the test with a suit charging it might contaminate water underground, fracture oil-bearing shale layers and produce gas that would be much more radioactive than normal gas. Colorado District Court Judge Henry E. Santo had rejected the arguments May 14 and authorized the AEC to proceed with the test.

Opponents of the blast were concerned that exploitation of the gas deposits in the Piceance Creek area would require an estimated total of 140-280 nuclear blasts, while 5,600-12,620 tests would be required to fully develop the gas fields under the combined area of Wyoming, Utah, Arizona, New Mexico and Colorado. Three hundred trillion cubic feet of gas were believed trapped in the five-state region.

A-bomb test link to cancer probed. A possible link between radiation fallout from a 1957 nuclear bomb test in Yucca Flats, Nev. and several cases of leukemia among soldiers who witnessed the blast was under study Dec. 1, 1977 by a coalition of government agencies. The National Center for Disease Control had initiated the study in April after two Army veterans who had contracted leukemia, Donald Coe, 44, and Paul Cooper, 43, filed disability claims against the U.S. They charged that their illnesses had resulted from the 44-kiloton explosion, code-named "Smokey."

The Pentagon Aug. 31 had supplied the CDC with a list of the 3,153 persons who had been issued film badges—regulation-required devices used to measure each person's degree of radiation exposure at an atomic bomb test. According to Dr. Glyn G. Caldwell, deputy chief of the center's cancer branch, 432 of those present had been located. Two cases of leukemia had been "definitely" linked to the 1957 blast and four other possible leukemia victims would "probably" be associated with the explosion, Caldwell said Dec. 13.

A House subcommittee held hearings Jan. 24 and 24, 1978 on the health effects of atomic tests on troops who had been near the test sites. It was told by scientists that the radiation exposure had led to cases of leukemia. Members of the panel—the health and environment subcommittee of the Interstate and Foreign Commerce Committee—criticized the Defense Department for failing to adequately monitor the later health records of those who attended the tests.

A Defense Department official told the subcommittee Jan. 25 that the Pentagon would make a major effort to put together the records of persons who had been exposed to the atomic blasts or their fallout.

An estimated 300,000 persons—military and civilian—had been exposed to radiation from 307 test explosions in Nevada and the Pacific between 1945 and 1962, the Washington Post reported Feb. 15.

The Defense Department Feb. 9 opened a toll-free telephone number in an effort to help contact people who had participated in the nuclear tests. The Pentagon Feb. 27 said that nearly 13,000 people had called in to report they had been present at one or more tests, and that 241 of those said they had cancer.

The Pentagon said it did not know whether 241 cases represented a normal or abnormal incidence of cancer for that group of people. There was no breakdown of the 241 cases into types of cancer, the Pentagon said.

A-test vet wins case—The Veterans Administration's Board of Veterans Appeals ruled Aug. 1, 1978 that a veteran who had developed leukemia some 20 years after he was exposed to radiation in the course of his military service had a service-related disability. The precedent-setting decision entitled Donald C. Coe to a higher pension than he was currently receiving.

Coe, a resident of Tompkinsville, Ky., had taken part in maneuvers conducted in 1957 at the Nevada site of a nuclear test a few hours after an explosion.

The appeals board decided that it was "reasonably probable" that the radiation Coe was exposed to then was a "competent causative factor" of the cancer that appeared 13 years after Coe retired from the Army.

The ruling was expected to lead other veterans to apply for increased benefits. About 2,400 former servicemen who had participated in similar maneuvers had reported recently to the Defense Department that they suffered from leukemia or some other form of cancer.

HEW confirms leukemia result—Government sources agreed early in 1979 that soldiers apparently had suffered the claimed effects from A-testing.

A study by the Department of Health, Education and Welfare confirmed that twice as many leukemia cases as expected had developed in ex-GIs exposed to low-level radiation while participating in a 1957 nuclear weapons test nicknamed Smoky, it was reported Jan. 29. And on Feb. 1, the Washington Post reported that a draft report of a scientific study by a Defense Department contractor concluded that soldiers at the Smoky test might have received twice the external radiation to their bodies that was shown by film badges worn at the time.

A-risk notice required—The U.S. Third Circuit Court of Appeals ruled Feb. 9, 1979 that government officials could be forced to notify servicemen of medical risks resulting from exposure to a nuclear bomb test in 1953.

But the appeals court upheld a federal district court ruling that the government was not financially liable for medical care of any soldiers affected by that exposure.

The ruling came in the case of Stanley Jaffee, a New Jersey pharmacist, who contended that he developed inoperable breast cancer as a result of his being required as a serviceman to witness an atomic test at Desert Rock, Nev.

The appeals court said that while the Army and other agencies might not have been aware of the dangers of radiation at the time of the test, they had become aware and "had failed to act" in warning exposed soldiers.

In refusing Jaffe's demand for government-provided medical care for his condition, the court cited the doctrine of "sovereign immunity," which protected the government and its officials from being sued without their consent. (A lower court had held that Jaffe lacked the standing to bring a class action, but had left open the question of whether he could seek individual damages from military officers for failing to warn him of the hazards of nuclear radiation.)

The Supreme Court May 21 upheld the appeals court decision by refusing to review it.

Low-Order Tests Planned—Declassified government documents revealed that the Nevada Test Site was never planned to be anything more than a facility for "a few relatively low-order detonations" and "only in event of an emergency," the Las Vegas Sun reported Dec. 18, 1978.

The Sun quoted Atomic Energy Commission Chairman David Lilienthal as saying that Gen. Dwight Eisenhower "strongly opposed" locating a nuclear testing facility in the U.S. during a June 1947 National Security Council meeting with President Harry S Truman present.

Truman ordered the go-ahead for a continental nuclear facility in November 1950, faced with the "emergency" of the Korean conflict. He approved the Nevada site in December 1950, before the Army Corps of Engineers had completed its studies on radiological safety factors.

Background—A Senate report provided data on soldiers involved in A-weapons tests:

> Beginning in 1945, and continuing until the Limited Test Ban Treaty is 1963, the United States exploded some 235 nuclear weapons in atmospheric tests. The Department of Defense (DOD) has recently estimated that approximately 250,000 DOD personnel participated in the testing program and that some 200,000 of these were uniformed personnel. Most of those persons were subsequently discharged from the Armed Forces and are thus veterans.
>
> The testing was heaviest in the mid-1950's. At certain tests, 3,000 to 4,000 troops were positioned near blast sites. On occasion, volunteer service personnel were placed in open

trenches as close as 2,000 yards to ground zero, and at one test six volunteers stood at ground zero under an air burst some 20,000 feet above them. At other tests, units were marched or taken by helicopter to ground zero after the explosion and put through simulated combat maneuvers to test their psychological and military responses to what had just occurred. Film badges and dosimeters intended to monitor individual radiation exposures were sometimes provided to only one individual in a unit rather than to each individual. Variations in the accuracy of monitoring techniques are known to have existed, and some types of radiation were not measured at all.

In the Committee's view, it is important to remember that this testing occured immediately following the use of atomic weapons during World War II and during the height of the Korean conflict and the "Cold War." During that period of great international tension, there was overwhelming national concern about the possibility of the United States being forced to use nuclear weapons. National security considerations were of paramount importance. Safety standards were generally set in accordance with the scientific knowledge of the day, which tended to minimize the risk of disability resulting from exposure to low levels of radiation...

The long-term health effects of exposure to "low levels" of ionizing radiation are not yet completely understood. It is clear that ionizing radiation causes an increased incidence of malignant tumors and can cause genetic damage. What is unclear is how much increased risk is caused by exposure to levels of radiation that are not "massive". It is also recognized that there is a long interval —the "latent period"—between radiation exposure and the subsequent development of malignancies. Without a clear scientific basis in fact, the issue of just compensation for conditions that develop in individuals who have been exposed to relatively low levels of ionizing radiation is a highly complex one.

Current national statistics indicate that approximately 62,500 of the 250,000 DOD personnel who participated in the nuclear weapons test program would be expected to develop some form of cancer during their lifetimes because of "natural" causes, and, of that number, some 40,000 would be expected to die of some form of cancer. At present, it is not possible to distinguish malignancies caused by radation from those caused by other hazards of "natural" causes. This further complicates the difficult factual context of the claims process. Thus, it is currently impossible to find a way to compensate only those individuals who develop cancer as a direct result of radiation exposure while serving the Armed Forces.

In recent years, the VA has received more than 600 claims for benefits from veterans who were nuclear weapons test participants and their survivors. Fewer than twenty claims have been granted for radiation-induced illness related to weapons testing. The claims process has clearly been made more difficult by problems caused by incomplete or missing records, documents that may be or have been classified, or records that are unavailable because of destruction in the 1973 fire at the St. Louis National Personnel Records Center.

A-test cancer link ignored. The Washington Post reported Jan. 8, 1979 that federal health officials had evidence as early as 1965 that excessive leukemia deaths were occurring among Utah residents exposed to radioactive fallout from atomic bomb tests at the Nevada Proving Grounds.

The evidence was in an unpublished study that was conducted by Edward S. Weiss and dated Sept. 14, 1965. The study was requested by the Post and obtained from the government under the Freedom of Information Act.

The U.S. Public Health Service, which ordered the study, apparently ignored its findings and withheld the report, which cited the cancer victims' "extended residence" in the area.

Officials of the Department of Health, Education and Welfare (HEW) were described Jan. 8 as "horrified" to learn from the Post request that an unpublished study existed.

HEW Secretary Joseph A. Califano ordered a search of federal health files for any other studies on adverse effects on health in Utah, it was reported.

Weiss said a week before the Post story appeared that his study found 28 leukemia deaths from 1950 to 1964 in the southwest Utah counties of Washington and Iron. Weiss said he had calculated that among the 20,000 residents only 19 cases should have occurred.

Weiss said the possibility of a link between the deaths and radioactive fallout should have been investigated further in 1965. But government documents revealed that Atomic Energy Commission officials had criticized the study, citing its relatively few cases of leukemia.

The AEC had refused to investigate the 1953 deaths of nearly 4,300 sheep after nuclear bomb tests in Nevada or to investigate the possibility of radiation damage to humans, Utah officials said Feb. 14.

Some 400 documents, most of them from the federal government, were released by Utah Gov. Scott M. Matheson's radiation committee.

The documents, discovered in the state archives in 1978, showed that Utah ranchers placed 18,000 sheep on winter grazing land in Lincoln County, Nev., near the Nevada Proving Grounds. When the sheep returned to Utah in the spring of 1953, ranchers noted that many were sick and dying.

Despite evidence of high radiation exposure, the AEC concluded in late 1953 that radiation had not caused the deaths.

Matheson said it had to be assumed that the radiation exposure levels for the sheep, up to 1,000 times the maximum amount of radioactive iodine allowed for humans, corresponded to those for humans in the area at the time of the tests.

Also on Feb. 14, the Deseret News (Salt Lake City) disclosed a study by Dr. Joseph Lyon, co-director of the Utah Cancer Registry, that concluded that children born in southern Utah in the 1950s, when the tests were held, died of leukemia at a rate 2½ times higher than the rate of those born before or after.

The News quoted Dr. Lyon as reporting that from 15 to 20 children died of cancer who would not have died if the tests had not been held. He refused to comment on the study Feb. 14.

Claims filed—Former Interior Secretary Stewart L. Udall and other lawyers filed 447 claims against the Energy Department between September 1978 and February 1979 in demands for hundreds of millions of dollars in damages for persons who said they or their relatives had contracted cancer or leukemia as a result of nuclear weapons testing.

The persons involved claimed that "negligent testing" from 1950 to 1966, failure to warn citizens of the hazards and other government shortcomings had "resulted in damage, injury and death."

In all, from 1951 until 1963, eighty-four above-ground nuclear devices were detonated at the Nevada Test Site (originally named the Nevada Proving Grounds), north of Las Vegas.

An Atomic Energy Commission publication during the period described persons living near the site as "active participants in the nation's atomic test program."

In 1955 the AEC wrote local residents: "At times, some of you have been exposed to potential risks from flash or fallout. You have accepted the risk without fuss, without alarm, without panic."

The claims were filed on behalf of residents of Utah, Nevada and Arizona.

Cancer high near weapons plant. Rep. Ted Weiss (D, N.Y.) discussed in the House of Representatives April 10, 1979 reports of high cancer rates in Colorado near a nuclear weapons plant. He said in a statement in the Congressional Record:

> A study conducted by Dr. Carl Johnson, county health director in Jefferson County, Colo., found that people living downwind from the atomic weapons plant in Rocky Flats, Colo., have substantially higher rates of cancer than other Colorado residents who are not exposed to the plant's plutonium emissions.
>
> Men living up to 13 miles downwind from Rocky Flats had a testicular cancer rate 140 percent higher than the norm for Denver-area men who do not reside within the plant's emission radius. Overall cancer rates—for both men and women—in the vicinity of the plant were 24 percent higher for males and 10 percent higher for females, according to the study.
>
> It is crucial to note, Mr. Speaker, that these findings directly contradict a 1977 environmental impact statement prepared by the former Energy Research and Development Administration. The ERDA report said the plutonium emissions from Rocky Flats had the potential to cause only one cancer death and one genetic defect among the 1.6 million people in the Denver area. But the Johnson study found that there have already been 501 unexpected cancer deaths downwind from the nuclear armaments plant.

Other Radiation Problems

Low-Level Radiation Risks Seen. A government study group said in a report released Feb. 27, 1979 that low level radiation might be more harmful than previously believed.

The White House Interagency Task Force on Ionizing Radiation advised Americans to be wary of exposure. But the group said more scientific research was needed to settle the issue.

Critics of federal radiation policy had contended that permissible levels of radiation exposure had been set too high, endangering the health of the public and nuclear industry workers.

Joseph A. Califano Jr., secretary of health, education and welfare, in releasing the report, promised to expand HEW's research into radiation. He also said HEW would move to reduce "unnecessary" human exposure to medical equipment such as X-ray and body-scanner machines.

Radiation exposure was associated with several types of cancer. But because it often took 20 to 30 years for many radiation-caused cancers to develop, there had been little data on the risks of low-level exposure.

A-Plant Communities Studied. A Pennsylvania State University survey released March 17, 1979 suggested that people living near atomic plants had little fear that the plants would hurt area property values. The study was prepared for the Nuclear Regulatory Commission.

The communities studied were within a 20-mile radius of Plymouth, Mass., Water ford, Conn., Oyster Creek, N.J., and Ontario, N.Y., all near the sites of atomic plants.

Hays Gamble, associate director of Penn State's Institute for Research on Land and Water Resources, said: "Judging from the fact that even the value of houses within view of a nuclear plant did not decline, most people in these areas apparently have little fear about health and safety."

Gamble added: "If many people really were worried, they wouldn't choose to live near a nuclear plant, and this would be reflected in the real estate market."

Researchers found in the four locations that a nuclear plant did not affect the sale prices of one-family homes within 20 miles, but appeared to spur growth because of lower taxes for residents.

Radioactive Leaks at Plants. The staff of the Nuclear Regulatory Commission (NCR) reported May 2, 1979 that at least 15 A-power stations had problems with coolant water pipes that leaked small amounts of radioactive water.

According to the NRC staff, six of the plants had extensive corrosion or cracking in pipes that carry radioactive water. The six were Surry No. 1 and No. 2 at Gravel Neck, Va.; Turkey Point No. 1 and No. 2 in Florida; San Onofre in California and the Palisades plant in Michigan.

The staff said nine plants had moderate or minor cracking: Millstone No. 2 in Connecticut; R. E. Ginna and Indian Point No. 1, both in New York; Point Beach No. 1 and No. 2 in Wisconsin; Maine Yankee; St. Lucie in Florida; Connecticut Yankee, and H. B. Robinson in South Carolina.

NRC staff member Darrell Eisenhut said the problem stemmed from a chemical reaction in the plants' steam generators, which caused pipes that were part of the primary cooling system to crack under the pressure of the corrosive buildup.

As a temporary solution, Eisenhut said, plants had been plugging pipes that developed leaks. At some of the plants as many as one-fourth of the pipes were out of use, he said.

Henry Kendall, a physicist at the Massachusetts Institute of Technology, said the leaks were a major unresolved safety issue. He claimed that under certain circumstances, the leaks could result in the blockage of water from the emergency system cooling the reactor core and lead to a serious accident.

Dispute over Radiation's Hazards. Rep. Edward P. Beard (D, R.I.) noted in a statement in the Congressional Record June 6, 1979 that in Congressional "attempts to reach a definitive basis for the consideration of radiation as an occupational hazard, we found a morass of conflicting opinions. . . ." He said:

Unlike any other occupational hazard, radiation effects cannot be seen by X-rays or any other diagnostic tool. It is possible for physicians to diagnose carcinoma, lung diseases, skin effects, and other disabilities caused by specific agents used in the workplace, but not radiation in humans. What is known is that low-level exposure to radiation can cause injury to cell structure, blood composition, bone marrow and other organs but science has not yet been able to pinpoint the specific cause of, say, pancreatic cancer as definitely due to radiation exposure. Despite this, certain standards for exposure to ionizing radiation in the workplace have been established and are supposed to be enforced by the Nuclear Regulatory Agency. I say "supposed to be" because, as we have recently seen in the case of the incident at Three-Mile Island in Pennsylvania, there is already enough evidence to show that many NRC regulations as to safety and health were not observed there and in other NRC-licensed installations. Testimony at our hearings reveals that there are serious radiation problems not being dealt with properly in the mines and mills that produce and refine uranium ore. Other testimony points to NRC rules and regulations being bent to suit particular situations. Most of the testimony offered by Government departments seems to be designed to protect the current operation of existing nuclear plants and to downgrade the hazards of occupational exposure to radiation. Even the National Cancer Institute bases its view of radiation hazards on an exercise in mathematical probability rather than even considering the extensive researches of responsible, independent scientists into the lives of thousands of workers who have been employed in nuclear reactor plants.

In addition to the hazards of ionizing radiation, there is no question that millions of workers are exposed every day in the workplace to a variety of radiation emanating from devices that make use of microwaves, extremely short radio waves, in such operations as heat-sealing, communication, melting, cooking and military applications. The microwave oven is the best-known instrument using these extremely high frequencies and from the testimony I have heard, the radiation levels set by the Food and Drug Administration are, at best, a guess at what the highest permissible level should be.

I do not believe there is any acceptable number of cancer deaths due to the fact that we need nuclear power. I do not subscribe to the philosophy of the nuclear-power industry that radiation is a hazard in the same class as fire or electricity. I do not believe that there is any acceptable mathematical computation that tells us x number of people are going to die of radiation-induced cancer as long as we have standards that are not realistic, Government agencies that are devoted to promoting nuclear power no matter what the consequences and public and industry officials who have resigned themselves to death and disability caused by radiation.

Rep. John W. Wydler said in a statement in the Congressional Record June 11 that "our dynamic society is shackling itself" to "the myth that nuclear energy presents unusual dangers from radiation." Wydler asserted that "nuclear energy results in less radiation exposure to the public than energy from coal and far less than from natural gas." He continued:

We, and our forefathers, have always lived immersed in a sea of natural radiation. It showers down upon us from the sky, is emitted from atoms in our own bodies, and is emitted by the soils below us and stones around us in our buildings. The fact that it is emitted by the soils and stones is the key to understanding the radiation exposures from coal. Although it is primarily carbon, coal is typical of other rocks and soils by containing minute quantiites of the radioactive elements uranium and thorium. Even though there are only a very few radioactive atoms for every million atoms of carbon, 1 million tons of coal are consumed each year in a single powerplant. That means that the tons of uranium and thorium contained in the coal are removed from their underground protection for humans and brought to the surface of the Earth. A small fraction is emitted by the smokestacks and settles down among us, producing a surface film of these radioactive elements on the Earth.

This surface film of radioactive elements from coal energy sounds frightening. But actually, radiation doses from coal or nuclear energy are among the least of the various radiation doses we all unavoidably receive. Coal energy results in an average of 0.1 millirem dose per year to the general public—the term millirem is a unit of radiation dose. Nuclear energy results in an average of one-third this dose. These small exposures should be compared to the approximately 100-millirem minimum dose received from a chest X-ray, or individually received each year from the unavoidable cosmic rays, body-generated radiation, and terrestrial radiation that I have mentioned. While remembering that radiation exposures from coal and nuclear energy are minute, we should recognize that the average radiation dose to the public from a single full-size powerplant is greater when it is coal-fired than when it is nuclear.

Although radiation from any source of energy is small, let us turn to the energy source that results in the far largest radiation exposures. This is natural gas. Natural gas originates underground in regions containing radon, which emits radiation. Radon is a gaseous daughter element of radium. Radon flows along in the natural gas pipes, but is not burned by the pilot lights and burners of the unvented cooking stoves in homes. Only part of the population has natural-gas stoves, but the average dose to the Nation is 10 millirem per year from this source. We see that natural gas results in a hundred times greater radiation dose to the public than coal, and still greater than from nuclear. Yet the doses from this highest-radiation energy source, natural gas, is less than one-tenth of the radiation dose that the public receives from natural sources.

In being objective, we must remember that radiation doses from energy are among the least of the man-caused doses. Radiation from the healing arts, principally medical X-rays, results in a national average of about 85 millirem per year, which is many times more than even from the high-radiation natural gas. So also is the increased radiation exposure from living in brick or stone houses, rather than wood. The bricks or stones contain the radiation-producing uranium and thorium. Normally, residency in brick houses adds about 50 millirem per year doses, but some of our very massive stone buildings here on Capitol Hill add much more.

We see that energy production is a small part of the radiation doses we receive and that nuclear is among the least of these. But this is a narrow view of the hazards from energy. The real concern about fatalities from the normal day in, day out, production of energy is actually about the pulmonary ailments from the nitrogen oxides and sulfur oxides from burning of fossil fuels, principally coal. A full-size coal-fired plant results in over a dozen, generally unidentified, deaths per year largely from this cause. In contrast, a nuclear plant might result in a single death from all causes in perhaps 2 years of operation. When all is considered, coal-powered electricity steadily kills, but nuclear rarely does.

THREE MILE ISLAND

Particularly in the aftermath of the Three Mile Island incident, it is appropriate to consider radiation exposures from accidents at nuclear plants. We accurately know the radiation doses from that accident, where now-corrected plant inadequacies resulted in very substantial releases of radioactive gases from within the reactor. As I recently explained, we well understand the effects of radiation. Thus we know that perhaps one unidentifiable person might get cancer from this radiation release. This was a bad radiation release, hopefully not to be repeated. The Congress now has the opportunity to know the harm to the public from a nuclear accident, particularly compared to the harm from properly operating energy alternatives. Perhaps one fatality will eventually result from the radiation released during the worst 3 days of the Three Mile Island accident, but gaseous emissions from the Nation's coal-fired plants during these same days will result in scores of fatalities. Thus, during these days, overwhelmingly more fatalities resulted from coal-plant normal operations than from this worst of nuclear accidents. Yet, ironically, news media were quiet about coal, but deluged us with frightening nuclear coverage.

Other Dangers

Danger in Pesticides

By the time 1970 ended, the use of the pesticide DDT (dichloro-diphenyl trichloroethane) had been virtually banned in the U.S. as a result of some eight years of controversy largely spurred by the late Rachel Carson in her prophetic book "Silent Spring." Controversy continued, however, over balancing DDT's undoubted beneficial effects against the equally undoubted harm it had done and could continue to do.

DDT pro & con. Some of the major arguments against DDT were summarized by Rep. Edward I. Koch (D, N.Y.) Feb. 20, 1970 in a letter to Harry W. Hays, director of the Agricultural Research Service's Pesticides Regulation Division. Koch wrote:

"... The implications of DDT for human health and environmental safety necessitate a complete ban on its use with the well-defined exception that in potential catastrophic insect infestation that would pose an imminent threat of human health disaster, widespread destruction of agricultural areas or extensive damage to a natural resource, DDT could be used for short periods of time in the event that no other less persistent insecticide was available in sufficient quantities....

"Available scientific findings have established that DDT is a potential cancer-producing agent. Some of these findings include the following:

"(1) As far back as 1947 the Food & Drug Administration found increased incidences of liver tumors in rats which were fed DDT.

"(2) On May 1, 1969, the National Cancer Institute reported that DDT added to the diet of mice quadrupled the frequency of tumors in the liver, lungs, and lymphoid organs.

"(3) Hungarian scientists reported similar findings concerning the relationship of DDT and the development of tumors and leukemia. A recent University of Miami Medical School study revealed that the bodies of persons who died of cancer contained more than twice the DDT concentration as persons who died of accidental causes.

"(4) We know that the DDT concentration in mothers' milk has been found to be more than twice as great as the concentration permitted in cow's milk sold for public consumption.

"DDT has polluted our waterways, contaminating fish which are later consumed as food. Persistent chemicals have been carried down rivers and streams into the lakes and oceans of the world. ...

"Effective and economical alternatives for pest control have been developed. The USDA presently lists effective alternatives for DDT for virtually every crop of which this most persistent pesticide is presently used...."

Attack on DDT. Michigan April 16, 1969 became the first state to ban the sale of DDT (dichloro-diphenyl trichloroethan). (The use of the controversial pesticide had been banned in Sweden in March and in Denmark in June.)

The Michigan Agriculture Commission decision barred licenses to chemical companies wanting to distribute DDT-bearing products. The commission, which had halted the sale of DDT for mosquito control in 1968, announced a limited ban on the use of DDT June 18. It said it had canceled DDT registrations except for control of mice, bats and body lice by professional applicators and by government officials for public health purposes.

In a 90-0 vote July 18, the Wisconsin Assembly voted to ban the sale and use of DDT in all but emergency situations, which would be declared as such by a three-member emergency board.

Jerry W. Fielder, California Agriculture Department director, had announced June 12 that the state would ban DDT and another long-lived pesticide, DDD, from homes and gardens beginning Jan. 1, 1970. He said: "We know no reliable evidence that these pesticides are directly harmful to man, but they do represent a hazard to man's natural environment, including fish and wildlife."

In a communication released July 9, Sen. Gaylord Nelson (D, Wis.) urged Secretary of Agriculture Clifford M. Hardin to order a national ban on aerial "dusting" with DDT and by any means in areas close to water. This should be a step toward the complete banning of DDT, Nelson said.

The U.S. Department of Agriculture announced July 9 that it had suspended the use of nine long-lasting pesticides, including DDT, in its pest-control programs pending a 30-day review. The nine pesticides belonged to the man-made family of chlorinated hydrocarbons, which were distinctive for their longevity and toxicity. (One of the most controversial pesticides suspended was dieldrin, which had been used at 56 civilian and military airports to avert insect infestation by airplanes from abroad.)

The federal Food & Drug Administration (FDA) in March had seized 28,150 pounds of Lake Michigan coho salmon, which had been brought from Oregon a few years previously. According to various reports, the salmon contained between 12 and 30 parts per million of DDT residues. The FDA had recommended permitting no more than 3.5 parts per million in fish shipped in interstate commerce. But the FDA announced April 22 that it had limited the permissible amount of DDT residue in fish shipped interstate to 5 parts per million.

Secretary of Health, Education & Welfare Robert H. Finch had announced April 21 that he had appointed a Commission on Pesticides & Their Relationship to Environmental Health to make a study of pesticides and their effect on humans. Dr. Emil M. Mrak, chancellor of the University of California at Davis, was named to head the commission. Finch said that "each American body" already had 12 parts per million of DDT in its fatty tissue. While the average daily U.S. individual consumption of DDT was only .7 of a milligram, or one-tenth of the maximum daily consumption the U.N. Food & Health Organization had called permissible, Finch pointed out that no amount was desirable.

Dr. M. G. Candau, director general of the U.N. World Health Organization (WHO), warned July 9 against restricting DDT in countries where the elimination of insect-born diseases was of major importance. He said: "We must not forget the enormous benefits insecticides have brought to humanity. . . . The record of the safety of DDT to man has been outstanding in the last 20 years, and its low cost makes it irreplaceable in public health at the present time."

DDT phaseout ordered—The Nixon Administration Nov. 20, 1969 ordered the use of DDT in residential areas ended within 30 days. It also decreed a virtual halt to the use of DDT elsewhere by 1971.

The plan to restrict DDT had been drawn up by the Department of Agriculture and the Department of Health, Education and Welfare (HEW). HEW Secretary Robert H. Finch had revealed the government's plan to curb the use of DDT Nov. 12.

The phaseout was ordered by Secretary of Agriculture Clifford M. Hardin following a meeting of the Environmental Quality Council at the White House. The immediate effect of the order would be to reduce the use of DDT by about one-third almost immediately.

A science adviser to President Nixon projected that the ban would "mean the end of 90 per cent or more of the DDT now in use."

U.S.S.R. bans DDT production—The Soviet Union said May 1, 1970 that it had banned production of DDT and was taking steps to restrict the use of other pesticides blamed for the killing of some rare wildlife.

In a letter printed in the newspaper Komsomolskaya Pravda in response to criticism leveled by the newspaper, the Ministry of Agriculture said "starting in 1970, it is forbidden to produce preparations of DDT for the protection of food and fodder crops."

Attack on other chemicals. Testifying before the New York State Environmental Health Subcommittee July 9, 1969, Dr. James T. Grace, director of Roswell Park Memorial Institute, said that research conducted by the institute indicated that certain chlorinated hydrocarbons, including DDT and several other pesticides, "clearly" produced cancerous tumors in mice. Although Grace did not directly link his research with cancer in humans, he said that lack of knowledge of cause and effect itself was a rational ground for caution in the use of "potent compounds with potent effects which are persistent and whose build-up becomes concentrated."

The Washington Post reported Aug. 4 that the FDA was making a survey of the pesticide level in grapes being sold in the U.S. The survey was a result of an Aug. 1 allegation by a California grape union spokesman that certain grapes contained the pesticide Alrin at 180 times the level judged safe for consumption.

President Nixon's science adviser, Lee A. DuBridge, announced Oct. 29 that a widely used herbicide, 2, 4, 5-T, would be restricted because of its potential harmful effects. DuBridge said the herbicide, used in Vietnam and the U.S., would be limited to areas remote from population and that the Agriculture Department would cancel registrations of 2, 4, 5-T for food crops beginning Jan. 1, 1970 unless the Food and Drug Administration had discovered a safe tolerance in and on foods.

It was reported later that 2,4,5-T and similar pesticides contained dioxin (TCDD, or tetra-chloro-dibenzo-dioxin), a suspected carcinogen, as an unavoidable contaminant.

Federal agencies moved April 15, 1970 to end the use of 2,4,5-T to kill weeds around homes, lakes and ponds and on food crops. The Defense Department simultaneously announced that the use of "agent orange"—a defoliant composed of 2,4,5-T and a related pesticide 2,4-D—was being suspended in Vietnam.

In separate announcements, the Agriculture, Health, Education & Welfare and Interior Departments said registration of 2,4,5-T in its liquid form would be suspended, making interstate sales illegal. According to the announcements, the action was taken because it was felt that the herbicide posed "imminent danger" to women of child-bearing years due to findings that it may produce "abnormal development in unborn animals." Non-liquid forms of the herbicide were ruled a potential hazard for use around the home or on food crops, but sales would not be banned until hearings and possible appeals could be completed.

None of the actions affected the uses of the herbicide on range, pasture, forest and other nonagricultural lands. Such uses accounted for most of the 2,4,5-T sold in the U.S.

The Defense Department said it would rely entirely on "agent white"—

composed of 2,4-D and a Dow Chemical Co. pesticide, picloram—to spray sparsely populated areas in Vietnam. The use of both "agent white" and "agent orange" had already been restricted to areas remote from the population.

The White House Dec. 26 announced plans for "rapid phase-out" of herbicide operations in South Vietnam. The order said "use of herbicides in Vietnam will be restricted to the perimeter of firebases and United States installations or remote unpopulated areas."

The White House said the directive would bring into line the policies governing the use of herbicides in Vietnam with the regulations controlling the domestic use of plant-killing agents.

The defoliation program in Vietnam was nearly 10 years old. During 1970, the armed forces in Vietnam had restricted herbicide operations that were aimed at destroying rice crops and heavy jungle foliage where enemy troops could hide.

EPA retreats on herbicide. The Environmental Protection Agency said June 24, 1974 that because of insufficient evidence of potential harm to humans, it would not press legal motions to ban the herbicide 2,4,5-T, widely used domestically and, according to some evidence, the possible cause of deaths following defoliation operations in South Vietnam.

The EPA said its legal challenges were being withdrawn because after more than three years of research, it had found that unreliable analytical techniques were being used.

According to an EPA spokesman, the study of 2,4,5-T and dioxin, one of its highly toxic components, would not be abandoned but resumed later using more reliable methods. Although dioxin was known to be toxic to laboratory animals, the minimum level at which it was believed harmful to humans was too low for conventional environmental measurements. The spokesman said that before legal action was taken against a suspected substance, it was standard EPA practice to establish that the substance was not only toxic in laboratory tests but also persisted in the environment in appreciable quantities and reached animals and humans.

Tainted chickens ordered killed. The Environmental Protection Agency (EPA) March 23, 1974 ordered the destruction of chickens found by the Agriculture Department to be contaminated with Dieldrin, an insecticide known to induce cancer in high concentrations.

While the Agriculture Department had first estimated that as many as 20 million birds were contaminated, the EPA lowered the maximum estimate to eight million, and after additional testing, the EPA said March 25 that the destruction might involve no more than two million, all grown by five Mississippi operators. Officials said it was unlikely that contaminated chickens had been marketed.

The Agriculture Department had detected the contamination during testing in late February; some chickens, the department said, showed concentrations of three parts per million, 10 times the maximum set by the EPA. Traces of Dieldrin had been found in vegetable fats used in chicken feed mixtures, it was reported March 28.

James O. Eastland and John C. Stennis, Mississippi's Democratic senators, introduced legislation March 26 to provide federal compensation to poultry producers whose products were kept from the market, and supplemental benefits to workers temporarily unemployed by plant closings.

4 more pesticides banned. The Environmental Protection Agency moved July 30, 1974 to ban the pesticides chlordane and heptachlor, which had been found to cause cancer in laboratory animals. EPA Administrator Russell Train said the human cancer hazard from the pesticides was "made even more alarming by evidence that human exposure begins in the mother's womb and continues without interruption throughout life."

The pesticides were used extensively for home, lawn and garden purposes and in agriculture on corn. Velsicol Chemical Corp. of Chicago, a subsidiary of Northwest Industries Inc., was the sole U.S. manufacturer.

Residue of the pesticides had been found in food and human milk, and in the organs of 10 infants stillborn in two Atlanta hospitals, the EPA noted. Both pesticides were chlorinated hydrocarbons which were not broken down in the environment and which could be passed up the food chain from animal to man.

Stocks in stores and homes would not be recalled, because of the impracticality, Train said, and he cautioned against unwise disposal. Either use it according to directions, he said, or bury it at least 18 inches underground away from any water source or wrap it and put it in the trash. He minimized the economic impact because there were many substitutes for the two pesticides.

Velsicol chairman and president Robert M. Morris said July 30 the sales of the pesticides were minor when compared with total sales and the company's concern was about "the loss of these valuable products to the agricultural community." They had been in use for "over 25 years without evidence of cancer or, when properly used, any other danger to man," he said. He criticized the ban as "a bureaucratic decision, not a scientific one."

The final order banning the pesticides' use for most purposes was issued by the EPA Dec. 24, 1974.

Citing evidence that two other pesticides, Aldrin and Dieldrin, could also cause cancer, the EPA Oct. 1 had ordered an immediate ban on further production for most uses.

The order allowed continued sale and use of existing stocks, a procedure which the EPA said would be safer than shipment to a disposal site. The order also exempted three minor uses of the pesticides: deep-ground insertion for termite control, root and top treatment for non-food plants and certain types of moth-proofing where escape into the environment would be unlikely.

The major uses (more than 90%)—insect protection for corn, citrus trees, onions and a few minor crops—would be banned.

Kepone case. Allied Chemical Corp. was fined $13.3 million Oct. 5, 1976 for polluting the James River with the toxic insecticide Kepone. Allied had pleaded no contest to 940 counts of violating federal water pollution control laws. Kepone had been found to be a carcinogen, in animals at least, and was said to cause a variety of ailments in human beings.

A fine of $3.8 million was assessed against Life Science Products Co., the now-defunct Kepone producer. Life Science had pleaded no contest to 154 charges of violating the federal pollution laws and to a conspiracy count.

The two owners of Life Science, William P. Moore and Virgil A. Hundtofte, who also had pleaded no contest, were given suspended five-year jail sentences by U.S. District Court Judge Robert R. Merhige Jr. Each was also fined $25,000 on one count and was given a suspended $25,000 fine on additional pollution charges.

The $13.3 million fine was the largest fine on record for violation of federal environmental standards, but Merhige reduced the fine Feb. 1, 1977 to $5 million.

The reduction was made after the company declared, in a hearing before Merhige on Jan. 28, that it would establish an $8-million nonprofit endowment fund for Virginia. The fund would be used to clean up pollution of the James River resulting from Kepone production.

Merhige previously had dismissed all criminal charges against Allied Chemical in the Kepone case.

Workers suffer Kepone poisoning—In the Kepone case, more than half the 110 workers at Life Science Products Co. in Hopewell, Va. were found to have high levels of Kepone in their blood. Some 28 were hospitalized, including the wife of an employe, with symptoms such as uncontrollable trembling, memory loss and possible sterility. Kepone also had been found to cause a significant increase in liver cancer in test animals.

The Kepone, an ant and roach pesticide, was processed by Life Science for Allied Chemical Corp. Life Science operated for 16 months before it was closed in July, 1975, the day after a visit from a state epidemiologist and the hospitalization of seven workers on the spot.

EPA head Train said Feb. 26 that Virginia officials had reported finding Kepone traces in fish in Chesapeake Bay and one of its tributaries, the James River, on which Hopewell was situated.

Train also disclosed Feb. 26 that small amounts of Kepone had been found in breast milk of some women—in nine of 298 samples—in Georgia, North Carolina and Alabama.

The source of this Kepone was related to Mirex, a chemical made by Allied Chemical and used as bait to kill fire ants. There was evidence Mirex broke down under direct sunlight and moisture into traces of Kepone. Some 100 million acres in nine Southern states had been treated with Mirex under an Agriculture Department fire-ant eradication program under way since 1962. Production of Mirex was suspended in July 1975, then discontinued.

DBCP curb. The EPA Sept. 19, 1978 proposed permanent restrictions on the use of DBCP, a pesticide found to cause sterility among workers and cancer in laboratory animals.

The restrictions were similar to those put into temporary effect in 1977.

The use of DBCP, or dibromochloropropane, would be barred outright in 19 food crops.

The pesticide would be permitted to be used on certain crops but only under strict conditions. The crops included soybeans, cotton, ornamental plants, grass and citrus and other fruits, such as peaches, grapes and pineapples.

Application in these cases would have to be by commercial personnel or specially trained workers wearing protective clothes and respirators.

The pesticide was no longer made in the U.S. but certain companies had been given permission to sell it, with the proper warning labels, for limited uses.

Environmental Developments

The widespread and rapid growth of pollution of every kind became increasingly obvious and a matter of developing concern during the closing years of the 1960s. This situation spurred action on all levels in 1969 and the first years of the 1970s. On the federal level, President Richard M. Nixon stressed a determination to control environmental pollution as he addressed Americans on "the summons" of the 1970s. A pressing issue in the pollution situation was the growing realization that many of the pollutants were causes of cancer.

Anti-pollution council. A cabinet-level advisory panel to combat environmental pollution was established by executive order of President Nixon May 29, 1969. Nixon, who would serve as chairman of the panel—the Environmental Quality Council—said the new group would function as a "focal point" of efforts to preserve "the availability of good air and good water, of open space and even quiet neighborhoods."

Vice President Spiro T. Agnew became vice chairman of the council, Dr. Lee A. DuBridge, the President's science adviser, its executive secretary. Other members were the Secretaries of Agriculture; Commerce; Health, Education and Welfare; Housing and Urban Development; Interior; and Transportation.

(The council was renamed the Cabinet Committee on the Environment Jan. 29, 1970.)

Environmental policy measure. In his first formal statement of 1970, President Nixon Jan. 1 stressed the urgency of mounting an effort against environmental pollution. The 1970s, he said, "absolutely must be the years when America pays its debt to the past by reclaiming the purity of its air, its waters and our living environment. It is literally now or never."

Nixon issued the statement as he signed the National Environmental Policy Act, which allowed establishment of a three-member Council on Environmental Quality that the President intended to have "occupy the same close advisory relation to the President that the Council of Economic Advisers does in fiscal and monetary matters."

The legislation (S1075) had been passed by the Senate Dec. 20 and the House Dec. 23, 1969.

Nixon Jan. 29 named Russel E. Train, 52, undersecretary of the interior and a leading conservationist, as chairman of the newly established Council on Environmental Quality. The President also appointed to the council Robert Cahn, 52, a Washington correspondent for the Christian Science Monitor whose series for the newspaper on national parks won a 1969 Pulitzer Prize, and Gordon J. F. MacDonald, 40, vice chancellor for research and graduate affairs at the University of California at Santa Barbara and chairman-designate of the Environmental Studies Board of the National Academy of Science.

The President said the council would develop and coordinate federal environmental programs and policies and would see that all federal activities "take environmental considerations into account." He also noted that the Cabinet Environmental Quality Council would be renamed the Cabinet Committee on the Environment.

State of the Union. President Nixon put before the Congress and the nation Jan. 22, 1970 the challenge of "perfecting" America. In his first State of the Union Message, delivered before a joint session of Congress, Nixon called the challenge "the summons" of the 1970s, when the moment had arrived "to harness the vast energies and abundance of this land to the creation of a new American experience" reflecting more "the goodness and grace of the human spirit."

The major focus of the address was on domestic problems, mainly on environmental pollution.

"In the next 10 years we shall increase our wealth by 50%," he said, but "the profound question is: Does this mean we will be 50% richer in a real sense . . .?" Or would it mean that in the coming decade 70% of the population would live "in metropolitan areas choked by traffic, suffocated by smog, poisoned by water, deafened by noise and terrorized by crime?" "Shall we surrender to our surroundings," he asked, "or shall we make our peace with nature and begin to make reparations for the damage we have done to our air, to our land and to our water."

Comprehensive new regulations were required, he said, to salvage the nation's air and water. "We can no longer afford to consider air and water common property, free to be abused by anyone without regard to the consequences," he declared. ". . . To the extent possible, the price of goods should be made to include the costs of producing and disposing of them without damage to the environment."

Democratic response—In response to the environmental proposals announced in the State of the Union message, Sen. Edmund S. Muskie (Me.) Jan. 23 presented a Democratic legislative program to bring pollution under control. Muskie, chairman of the Senate Subcommittee on Air and Water Pollution and author of most of the antipollution legislation currently enacted, said the "rhetoric of concern" in President Nixon's address was "excellent" but that Mr. Nixon's concern for environmental problems would be judged "in the last analysis" on Administration programs proposed and money requested.

Muskie's own antipollution program called for $15.5 billion in federal spending over the next five years to be matched by at least an equal outlay in state and municipal funds in addition to large contributions from private industry. The program, outlined at the news conference in Washington, D.C., included some legislation already in committee and other proposals to be introduced.

The senator called for $12.5 billion as the federal contribution to a $25 billion five-year program to control water pollution. Other proposals included appropriations to improve air quality and to provide solid waste disposal and noise abatement programs.

Administration organizes. A variety of actions were taken by Nixon Administration officials in January 1970:

■Secretary of State William P. Rogers announced Jan. 13 the creation of an Office of Environmental Affairs within his department to be headed by Christian A. Herter Jr., son of the former secretary of state. Rogers said Herter would be his special assistant for environmental affairs. Rogers said the appointment marked the Nixon Administration's recognition that environmental problems were international in scope.

■A study board of the National Academy of Sciences recommended Jan. 21 that a board of environmental affairs be set up within the President's office to direct the battle against pollution at a high government level. The panel made eight other recommendations in what was described as a "background paper . . . to provide a basis on which the board will make recommendations for effective approaches and institutional mechanisms for dealing with environmental problems."

Nixon seeks compliance & cooperation. President Nixon acted in early February 1970 to get federal compliance and political cooperation with anti-pollution efforts:

■Nixon issued an executive order Feb. 4 directing all federal agencies to comply with state water and air pollution standards by the end of 1972. In a statement accompanying the order, the President pledged $359 million to help the agencies eliminate pollution caused by federal projects and installations. The order provided for the establishment of strict federal pollution standards for a government installation if the state standards were nonexistent or too lenient.

■President Nixon Feb. 6 asked for an end to "sterile discussions" between Republicans and Democrats "as to who really deserves the credit for discovering the issue of dealing with pollution." The President said that the problem demanded the cooperation of the federal and state governments, both parties and private individuals. Nixon made his remarks in Chicago where he had gathered members of his Administration for a meeting of the Cabinet Committee on Environment.

President's message to Congress. In his first special message to Congress in 1970, President Nixon Feb. 10 presented a program to improve the nation's environment by controlling water and air pollution, improving means for disposing of solid wastes, increasing park and recreational facilities and coordinating federal and private industry programs that deal with environmental problems.

President Nixon proposed that the federal government assume more responsibility for establishing and enforcing national standards for clean water and air. He asked for precise water quality standards to control pollution of the nation's waterways by municipal or industrial waste. He also proposed that the federal government establish national air quality standards and require states to prepare plans within one year to meet those standards.

Specific requests Nixon proposed a $10 billion program to build municipal waste treatment plants and asked Congress to authorize $4 billion in fiscal 1971 to cover the federal share in funding the program, to be allocated at a rate of $1 billion a year for the next four years.

To deal with automobile pollution, the President asked Congress to authorize the secretary of health, education and welfare to regulate fuel composition and additives.

The President recommended that Congress extend and broaden the 1965 Solid Waste Disposal Act, which was to expire in 1970.

Environment quality act. An Environmental Quality Improvement Act of 1970 became law April 3, 1970, as President Nixon signed it. The measure provided for the creation of an Office of Environmental Quality in the Executive Office of the President.

The new agency's duties would be to provide the professional and administrative staff for the Council on Environmental

Quality and to work with the federal agencies and departments in all matters affecting environmental quality.

State action. State officials and agencies, through statements and actions taken throughout 1970, displayed their concern over the pollution issue.

A number of state governors stressed environmental problems in messages to legislatures. Gov. Ronald Reagan (R, Calif.) told the California Legislature in Sacramento Jan. 6 that "the good life will be no good at all if our air is too dirty to breathe, our water too polluted to use, our surroundings too noisy and our land too cluttered and littered to allow us to live decently." He proposed a program Jan. 22 that would "provide the teeth needed" to enforce the state's "already tough controls on smog." Gov. Nelson A. Rockefeller (R, N.Y.), in his annual message to the state legislature in Albany Jan. 7, urged the creation of a new department of environmental conservation that would combine the conservation and pollution control responsibilities of a number of New York agencies.

In Vermont, the legislature adopted several environmental control bills April 5 that had been requested by Gov. Deane C. Davis. The legislation was designed to curb stream and river pollution and control the use of pesticides.

Governors of 17 Southern and border states joined May 7 to form the Southern Regional Environmental Conservation Council, which would work out multistate compacts and agreements to fight pollution. The council, largely the work of Gov. Winthrop Rockefeller (R, Ark.) and Gov. Arch A. Moore Jr. (R, W. Va.), was planned as an arm of the Southern Governors Conference.

Don S. Smith of Little Rock, Rockefeller's representative on the council, said May 9 that one of the group's first concerns would be to persuade Washington to enact an "umbrella compact" that would authorize states to work out specific ecological problems by entering into multistate agreements.

Illinois Gov. Richard B. Ogilvie, in St. Charles, Ill. for a nationwide meeting of state attorneys general, signed an environmental protection bill June 29 that he called the most comprehensive in the nation. The law, presented at the St. Charles meeting as a model for other states, set up three Illinois agencies to protect the environment—one with enforcement and investigative duties, one to set pollution standards and regulations and a third to act as a research and advisory unit. The act gave the state attorney general authority to seek broad court rulings against polluters and abolished special exemptions to pollution regulations granted by localities.

Michigan Gov. William G. Milliken July 27 signed a law permitting Michigan citizens to file antipollution suits against industries, state agencies or other citizens. Milliken said Michigan was the only state with a law to assure citizens legal standing in court to bring such suits, and he urged governors of other states to support similar legislation.

Milliken signed a companion bill Aug. 26 to monitor and regulate waste discharge into Michigan waters. The bill required industries to file annual reports on potentially hazardous waste discharges and set up a fee schedule to be paid by businesses under surveillance for pollution.

Ballots in 12 states in Nov. 3 elections included environmental proposals, mostly antipollution bond issues. Of 20 measures on the ballots, only four propositions were defeated.

Bonds to finance sewage treatment and other antipollution programs were approved in Alaska ($11 million), California ($250 million), Illinois ($750 million) and Washington ($25 million). Florida voters authorized increased bond insurance to finance sewage facilities.

"Environmental bill of rights" constitutional amendments were approved in Rhode Island and Virginia.

Industrial council formed. President Nixon, by executive order April 9, 1970, established a National Industrial Pollution Control Council to advise him and the Council on Environmental Quality "on

Curbing Dangers in the Air

Industries, power plants, furnaces, incinerators—these and other so-called "stationary sources" add enormously to the pollution of the air. In highly industrialized areas, such pollution can quite literally make breathing hazardous to health, and can cause unforeseen atmospheric and meteorological problems as well.

Increasingly, industry itself has been adopting ambitious pollution-control programs, and state and local authorities have been setting and enforcing stricter anti-pollution standards. But they have not gone far enough or fast enough, nor, to be realistic about it, will they be able to without the strongest possible Federal backing. Without effective government standards, industrial firms that spend the necessary money for pollution control may find themselves at a serious economic disadvantage as against their less conscientious competitors. And without effective Federal standards, states and communities that require such controls find themselves at a similar disadvantage in attracting industry, against more permissive rivals. Air is no respecter of political boundaries: a community that sets and enforces strict standards may still find its air polluted from sources in another community or another state.

. . .

—*I propose that designation of interstate air quality control regions continue at an accelerated rate, to provide a framework for establishing compatible abatement plans in interstate areas.*

—*I propose that the Federal government establish national emissions standards for facilities that emit pollutants extremely hazardous to health, and for selected classes of new facilities which could be major contributors to air pollution.*

In the first instance, national standards are needed to guarantee the earliest possible elimination of certain air pollutants which are clear health hazards even in minute quantities. In the second instance, national standards will ensure that advanced abatement technology is used in constructing the new facilities, and that levels of air quality are maintained in the face of industrial expansion. . . .

—From President Nixon's special environmental message to Congress Feb. 10, 1970.

programs of industry relating to the quality of the environment."

Nixon appointed Bert S. Cross, chairman of the board and chief executive officer of the Minnesota Mining & Manufacturing Co., as chairman of the new industrial council. Willard F. Rockwell Jr., chairman of the board and president of North American Rockwell Co., was named vice chairman.

New agency created. President Nixon, in a message to Congress July 9, 1970, proposed that most federal pollution control functions be united in one independent agency, to be called the Environmental Protection Agency (EPA). In a major reorganization of government units dealing with the environment, the President also proposed creation of a National Oceanic and Atmospheric Administration (NOAA) to provide "a unified approach to the problems of the oceans and atmosphere."

The EPA and NOAA became government agencies after the Oct. 2 deadline for Congressional veto of Nixon's reorganization proposal had passed with neither house of Congress vetoing the plans. No veto effort was made in the Senate, and a disapproval resolution in the House was rejected Sept. 28 by voice vote.

Stating that the government's "environmentally related activities have grown up piecemeal over the years" and that "the time has come to organize them rationally and systematically," Nixon July 9 had offered the plans under his executive reorganization authority.

Senate confirms EPA director. The Senate confirmed the nomination of William D. Ruckelshaus as director of the new Environmental Protection Agency by voice vote Dec. 2, 1970, the same day that the agency began operations. Ruckelshaus, formerly an assistant attorney general in the Justice Department's civil division, had been named by President Nixon to head the EPA Nov. 6, and the nomination was submitted to the Senate Nov. 16.

Pollution control costs projected. The President's Council on Environmental Quality, in its second annual report to Congress, said Aug. 6, 1971 that it would cost at least $105 billion to meet 1975 pollution control standards. The report, which said the investment would save higher costs in health care and damage to the environment, said the expense was "well within the capacity of the American economy to absorb."

President Nixon was less optimistic in a letter accompanying the report. He warned against seeking "ecological perfection at the cost of bankrupting the very taxpaying enterprises which pay for the social advance the nation seeks." He asked for a realistic approach to environmental problems and—citing the effects of pollution abatement on jobs, prices and foreign trade—said the question of "how clean is clean enough can only be answered in terms of how much we are willing to pay and how soon we seek success."

Russell E. Train, chairman of the council, told a press conference that industry's pollution control costs would be "far lower than the normal wage increases we deal with each year, lower than the costs of occupational health and safety, social security and other things we've built into the economy over the years."

The council said the main economic problems would be transitional, resulting from the closing of smaller and older plants. But it said, "to say that environmental controls will hurt business and industry is to confuse the interests of existing firms with the health of commerce as a whole."

The council's 360-page report said estimating costs of environmental controls was "hazardous" since evidence of pollution costs was "rudimentary" and estimates of control costs depended upon standards not yet set and techniques still being developed. The council estimated that air pollution alone probably cost the nation $16 billion a year in health costs, damage to crops and trees and in lowered property values.

The estimated $105 billion in pollution control costs through 1975 broke down to $23.7 billion for air pollution control,

$38 billion for water and $43.5 billion for solid waste.

Gerald R. Ford became President of the U.S. Aug. 9, 1974. Six days later, in his first major pronouncement on ecological issues, he asserted that there must be a compromise between the nation's economic and energy needs and environmental considerations.

Ford scores no-growth approach. In his first environmental policy message, President Ford said Aug. 15 that the "zero economic growth" approach to conserving natural resources "flies in the face of human nature" and must be compromised to meet economic and energy needs.

Ford's message was delivered at the Expo '74 fair in Spokane, Wash. by Interior Secretary Rogers C. B. Morton.

Ford said the previous winter's energy crisis had demonstrated the need for more coal mining, offshore oil exploration, oil shale development and nuclear power plant construction.

Rejecting the zero-growth argument that economic expansion and a clean environment were inconsistent, Ford said expansion was necessary to rebuild cities, improve transportation systems, generate employment and fund important environmental programs already under way.

Ford contended that meeting energy needs did not mean "that we are changing our unalterable course to improve the environment, and it doesn't mean that we are retreating or giving up the fight." He added, however, that "it does mean stretching the timetable in some cases," adjusting some long-range goals "to accommodate the needs of the immediate present," and some "trade-offs."

Ford noted that in the last five years the U.S. had launched "the greatest environmental clean-up in history," but that the energy situation had added a "critical new element in the environmental equation." Full energy production would "entail environmental costs or risks of one kind or another," Ford said, "but we must all be prepared to bear those costs."

High costs seen. In its fifth annual report, submitted Dec. 12, 1974, the White House Council on Environmental Quality (CEQ) estimated overall national expenditures for pollution control would total $325 billion during 1973–1982, more than $50 billion above the estimate of costs during the 1972–1981 decade.

According to the report, prospective expenditures for pollution control efforts attributable only to federal laws would total $194.8 billion for the 1973–1982 decade, including both capital and operating costs. This would represent a cost of about $80 a citizen by 1976, or about 2% of the average family income, the council said. The $80 figure was about double the 1973 level.

The higher cost findings were attributed to inflation, revised estimates of equipment needs and movement into a higher cost period in the abatement program.

Despite the higher cost estimates, the CEQ said costs "still are not expected to have any significant general economic impact" on growth, inflation or unemployment. The report also stated that "a rigid linkage between energy growth and economic growth is no longer accepted as self-evident."

In the report, President Ford said the nation cannot "achieve all our environmental and all our energy and economic goals at the same time," but he called for a "balance" between them and rejected "the extremes."

According to CEQ Chairman Russell W. Peterson, the nation had made only "modest advances" in slowing increasing air pollution that accompanied population and industrial growth between 1940 and 1970.

Pollution down, costs up. The White House Council on Environmental Quality Feb. 27, 1976 issued a report to Congress recognizing a decline in pollution of air and water in the U.S. The report increased its estimate of the cost of federally mandated pollution abatement to $217.7 billion for the decade 1974–83.

The council reported a limited water clean-up—"an improving trend" toward fewer illegal discharges and a decline in the number of monitored areas adjudged to have "very poor" and "severe" water quality problems. The report noted that polluting runoffs of pesticides and other foreign ingredients into waterways had been difficult to control.

After a substantial rise in air pollutant emissions from 1940 to 1970, the council reported, particulate matter had subsided since 1970 29%, sulphur dioxide 8%, carbon monoxide 12% and hydrocarbons 5%. A 10% increase in nitrogen oxide emissions—from cars, electric power plants and factories—was reported for the period 1970 to 1975.

The council said California continued to have the most severe car pollution problems.

The report stressed the environmental link to cancer. It estimated that from 60% to 90% of cancer came from environmental causes, such as exposure to chemicals in workplaces, cigarette smoking and solar and cosmic radiations.

In warning about possible chemical contamination of the environment, the council said "the sheer number of chemical compounds, the diversity of their use and the adverse effects already encountered from some make it increasingly probable that the chemical contaminants in our environment have become a significant determinant of human health and life expectancy."

Jimmy Carter was sworn in as President of the U.S. Jan. 20, 1977. In its early actions and statements on the pollution issue, the Carter Administration seemed to steer a center course.

Scientists' report criticizes EPA. A scientific appraisal of the Environmental Protection Agency March 21, 1977 found it lacking in legislative guidance and scientific expertise.

The report, released by the National Academy of Sciences, said the agency was "dependent on the industries it regulates for much of the technical and economic information it uses in decision making." The report called for more scientific input in the agency's operations.

The report also charged that there were "significant gaps in environmental monitoring" done by the EPA and that the agency lacked speed and flexibility in moving against violators of environmental regulations.

The study did not fault the agency's attempt to carry out the wishes of Congress but found that many obstacles interfered with the EPA's mission.

Diet & Nutrition

Danger in improper diet? Dr. Arthur Upton, director of the National Cancer Institute, testified before the Senate Agriculture Committee's Subcommittee on Nutrition Oct. 2, 1979 that, tentatively, there seemed to be reason to to suspect that improper diet could increase the danger of cancer. He said:

> Although no direct cause-effect relationship has been observed for nutrition and cancer in humans, numerous scientific studies suggest that dietary factors may affect the risk of the disease. Because many other variables also influence the occurrence of cancer, the exact role that diet plays remains unclear. The National Cancer Institute has undertaken a number of activities to explore the role of diet in the causation of cancer, but until definitive results of such studies become available, only tentative inferences are possible. Based on the incomplete evidence now at hand, the following would appear to be prudent interim principles:
>
> In general, excessive body-weight should be avoided by maintaining a balance between caloric intake and proper exercise. The appropriate balance should be determined by each person in consultation with his or her physician, depending on body build and medical status.
>
> To facilitate control of body weight, and in view of the suggestive association between fat consumption and the risk of cancer, a high intake of fat should be avoided.
>
> A generous intake of dietary fiber would seem prudent, based on the reduced incidence of bowel cancer in human populations and experimental animals that has been associated under certain conditions with a high intake of dietary fiber.
>
> In addition to providing the minimal daily requirements of vitamins, minerals, fatty acids, and protein, the diet should be well balanced, including ample fresh fruits and

vegetables. Such a diet, on the basis of present knowledge would not ordinarily be expected to require supplementation with additional minerals, vitamins, or other factors.

Alcoholic beverages should be consumed only in moderation, in view of the high correlation between heavy alcohol consumption and an increased risk of certain types of cancer.

. . .

Diseases of the intestines, including appendicitis, diverticulosis, colonic polyps and colon cancer have been noted to occur with relatively low frequency in populations ingesting large amounts of fiber. These populations are usually found in less industrialized countries. When individual differences have been investigated between geographic areas, a high fiber intake has been correlated with larger, softer stools, more frequent defecation, and more rapid intestinal transit times. It has been theorized that these effects could result in a decreased duration of exposure of the colonic mucosa to carcinogens in the feces, as well as a relative decrease in the concentration of such carcinogens in the feces.

With the epidemiologic data as a basis, a number of researchers began investigating the fiber-cancer correlation in the laboratory. In one such study, rats were previously treated with a digestive tract carcinogen and then fed different amounts of cellulose. Those rats fed the least amount of fiber developed more intestinal tumors. In addition, the observed number of tumors decreased with the increase in dietary bulk. In other studies, increased dietary fiber resulted in a decrease in mutagenic activity in human feces.

Possible effects of dietary fiber on the enterohepatic circulation of bile salts may also occur. Since bile salts and fat degradation products have been implicated as colon carcinogens, binding or dilution of these by fiber may be of significance.

. . .

A theory, currently held by many cancer investigators is that the increase in cancer rates observed in animals on high-caloric diets may be due to the increase in fat in the diet rather than to the increase in total food consumption. A recent series of experiments showed that rats fed diets containing unsaturated fatty acids, like those found in olive oil and sunflower oil, had a greater number of cancers than those fed more saturated types of fat, such as butter and coconut oil. In human populations, both breast cancers and colon cancers have generally been associated with the level of consumption of animal fat, which is mainly saturated.

Several theories to explain the mode of action of dietary fat in carcinogenesis have been suggested in recent years. The most widely held is that fat in the diet has a "promotional" effect on the development of cancer. In other words, it does not cause cancer directly but somehow influences metabolic processes of normal cells to make them more susceptible to the development of cancer caused by other agents. It has also been proposed that fat—whether unsaturated or saturated—may act as a solvent to enhance the effect of other carcinogens. Fats also are known to change the metabolism of many tissues in humans, possibly affecting the relation of various hormones to tissue growth. The case for this is strongest for breast cancer, where hormonal environment has been shown to influence susceptibility to cancer.

Breast cancer strikes more women in the United States, Canada and Western Europe than any other form of cancer. Yet it is comparatively rare throughout the developing world. Some scientists have suggested that the fat content of today's diet in the industrialized countries alters the body's balance of sex hormones, which in some as yet undetermined way increases susceptibility to breast cancer.

Although Japanese women living in Japan seldom develop breast cancer, their risk of the disease increases when they move to the United States. Likewise, some populations within the U.S. have lower breast cancer rates. The Seventh Day Adventists are an example. One thing that the native Japanese and the Adventists have in common is a 20 to 50 percent less intake of fat in their diet than the general population of the United States.

Research on the initiation of mammary cancer in animals has supported this association. Despite differences in type or quality of fat or various elements of experimental design, scientists have found consistently that a high intake of dietary fat increased the development of mammary cancer in rodents.

. . .

Cancer of the colon and rectum accounts for some 15 percent of the total cancer burden in the United States, and is second only to lung cancer in the number of deaths each year. Like breast cancer, colo-rectal cancer is much more common in the developed Western countries than in less developed areas of the world, and the high levels of fat in the Western diet may conceivably be a factor. Some investigators have postulated that the low levels of fiber in the Western diet may also be important.

Current research indicates that a diet high in fat increases the amounts of bile acids and sterols excreted during digestion. These normal breakdown products may conceivably be converted into carcinogens by bacteria which are normally present in the colon.

. . .

Lean or underfed animals have been found to have a decreased incidence of spontaneous and induced tumors, as compared with normally fed controls. Recently, an expert panel convened by the American Society of Clinical Nutrition and the Association of American Physicians concluded that obesity increases the risk of death from heart disease and cancer; however, the panel noted that few controlled studies have been done on human populations, and that it is too early to establish a definite correlation between total caloric intake and the risk of developing cancer. Several studies have shown a relationship between obesity and at least two forms of cancer in women: cancer of the breast and cancer of the endometrium.

A number of substances that are mutagenic or carcinogenic for animals are present as natural constituents or contaminants of certain foods. Examples include safrole, various flavanoids, cycasin, and mycotoxins. The contribution of such substances to the human cancer burden remains to be determined. In general, ordinary foods have not been studied thoroughly for carcinogens.

There is no conclusive proof that alcohol alone causes cancer in either animals or humans. But scientific evidence strongly suggests that excessive intake of alcohol, especially in combination with smoking or dietary deficiencies, may lead to cancer.

A number of cancers are more prevalent among heavy alcohol drinkers, including cancers of the esophagus, mouth, throat, larynx and liver. Alcohol and tobacco are both well established as strong risk factors for cancers of the mouth and throat.

Among its other effects, alcohol is an irritant to the lining of the throat, esophagus and stomach. When combined with the physical and chemical insults of tobacco smoke, alcohol may promote abnormal cell proliferation at those sites. Nutritional and immunological deficiencies are commonly associated with or exacerbated by excess alcohol ingestion.

Index

A

ABBOTT Laboratories (Chicago)—84, 91
ABRAHAM, Carl—161, 169
ACRYLONITRILE (ACN)—35, 112-3
ACTH (adrenocorticotropic hormone)—126
ADAMO Wrecking Co. (Mich.)—24
AEROSALS & Ozone Threat—74-6
'AGENT orange' (2,4,5-T)—185-6
'AGENT white' (2,4-D)—185-6
AGNEW, Spiro T.—188
AGRICULTURE, Department of—91, 93-6, 110, 184-6
AIRCRAFT—46, 51, 70, 150. SST controversy—71-4
AIR Pollution—18-26, 33, 45, 191, 193-5. Aerosols & ozone threat—74-6. Aircraft—46, 51, 70-4; SST controversy—71-4. Auto-emission controls—43-50, 54, 59-61, 63-5, 70-1, 192, 195; catalyst controversy—49-50, 54-5, 59-60; truck exhausts—70-1. Cleanup progress—46-7, 55-61, 63, 66-70, 195. Energy crisis effect—55-60, 64-71, 194. Europe—64. Federal controls & trade-offs—43-63, 65-71, 75-6, 192-5. Penalties—70. Sulfur fuel & scrubbers—52, 55-8, 64-9. Transportation controls—47, 49, 56
AIR Quality Act (1967)—45
ALABAMA—15, 50, 53, 69, 188
ALASKA—175, 191
ALBERTO-Culver Co.—113
ALCOHOL & Alcoholism—112
ALDRIN—185, 187
ALLEN, Rep. Clifford (D, Tenn.)—153-4
ALLIED Chemical Corp.—13, 187-8
ALPHA-Naphthylamine—14
AMCHITKA (Aleutian Islands)—175
AMERICAN Apparel Manufacturers Association—36
AMERICAN Association for the Advancement of Science—107, 154
AMERICAN Brands, Inc.—105
AMERICAN Cancer Society—105, 108-9, 122, 137
AMERICAN Council of Life Insurance—110
AMERICAN Diabetes Association—84, 89
AMERICAN Electric Power System—55
AMERICAN Health Foundation—88
AMERICAN Heart Association—89
AMERICAN Home Products Corp. (N.Y.)—97
AMERICAN Iron & Steel Institute—53
AMERICAN Journal of Obstetrics & Gynecology—130-1
AMERICAN Medical Association (AMA)—111, 124
AMERICAN Medical Association, Journal of the—90, 103, 106-7, 125-7
AMERICAN Motors Corp.—61, 65
AMERICAN Petroleum Institute—35, 57, 68
AMERICAN Physical Society—150
AMERICAN Textile Manufacturers Institute—36
ANACONDA Co.—54
ANC (Acrylonitrile)—35, 112-3
ANDERSON, Gov. Forrest H. (Mont.)—54
ANDERSON, Dr. H. A.—10
ANDERSON Hospital & Tumor Institute, M.D., (Houston, Tex.)—137
ARIZONA—58, 125, 172, 179
ARIZONA Public Service Co.—58
ARKANSAS—191
ARMCO Steel Corp.—21
ARMY, Department of—176-9
ARSENIC—10, 12, 33
ASBESTOS—10, 12-3, 18-26
ASH, Roy L.—145
ATLANTA—23
ATLANTIC Richfield Hanford Co.—173
ATOMIC Energy Act (1954)—173
ATOMIC Energy Commission (AEC): A-waste disposal—171-4; leaks—172-3. A-weapons &

tests—174–6. Radiation hazards & reactor safety—139–42, 146–8; licensing—149; violations—147–8
ATOMIC Industrial Forum—143, 159
ATOMIC Scientist (magazine)—9
AUERBACH, Dr. Oscar—103, 105
AUSTIN, Tex.—171
AUSTRIA—64
AUTOMOBILES & Auto Industry: Antitrust suits—44. Emission controls—43–50, 54, 59–65, 70–1, 195; catalyst controversy—49–50, 54–5, 59–60. Gas economy & rationing—47–8, 59. Transportation controls—49, 56, 62. Truck exhaust controls—70–1
AYERST Laboratories—127–8
AYVAZIAN, Dr. L. Fred—126

B

BABCOCK & Wilcox—160, 164–6, 169
BAILAR 3rd, Dr. John—135
BALTIMORE—11, 148, 174
BALTIMORE Gas & Electric Co. (Calvert Cliffs, Md.)—148
BATES, Richard R.—80
BATTELLE Pacific Northwest-Laboratories—154
BAYLISS, David L.—10
BAYLOR School of Medicine—89
BAZELON, Judge David L.—152
BEARD, Rep. Edward P. (D, R.I.)—180–1
BEDFORD, Mass.—17
BEER—112–3
BENZENE—10, 34
BENZIDENE—14
BERNERO, Robert—167
BERTELL, Rosalie—167
BETA-napthylamine—12
BINGHAM, Dr. Eula—35
BIRMINGHAM, Ala.—53, 69
BIRMINGHAM, University (England)—154
BIRTH Control—132–4
BISCHLOROMENTHYL (BCME)—10, 32
BLACKMUN, Justice Harry A.—24
BLACKS—119–20
BLOKHIN, Dr. Nikolai N.—138
BOHANON, Judge Luther—124
BOSTON—23, 56, 133, 154–7
BOSTON Globe (newspaper)—154–7
BOWEN, Gov. Otis—125
BOWMAN, Ralph S.—124–5
BRADFORD, Robert W.—124–5
BRENNAN, Gov. Joseph E. (Me.)—112
BRENNAN Jr., Justice William J.—24
BRIDENBAUGH, Dale G.—150
BRIDGEPORT, Conn.—17
BRISTOL-Meyers Co.—113
BRITISH Aircraft Corp.—72
BRODEUR, Paul—19–20
BROGAN, John J.—44
BROOKHAVEN National Laboratory—64
BROWER, David—143
BROWN, Jr., Gov. Edmund G. (Calif.)—163–4, 166, 171
BROWN & Williamson Tobacco Corp.—105
BULLETIN of the Atomic Scientists (magazine)—4
BURGER, Chief Justice Warren E.—94
BURGESS, Anna—134
BURNEY, Dr. Leroy E.—103
BURNS, Gov. John A. (D, Hawaii)—47
BUTZ, Earl L.—95–6
BYRNE, Gov. Brendan—125

C

CADILLAC, Mich.—97–8
CAHN, Robert—189
CAIRNS, Thomas—82
CALDWELL, Dr. Glyn G.—176
CALIFANO Jr., Joseph A.—9, 23–4, 109, 111, 169, 178, 180
CALIFORNIA—17, 44, 47–8, 56, 58, 60–2, 98, 100, 106, 123–4, 141, 150–2, 163–4, 180, 184, 191
CALIFORNIA Medical Association—123
CALLAGHAN, James—74, 170
CALORIE Control Council—84
CANADA—21–2, 33, 84–5, 88–9, 96, 126, 173
CANDAU, Dr. M. G.—184
CAREY, Gov. Hugh L. (D, N.Y.)—26
CARSON, Rachel—183
CARTER, Jimmy—26–8, 37, 63–5, 74, 87, 163, 195
CEDAR River (Iowa)—29
CEMENTON, N.Y.—171
CENTER for the Study of Responsive Law—45, 91
CENTIFANTO, Dr. Ysolina M.—137
CER Geonuclear Corp.—176
CERTIFIED Color Manufacturers Association—94
CHAPMAN, Judge Robert F.—36–7
CHARLES City, Iowa—29
CHARLESTON, S.C.—98
CHARLESTON, W.Va.—98, 102
CHEMICAL & Atomic Workers International Union (AFL-CIO)—141
CHESAPEAKE Bay—188
CHICAGO—18, 49, 56, 60, 67, 126, 130, 149, 174
CHICAGO University—130
CHINA, People's Republic of—175
CHINA Syndrome, The (film)—162
CHLORDANE—186–7
CHLOROFORM—112
CHLOROPRENE—10
CHROMIUM—10, 12
CHRYSLER Corp.—44, 48, 61–2
CHURCH, Sen. Frank (D, Ida.)—171–2
CIGARETTE Smoking—1, 5, 7, 43, 88, 103–12, 195. Anti-smoking campaign—109-12. British report—105–6. Controls & controversy—103–10. Japanese report—106. Legislation—104. Surgeon General's report—103–4, 111
CIMARRON plutonium plant (Okla.)—158–9
CINCINNATI—100, 123
CINCINNATI University—123
CITIES: Air pollution—50–1; curbs—51, 53, 56, 62, 67–70; quality surveys—43, 69–70; transportation controls—49, 56, 62. Asbestos in drinking water—23. Auto-emissions controls—49, 60. Highest cancer death rates—11. Water supplies & contaminants—23, 98, 100
CIVIL Aeronautics Board—109
CLAIROL—113–4
CLEVELAND—11, 66, 70
CLEVELAND Electric Illuminating Co.—66–7

CLEAN Air Act (1970)—24, 46, 48–9, 51, 54, 56–7, 60, 62. (1977)—68
COAL—55–8, 64–9, 171, 181–2
COCA-Cola Co.—84–5
COE, Donald—176–7
COHEN, Wilbur J.—140
COKE Oven Emissions—33–4, 36
COLEMAN, William T.—73
COLORADO—50, 53–4, 98, 140, 172, 174
COLTON, Dr.—157
COLUMBIA, District of—43, 48, 50–1, 57, 112–3, 152
COLUMBIA University (N.Y.)—137, 146, 171
COLUMBUS, Ohio—66
COMMERCE, Department of—111–2
COMMONWEALTH Edison Co. (Ill.)—141, 148
CONCORDE (supersonic transport)—73
CONGRESS: Air pollution cleanup bill—45–6; auto-emission control delay–63; catalyst controversy—49–50; coal conversion—56–7. Anti-cancer drive—117–8. Anti-pollution policy—189, 193. Cigarette smoking—104. Dietary studies—195–7. FDA & experimental drugs—127–8. Food additives—71, 80–2; DES ban—94, 96; nitrites—93. Radiation & atomic power—139, 148, 150–1, 153–4, 157, 171, 181–2; A-tests—176–8; A-waste disposal problems—171–2; plutonium air transport curbed—150; Three Mile Island—161, 164, 166, 168–9. Toxic substances bill—17–8. Water quality bill—99–100
House of Representatives—81–2; 135; Agriculture Appropriations subcommittee—81; Commerce Subcommittee on Oversight & Investigations—26–7; Energy & the Environment, Interior subcommittee on—161; Environmental Quality, Council on—72; Government Operations, Committee on—83; Interior & Insular Affairs Committee—168
Senate—71–2, 80–1, 87–90, 96, 177–8; Energy, Nuclear Proliferation & Federal Services, Government Affairs subcommittee on—169; Environment subcommittee—15; Executive Reorganization & Government Research subcommittee—127–8; Health Committee—95; Human Resources Committee—166; Judiciary Committee—27; Monopoly subcommittee—132–3; Nutrition, subcommittee on—195–7; Nutrition & Human Needs, Select Committee on—71; Public Works Committee—46, 49–50; saccharin ban delayed—87–90; SST—71–2; Transportation subcommittee of the Appropriations Committee—72
CONNECTICUT—17, 50, 55, 60
CONNECTICUT Yankee nuclear power plant—180
CONSOLIDATED Coal Co. (Ohio)—66–7
CONSOLIDATED Edison Co.—56, 151–2
CONSUMER Products—2, 35–6. Dyes—93–4, 113–4. Hair dryer recall—26. Microwave ovens—181. Tris treated garments—35–6
CONSUMER Product Safety Commission (PSC)—26, 30, 37, 75–6, 107
CONSUMER Protection & Environmental Health Service—98–9
CONSUMERS Union—91
COOPER, John A.—80
CORNELY, Dr. Paul—119
COSMAIR Inc.—113
COSMETICS—31, 85, 94, 113–4
COSMETIC, Toiletry & Fragrance Association—113
COSTLE, Douglas M.—27, 63, 68, 70
COURTS: Air pollution—48–53, 58, 62–7, 69, 74. Antitrust suits—44. A-plants & radiation safety—140, 142–3, 146, 149, 158–9; NCR licensing process—152. A-tests—175, 177. Food additives: Nitrites—91; DES ban—95–6; Red dye no. 2 ban—94. Industrial & chemical hazards—21–2, 30–1; asbestos rulings—21–3; kepone case—187–8; water pollution—21–2, 101–2, 187–8. Medical treatment controversies—123–5, 129–30. PBB case—97–8. Plastic bottles challenged—112–3. Tris ban—36–7
CULVER, Sen. John C. (D, Ia.)—29
CUMBERLAND Packing Corp.—84
CYCLAMATES—83, 91

D

DACH, Leslie—136
DALTON, Mich.—29
DAVID Jr., Dr. Edward E.—115
DAVIS, Gov. Deane C. (Vt.)—191
DAVIS, Dr. Hugh J.—132–3
DAWES Laboratories, Inc. (Chicago)—97
DBCP (dibromochloropropane)—188
DDT (dichloro-diphenyl trichloroethane)—183–5
DECARBAZINE (DTIC)—125–6
DEFENSE, Department of—176–8, 185–6
De GUIRINGAUD, Louis—74
DELANEY, Rep. James J. (D, N.Y.)—71, 81, 85
DELAWARE—51, 125
DELUTH, Minn.—21–2
DENMARK—64, 170, 184
DENTISTRY—135
DENTON, Harold—163–7, 169
DENVER, Colo.—53–4, 70, 174
DEPO-Provera—134
DES (diethylstilbestrol)—94–7, 129–31, 133–4
DESERET News (Utah newspaper)—179
DETROIT—11, 48–9, 71
DEVITT, Judge Edward J.—22
DIABETES—84–6, 89–90
DIELDRIN—184, 186–7
DIET & Nutrition—195–7. See also FOOD & Food Additives
DIOXIN (TCDD)—185–6
DISTRICT of Columbia—43, 48, 50–1, 57, 112–3, 152
DJERASSI, Dr. Isaac—126
DMOCHOWSKI, Dr. Leon—137
DOCKING, Gov. Robert B. (Kan.)—172
DOW Chemical Co.—140, 186
DRESDEN nuclear power plant (Chicago)—141
DRINKING Water & Chemical Contaminants—17, 23, 29, 98–103. EPA filtration system proposal—102. Fluoridation—113. Industrial pollution cleanup costs—100–2

DRUGS—85, 123. Birth control pill—132–4. Blood pressure drug—136. Depo-Provera—134. DES & cancer in women—129–31, 133–4. Estrogen hormones—131–2. Medical treatment & research—See under 'M.' Psoriasis therapy—136. Red Dye No. 2—94. Sleep aids & nose sprays—136. See also specific drug
DTIC (imidazole carboxamide)—125–6
DuBRIDGE, Dr. Lee—43–4, 185, 188
DUKE University Medical Center—138
DURKIN, Sen. John (D, N.H.)—155
Du PONT de Nemours & Co., E.I.—10, 14, 30, 32
DUSTIN, Dr. Harriett—89
DYES—93–4, 113–4

E

EAST Germany (German Democratic Republic)—64
EASTLAND, James O.—186
EDELMAN, Harlan—125
EDWARDS, Dr. Charles C.—15, 71, 83, 95, 129, 133
EISENHOWER, Dwight D.—177
EISENHUT, Darrell—165, 180
ELI Lilly & Co.—130, 133
ELKINS, Charles L.—145
EMORY University (Atlanta)—137
ENERGY, Department of—69, 155–8, 173–4, 179
ENERGY Research & Development Administration (ERDA)—173, 179
ENERGY Supply & Environmental Coordination Act (1974)—56–7
ENRIGHT, Judge William B.—125
ENVIRONMENT, Cabinet Committee on the (U.S.)—188–9
ENVIRONMENTAL Defense Fund (EDF)—58, 91, 100, 113–4, 136
ENVIRONMENTAL Pollution:
Air pollution: aerosol & ozone threat—75–6; aircraft smoke curbs—46, 51, 70–4; auto emissions—46–50, 54, 56–65, 70–1, 195; Federal controls—43–50, 54, 59–61, 63–5, 70–1, 192, 195; sulfur fuel & scrubbers—52, 55–8, 64–9. Atomic worker exposure—139–46, 149, 151, 153–8, 180–1; low-level radiation study—154–7
Cancer incidence & death rate—4–14, 35, 43; animal tests & controversy—3–4, 82–9. Cigarette smoking—1, 5, 7, 43, 88, 103–12, 195. Consumer products—2, 26, 35–6, 93–4, 113–4, 181. Court actions—See COURTS
Diet & life style—5, 7, 195–7. Drinking water—17, 23, 29, 98–103, 113
Food additives—2, 7, 71, 77–91; nitrites—81, 91–3; Sweeteners—83–91. Food & chemical contaminants—See FOOD. Diet & Additives
Industrial wastes, occupational hazards & toxic substances—1–2, 4–5, 9–41; acrylonitrile—35; arsenic—33; asbestos—10, 12–3, 18–26; benzene curbed—34–5; cover-up charged—12–4; dump sites & water pollution—26–9, 99–103; inventory of chemicals rule—30; miners—4; most hazardous industries—10–1; occupational hazards—10, 30; PCBs—16–8; pesticides—13, 187–8, 195; plastics, dyes & fire-resistant fabrics manufacturing—10; vinyl chloride—31–3
ENVIRONMENTAL Protection Agency (EPA)—3, 193, 195. Air pollution curbs—45–7, 51–63, 66–8, 70; aerosol curbs—75–6; aircraft smoke curbs—70; auto emissions—46–8, 54, 56–61, 63, 65, 71; catalyst controversy—49–50, 59–60; SST—72; sulfur fuel & scrubbers—52, 58, 68–9; transportation controls—49, 56, 62; truck exhausts—70–1. A-power & radiation controls—141, 145–7, 149; waste disposal—172, 174
Industrial wastes & toxic substances—27–9, 31, 99; asbestos—18–26; drinking water—100–3; inventory of chemicals—30; PCB curbs—16–8; water pollution cleanup costs—100–1
Pesticides & herbicides—186–9
ENVIRONMENTAL Quality, Council on—69–70, 188–9, 193–5
ENVIRONMENTAL Quality Improvement Act—190–1
EPHRAIM McDowell Community Cancer Network (Lexington, Ky.)—121
EPSTEIN, Dr. Samuel S.—4, 9, 11
ERLEWINE, John—172
ESCONDIDO, Calif.—17
ESPOSITO, John C.—45
ETHYLENE Dibromide (EDB)—33
ETZWILER, Donnell—89
EUROPE—64
EVALUATION of Low Levels of Environmental Chemical Carcinogens, Ad Hoc Committee on the—71–81
EVANSVILLE, Ind.—100

F

FALK, Hans L.—80
FALLDIN, Thorbjorn—170
FEDERAL Aviation Administration—73
FEDERAL Bureau of Investigation (FBI)—158
FEDERAL Energy Administration (FEA)—56–7, 59
FEDERAL Radiation Council—141
FEDERAL Trade Commission—104–5
FEDERAL Water Pollution Control Act—101–2
FEDERATED Department Stores, Inc.—37
FIELDER, Jerry W.—184
FINCH, Robert H.—43, 46, 184–5
FINLAND—64
FISH—15, 17–8, 184, 188
FLANNERY, Judge Thomas A.—101
FLORIDA—84, 112, 180, 191
FMC Corp. (Charleston, W.Va.)—102
FONDA, Jane—171
FOOD, Diet & Additives—2, 71. Alcoholism—112. Artificial sweeteners—81, 83–91, 125. Court actions—See COURTS. DES—94–6. Dietary studies—195–7. Drinking water—17, 23, 29, 98–103, 113. Federal controls on chemicals in food—112. Fish—15, 17–8, 184, 186, 188. Food coloring—93–4. Meat—94–8, 113. Microwave ovens—181. Nitrites & nitrates—81, 91–3. PBB

contamination—96–8. Pesticides—184, 186, 188. Plastic bottles—112–3. Scientific reports & recommendations—77–81, 92–3, 195–7. TCE ban—112. 'Threshold dose' theory—81–2
FOOD, Drug & Cosmetic Act (1958)—71, 81, 85, 87, 89, 95
FOOD & Drug Administration (FDA)—15, 31. Aerosol ban—75–6. Birth control drugs—134–5; Depo-Provera—134; DES—129, 131, 133. Blood pressure drug—136. Chloroform—112. Dyes—114. Experimental drugs—127–9. Food additives—71, 82; artificial sweeteners—83–91; DES ban—95–6; food coloring—93–4; nitrites—91–3. Laetrile—123–5. Pesticides—184, 186, 188. Plastic bottles—112–3. Sleep aids & nose sprays—136. Radiation hazards—164; microwave ovens—181. TCE—112, 114.
FORD, Betty—122
FORD, Daniel—146–9
FORD, Gerald R.—17, 59–60, 100, 150, 194
FORD Foundation—152–3
FORD Motor Co.—44, 48–9
4-AMINODIPHENYL—34
4 methoxy-m-phenylenediamine (4MMPD)—113–4
FRALEY, Dr. Elwin—137
FRANCE—64, 72–74, 132, 139, 170, 173, 175
FRAUMENI Jr., Joseph F.—4–5
FREDRICKSON, Dr. Donald S.—88, 90
FREEDOM of Choice in Cancer Therapy Inc., Committee for—124–5
FREEDOM of Information Act—149
FREEMAN, Richard—69
FRI, Robert W.—49
FRIENDS of the Earth (environmental group)—143

G

GALVESTON, Tex.—49
GAMBLE, Hayes—180
GARN, Sen. Jake (R, Utah)—65
GARY, Ind.—52
GAS, Natural—175–6, 181–2
GENERAL Accounting Office (GAO)—30, 93–4, 113–4, 127–9
GENERAL Electric Co.—17–8, 150
GENERAL Energy Corp.—66
GENERAL Hospital (Boston)—129
GENERAL Motors Corp. (GM)—44, 48, 59, 71
GENERAL Service Administration (GSA)—44–5
GEOLOGICAL Survey, U.S.—172
GEORGIA—50, 58, 188
GEORGIA Institute of Technology (Atlanta)—135
GERMAN Democratic Republic (East Germany)—64
GERMANY, Federal Republic of (West Germany)—64
GERUSKY, Thomas—162
GILBERT, Ethel—154
GINNA nuclear power plant, R.E. (N.Y.)—180
GIOTTO, Antonio M.—89
GIRAUD, Andre—170
GOFMAN, Dr. John—141, 158
GOLDENBERG, Dr. David—121
GOODMAN, Leo—141
GOODRICH, William W.—83
GORI, Dr. Gio B.—2, 71, 108
GOULD, William R.—58, 143
GRACE, Dr. James T.—185
GRAND Junction, Colo.—172
GRAVEL, Sen. Mike, (D, Alaska)—169–70
GRAVEL Neck nuclear power plant (Va.)—180
GREAT Britain—15, 64, 72, 105–6, 132, 134, 170, 173
GREEN, Mark—31–2
GREEN, Parnell—95
GREENBERG, Daniel S.—7
GREEN Livestock Co. (Layton, Utah)—95
GRIFFIN, Sen. Robert P. (R, Mich.)—46
GROUP Against Smokers' Pollution (GASP)—112
GUAM—50
GUY Jr., Ralph B.—49

H

HADEN 2d, Charles H.—102
HAMMOND, Dr. E. Cuyler—20, 105
HANDLER, Dr. Philip—80–1
HANFORD Atomic Reservation (Wash.)—154, 156–8, 173
HANNAN, Daniel—52
HART, Sen. Gary (D, Colo.)—164
HART Jr., Judge George L.—36, 142
HARVARD University—74–5, 89, 107
HATCH, Sen. Orrin (R, Utah)—65
HAWAII—47, 67–8
HAYDEN, Tom—171
HAYES, Danis—141
HAYS, Harry W.—183
HEALTH, Department of (Colo.)—174
HEALTH, Education & Welfare, Department of (HEW)—111, 131, 178–80, 83. Air pollution—43, 45–6. Alcoholism—112. Anti-cancer drive—117. Cigarette smoking—109, 111. Drinking water—98. Occupational dangers—9, 23–4, 30, 32, 37–41. Pesticides—184–5. Radiation—166, 169; A-tests—117
HEALTH Research Group—109–10, 112, 130
HENDRIE, Joseph M.—161–3, 166, 168–9
HEPTACHLOR—186
HERBST, Dr. Arthur L.—130–1
HERMANSDORFER, Judge H. David—66
HERTZ, Dr. Roy—133
HESS & Clark (N.Y.)—97
HEXAMETHYLPHOSPHORAMIDE (HMPA)—33
HIGGINSON, Dr. John—7, 120
HILBISH, John—164
HIRAYAMA, Dr. Takeski—106
HIROSHIMA (Japan)—144
HODGKINS Disease—119
HOFFMANN-LaRoche, Inc.—125
HOLIFIELD, Rep. Chet (D, Calif.)—139
HOLLINSHEAD, Dr. Ariel C.—137
HONOLULU—67–8
HOOKER Chemicals & Plastics Corp.—26–7
HOOVER, Robert—4

HOUSTON, Tex.—49
HUBBARD, Richard B.—150
HUDSON River (N.Y.)—17–8, 102
HUEPER, Dr. Wilhelm—14
HUMBOLDT Bay atomic power plant (Calif.)—141
HUMPHREY, Sen. Gordon J. (R, N.H.)—157
HUNDTOFTE, Virgil A.—187
HUNGARY—64
HUTCHESON Jr., Dr. Robert—134

I

ILLINOIS—17, 56, 141, 148–9, 171, 191
IMIDAZOLE Carboxamide (DTIC)—125–6
IMPERIAL Chemical Industries Dystuffs Division—14
INDIA—136, 151
INDIANA—17, 52–3, 125
INDIAN Point nuclear power plant (N.Y.)—151–2, 180
INDUSTRIAL Pollution—See 'Industrial wastes, occupational hazards & toxic substances' under ENVIRONMENTAL Pollution
INGRAHAM, Dr. Hollis S.—129
INMAN, William P.—83
INSTITUTE for Medical Research (Camden, N.J.)—136
INTERAGENCY Task Force on Ionizing Radiation—180
INTERNATIONAL Agency for Research on Cancer—3
INTERNATIONAL Association of Machinists & Aerospace Workers—157
IOWA—29
IRELAND—64
ISSELBACHER, Dr. Kurt J.—89
ISSENBERG, Phillip—93
ISSUES & Answers (TV program)—164
ITALY—64, 137, 170

J

JABLON, Seymour—154
JAFFEE, Stanley—177
JAMES River (Va.)—13, 187–8
JAPAN—106, 144, 170, 173
JENNINGS, Dr. John—129
JOHNS, Henry Ward—18–20
JOHNS Hopkins University—88–9, 132
JOHNS-Manville Corp.—13, 18–9
JOHNSON, Dr. Carl—179
JOHNSON Jr., Charles C.—98–9
JORDAN, Dr. Walter H.—153
JOURNAL of the National Cancer Institute—2
JUSTICE, Department of—23, 44, 128
JUVENILE Diabetes Foundation—89

K

KANSAS—98, 172
KAUFMAN, Chief Judge Irving R.—74
KELLEN, Robert M.—84
KENDALL, Dr. Henry—147, 180
KENNEDY, Dr. Donald—85, 87, 123
KENNEDY, Sen. Edward M. (D, Mass.)—88–9, 95, 166, 171
KENNEDY, John F.—123
KENNEDY, Richard T.—168
KENNEDY International Airport (N.Y.)—73–4
KENTUCKY—66, 69
KEPONE—13, 17, 187–8
KERR-McGee Corp. (Crescent, Okla.)—149, 158–9
KESSLER, Dr. Irving—88–9
KHANDEKAR, Dr. Janardan D.—125
KISTNER, Dr. Robert W.—132–3
KLEPPE, Thomas S.—58
KLIGERMAN, Dr. Morton—126
K-MART Apparel Corp.—37
KNAPP, Judge Dennis R.—30
KNEALE, George—154
KNOXVILLE, Tenn.—69
KOCH, Rep. Edward I. (D, N.Y.)—183
KOHNSTAMM & Co., H.—94
KOTIN, Paul—80
KREBS Jr., Ernst T.—123–4
KREBS Sr., Ernst—123–4
KRESGE Co., S.S.—37
KUCHERA, Dr. Lucile K.—133
KUNZIG, Robert L.—44

L

LABOR, Department of—10, 19, 23–4, 30–1, 33–5
LAETRILE—123–5
LALONDE, Marc—96
LANCET, The (British medical journal)—89, 97, 138
LECHOWICH, Richard V.—93
LEDERLE Laboratories—128
LEE, Dr. Philip R.—117
LEESE, Paul—163
LEMEN, Richard A.—10
LEVINE, Saul—147
LIFE Science Products Co.— 87
LIGGETT & Myers, Inc.—105
LIJINSKY, William—80
LILIENTHAL, David—177
LITTLE, Dr. John B.—107
LITTLE Rock, Ark.—67
LIVESTOCK—94–8
LOEWS Corp.—105
LONG Beach, Calif.—67
LORD, Judge Miles W.—21
Los ANGELES—44, 47, 49, 56, 60–1, 67, 70, 84, 131
LOUISIANA—50, 100
LOVE, Gov. John A. (Colo.)—55, 172
L-PHENYLALANINE mustard (L-PAM)—122
LYING-In Hospital (Chicago)—130
LYON, Dr. Joseph—179
LYONS, Kansas—172

M

MacDONALD, Gordon J. F.—189
MACK, Dr. Thomas M.—131

MACY & Co., R. H.—37
MAGNUSON, Sen. Warren G. (D, Wash.)—118
MAGRUDER, William M.—72
MAHONEY, Richard J.—6-7
MAINE—112, 154-7, 180
MAINE Yankee nuclear power plant—180
MALLIK, Harold—52
MANCUSO, Dr. Thomas—154, 157-8
MANSFIELD, Sen. Mike (D, Mont.)—118
MANSFIELD, Judge Walter R.—62
MARKS, Dr. Lawrence—128-9
MARSHALL, Ray—34
MARTELL, Dr. E. A.—140
MARYLAND—11, 43, 49-50, 148
MASON, Thomas J.—4
MASSACHUSETTS—17, 50, 55, 92, 129, 131, 133, 154-5
MASSACHUSETTS Institute of Technology (MIT)—92, 180
MATHESON, Gov. Scott M. (Utah)—179
MATTSON, Roger J.—168
MAYO Clinic Medical School—90
MAZZOCCHI, Anthony—141
McCOY Elkhorn Coal Corp. (Ky.)—66
McDERMOTT, James H.—98
McDONALD, Dr. James E.—71-2
McDONNELL Douglas Corp.—46
McGAHN, Joseph L.—125
McGILL, William J.—171
McINTYRE, Sen. Thomas (D, N.J.)—155
McKAY, Frank—4
McNAUGHTON, Andrew R. L.—125
McNAUGHTON Foundation—124-5
MEAD Corp.—27
MEAD Johnson Co.—134
MEAT & Meat Products—91-3. Canadian import curb—96. DES in livestock—94-7. Hamburgers—113. Nitrites—91-3. PBB contamination—97-8
MEDICAL Treatment & Cancer Research: Anesthetic gases—30-1. Birth control pills—132-5. Blood pressure drugs—136. Bone cancer drug—126. Breast surgery controversy—122-3. Cancer death & survival rate—119-20; detection developments—122-3, 125-6, 135; DES—129-31, 133-4. Estrogens—131-2. FDA & experimental drugs—127-9. Krebiozen ban—123. Laetrile—123-5. Melanoma drug—125-6. Neutron beam—126. "Pion" therapy—126. Psoriasis therapy—136. Radiation hazards—153-7; A-bomb tests—140, 153, 174-9; X-rays—2, 6, 135-6, 139, 144, 180-2. Sleep aids & nose sprays—136. U.S.-Soviet exchange—138. Virus link—136-8
MELANOMA—11, 125-6
MEMPHIS, Tenn.—69
MERCK, Sharp & Dome Research—128-9
MERHIGE Jr., Judge Robert R.—187
MERRELL-National Laboratories—128
METALS & Mining—10, 12, 21-2, 52-4, 60, 64, 66, 140-1
METHAPYRILENE—136
METHOXYPSORALEN—136
METROPOLITAN Edison Co. (Pa.)—159-66
METZENBAUM, Sen. Howard (D, Ohio)—66
MEXICO—124-5
MIAMI—84
MICHIGAN—11, 18, 21, 29, 50, 97-8, 130, 133, 152, 180, 184, 191
MICHIGAN, Lake—18, 53, 149
MICHIGAN Chemical Co.—97-8
MICHIGAN University—75, 133
MIDLAND, Mich.—152
MILLER, Rep. George (D, Calif.)—11-2
MILLER, Robert B.—139
MILLIKEN, William G.—191
MILLSTONE nuclear power plant (Conn.)—180
MINK, Patsy—130
MINNEAPOLIS—21-2, 140
MINNESOTA—15, 21-2, 140
MINOR, Gregory C.—150
MISSISSIPPI—50, 186
MISSISSIPPI River—100
MITRE Corp.—152
MOLONEY, Dr. John B.—138
MONARCH Nugrape (Doraville, Ga.)—94
MONDALE, Sen. Walter F. (D, Minn.)—19-20
MONTANA—54
MOORE Jr., Gov. Arch A. (W.Va.)—55
MOORE, Dr. Condict—106
MOORE, Dr. Dan H.—136
MOORE, William P.—187
MOORMAN, James W.—27
MORGAN, Dr. Karl Z.—135, 167
MORRIS, Robert M.—187
MORRIS, Inc., Philip—105
MOSS, Sen. Frank (D, Utah)—107
MOSS, Laurence I.—52
MRAK, Dr. Emil M.—184
MUIR, Dr. Calum S.—120
MUSKIE, Sen. Edmund S. (D, Me.)—45, 189
MYERS, Dr. Brooks—137

N

NADER, Ralph—45, 91, 112, 143, 147, 171, 173
NAGASAKI, Japan—144
NAJARIAN, Thomas—154-5, 157
NAPLES, University of (Italy)—137
NASHVILLE, Tenn.—69
NATIONAL Academy of Engineering—54
NATIONAL Academy of Sciences (NAS)—6, 54, 72-3, 75, 79-81, 83-4, 86, 93, 129, 171-2, 190, 195
NATIONAL Air Pollution Control Administration—46
NATIONAL Cancer Institute (Canada)—86-7
NATIONAL Cancer Institute (U.S.)—3-4, 9, 71, 89, 95-6, 113-5, 119, 123, 135-8, 144, 183
NATIONAL Center for Disease Control—176
NATIONAL Center for Toxicological Research—82
NATIONAL Council on Radiation Protection (NCRP)—141
NATIONAL Environmental Policy Act—188
NATIONAL Heart, Lung & Blood Institute—108
NATIONAL Indian Brotherhood—33
NATIONAL Institute of Environmental Health Sciences—9

NATIONAL Institute of Occupational Safety & Health (NIOSH)—3, 9–10, 30–1, 33, 114
NATIONAL Institute on Alcohol Abuse—112
NATIONAL Institutes of Health—88, 90, 100, 115, 117–8, 125–6, 130, 137
NATIONAL Intervenors (environmental group)—142–3
NATIONAL Oceanic & Atmospheric Administration (NOAA)—193
NATURAL Resources Defense Council—48, 69, 75, 112–3
NAUTILUS (nuclear submarine)—5–6
NAVAL Research Laboratory (Wash.)—126
NAVY, Department of—154–8
NELSON, Sen. Gaylord (D, Wis.)—80–1, 87, 89–90, 93–4, 132–3, 184
NETHERLANDS—64, 86
NEVADA—125, 174, 178–9
NEWARK, N.J.—56
NEWBERNE, Dr. Paul M.—92–3
'NEWBERNE Report on the Effect of Dietary Nitrite in the Rat'—92–3
NEW England Journal of Medicine—89, 109, 113, 131–2, 136
NEW Hampshire—50
NEW JERSEY—35, 43, 47, 50, 55–6, 60, 125, 152, 174
NEW Mexico—172
NEW Orleans—67, 98, 100
NEWSWEEK (magazine)—64
NEW York—11, 17–8, 26–7, 55–6, 60, 62, 73–4, 84, 98, 102, 124, 129, 146, 151–2, 171, 174, 180, 191
NEW York Academy of Sciences—71, 80–1
NEW York Coffee & Sugar Exchange—85
NEW York Public Interest Research Group—102
NEW York Stock Exchange—85
NEW York Times (newspaper)—74
NIAGARA Falls, N.Y.—21, 26–7
NICKEL—10
NIXON, Richard M.—44–5, 55–7, 72, 99, 104, 115–7, 184, 188–93
NORTH Carolina—15, 50, 112, 188
NORTH Dakota—50
NORTHERN Indiana Public Service Co.—149
NORTHERN States Power Co.—140
NORWAY—64
NUCLEAR Regulatory Commission (NRC): A-plants—148, 161, 164–9. Communities study—180. Offshore A-plant—152. Plutonium air transport curbed—150. Three Mile Island—161–9

O

OBEY, Rep. David R. (D, Wis.)—81–2
OCCIDENTAL Petroleum Corp.—26–7
OCCUPATIONAL Health & Safety Administration (OHSA)—19, 23–4, 30, 35
OFFICE of Technology Assessment—86
OGILVIE, Gov. Richard B. (Ill.)—191
OHIO—11, 60, 65–7, 100, 102
OHIO Edison Co.—66
OIL, Chemical & Atomic Workers International Union (AFL-CIO)—141, 149, 158
OKLAHOMA—125, 149, 158–9
OREGON—50, 75, 172, 184
ORTHO Pharmaceuticals—134
OWEN, Judge Richard—37
OZONE Threat—71–6

P

PADUCAH, Ky.—69
PALISADES nuclear power plant (Mich.)—180
PALUMBO, Dr. P. J.—90
PAPER mills—67–8
PAVLOV, Dr. Alexander S.—120
PBB (polybrominated biphenyls)—97–8
PCBs (polychlorinated biphenyls)—15–8
PENNEY Co., Inc., J. C.—37
PENNSYLVANIA—11, 54–5, 159–69, 174
PENNSYLVANIA State Institute for Research on Land & Water Resources—180
PENNSYLVANIA State University—180
PENTAGON, The—176
PEPSICo, Inc.—84–5
PERKINS, Bill—159
PESTICIDES & Herbicides—13, 99–100, 183–8, 195. DDT & other cholorinated hydrocarbons—183–8. Kepone—187–8
PETERS, James A.—80
PETERSBURG, W. Va.—102
PETERSON, Esther—141
PETERSON, Russell W.—194
PETERSON, Judge William—97
PETROLEUM & Petroleum Industry—10, 12, 50, 55, 99
PHARMACEUTICAL Industry—130, 132–3
PHILADELPHIA—11, 23, 54, 58, 60
PHILADELPHIA Electric Co.—58
PICLORAM—186
PINES, Wayne—136
PITTSBURGH, University of—157
PLUTONIUM—146, 149–50, 152, 158–9, 179
POINT Beach nuclear power plant (Wis.)—180
POLAND—64
POLLACK, Judge Milton—74
POLLARD, Robert D.—151–2
POLYCHLORINATED Biphenyls (PCBs)—15–8
PORTAGE, Ind.—149
PORT Authority of New York & New Jersey—74
PORTSMOUTH Herald (Maine newspaper)—157
PORTSMOUTH Naval Shipyard (Maine)—154–7
PORTUGAL—64
POTT, Percivall—4
POULTRY—15, 18, 186
POWELL, Jody—74
PRATT, Judge John H.—143
PRATT & Whitney—46
PRICE, Rep. Melvin (D, Ill.)—155
PRIORI, Dr. Elizabeth S.—137
PROXMIRE, Sen. William E. (D, Wis.)—9–10, 71–2, 94
PUBLIC Citizen, Inc.—130
PUBLIC Health Service, U.S.—3, 178
PUBLIC Service Electric & Gas Co. (N.J.)—152

PUEBLO, Colo.—98
PUERTO Rico—18, 50

Q

QUARLES, Jr., John R.—52-3, 62-3
QUINN, Thomas—61

R

RADIATION Council, Federal—172, 174
RADIATION Hazards—107. A-reactors & safety—139-50, 152-7, 180; A-engineers resign re safety—150-2; A-submarine—6; licensing—149, 152; offshore plant—152; plants near populated areas—149; plutonium air transport curb—150; safety report—146-7; Three Mile Island plant—159, 170-1, 181-2; waste disposal—142, 149, 152, 171-4; worker exposure & low-level dangers—151, 153-7. A-weapons & tests—140, 153, 174-9. Other radioactive dangers—2, 5-6, 139, 144
RADIOLOGICAL Health, Bureau of—172
RADIO & TV—104
RALSTON Purina Co.—18
RAMEY, James T.—140
RANDOLPH, Sen. Jennings (D, W.Va.)—45
RASMUSSEN, Dr. Norman C.—147
RAUSCHER Jr., Dr. Frank J.—95-6, 118, 120, 122, 135
RAY, Dixy Lee—145-6, 148-9, 173
REAGAN, Gov. Ronald (R, Calif.)—191
REAL, Judge Manuel L.—44
REED, Nathaniel P.—16-7
REHNQUIST, Justice William H.—24
REID, Rep. Ogden R. (R, N.Y.)—17, 94
REPUBLIC Steel Corp.—21
RESEARCH Triangle Institute—10-1
RESERPINE—136
RESERVE Mining Co. (Silver Bay, Minn.)—10, 21-2
REVLON, Inc.—113
REYNOLDS Tobacco Co., R.J.—105
RHODE Island—43, 55, 191
RHODES, Gov. James (Ohio)—66
RHODIA, Inc. (N.Y.)—97
RIBICOFF, Sen. Abraham A. (D, Conn.)—127-9
RICHARDSON, Elliot L.—141
RICHARDSON, Dr. John A.—124-5
RICHMOND, Dr. Julius—108, 111
RICKOVER, Adm. Hyman G.—5, 155
RIMER, Irving—121-2
RITTENHOUSE, Philip L.—142
ROBBOY, Dr. Stanley J.—131
ROBINSON, James—71
ROBINSON Jr., Judge Aubrey—94
ROBINSON nuclear power plant, H.B. (S.C.)—180
ROCHESTER Medical Center, University of—126-7
ROCKEFELLER, Gov. Nelson A. (R, N.Y.)—191
ROCKY Flats atomic bomb plant (Colo.)—140
ROGERS, William P.—190
ROSENBAUM, Ruth—121-2
ROSENBERG, Howard R.—80
ROSENHEIM, Lord—106
ROUMELL, Judge Thomas—130
ROYAL College of General Practitioners (Great Britain)—134
ROYAL College of Physicians—105-6
RUCKELSHAUS, William D.—46-8, 50, 72, 99-100, 193

S

SABIN, Dr. Albert B.—138
SACCAHARIN—81, 83-90
SACRAMENTO—56
SAFFIOTTI, Umberto—80
ST. LOUIS—70
ST. LUCIE nuclear power plant (Fla.)—180
SALAMAN, Frank—124-5
San BERNARDINO, Calif.—98
SanDIEGO—56, 58, 106
San DIEGO Gas & Electric Co.—58
San FRANCISCO—23, 49, 56, 100
San JOAQUIN Valley, Calif.—56
SANSOM, Robert L.—56
SANTO, Judge Henry E.—176
San ONOFRE nuclear power plant (Calif.)—180
SCHLESINGER, James R.—141-3, 175
SCHMIDT, Alexander M.—81, 94
SCHNEIDER, Dr. Howard A.—117
SCHNEIDERMAN, Marvin—80
SCIENCE (scientific journal)—4-5, 75, 107, 137
SCIENCE News (magazine)—154
SEARLE & Co., G. D.—134
SEATTLE—23
SEIDERS, Glenn A.—165
SELIKOFF, Dr. Irving J.—13, 20, 97, 141
SELLERSBURG, Ind.—17
SHERWIN-Williams Co. (Cleveland)—84
SHULMAN, Dr. Morton—21-2
SIERRA Club (conservationist group)—57, 69, 147
SILKWOOD, Karen—158-9
SLOAN-Kettering Cancer Center (N.Y.)—124, 137
SMELTERS—52, 54, 65
SMITH, Don S.—191
SMITH, Dr. Kenneth—13
SOFT-Drinks—112-3
SOUTH Africa—170
SOUTH Carolina—37
SOUTH Dakota—50, 172
SOUTHERN California, University of—131
SOUTHERN California Edison Co.—58
SOUTH Texas Nuclear Project—171
SOVIET Academy of Medical Science—138
SPAIN—64
SPEICE, Neal—171
SPOKANE, Wash.—67-8
SPORT Fisheries & Wildlife, Bureau of—172
SPRING Mills, Inc. (S.C.)—37
SQUIBB & Sons, E.R.—128-9
STATES & State Actions: Aerosal ban—75. Air pollution—43-55, 57-8, 60-2, 65-7; auto emissions—43, 47-50, 54, 60-2; SST-73-4; transportation-controls—56. Anti-smoking

laws—112. Artificial sweeteners—125. Cancer death rate—35, 43, 100. Drinking water & chemical contaminants—23, 98, 100. Environmental quality laws—191. Industrial waste—21-3, 26-7, 29, 172-4. Laetrile controversy—123-4. PBB contamination—97-8. Pesticides & herbicides—183, 187-8. Radiation hazards & A-plants—150, 146, 149-50, 152, 171; offshore A-plant—152; A-wastes disposal—172-4
STEEL—21, 52-3, 60
STEGER, Judge William—23
STEINFELD, Jesse L.—107
STENNIS, John C.—186
STERNGLASS, Dr. Ernest J.—161-2, 167
STEVENS, Justice John Paul—24-5, 101-2
STEWART, Alice—154
STEWART, Justice Potter—24
STUNKARD, Dr. Albert J.—89
SUGIURA, Dr. Kanematsu—124
SULVER Bay iron ore processing plant (Minn.)—21-2
SUPERIOR, Lake—21-2
SUPERSONIC Transport (SST)—71-4
SUPREME Court, U.S.—22, 24-5, 31, 58, 101-2, 123, 146, 175, 177
SURGEON General, U.S.—71
SUSQUEHANNA River—162, 166
SWEDEN—64, 170, 173, 175, 184
SWIFT & Co. (Minn.)—1, 15
SWITZERLAND—64
SYNTEX Laboratories—132, 134
SYRACUSE, N.Y.—106

T

TACOMA, Marilyn—97-8
TACOMA, Roy M.—97-8
TALBOTT, Dr. John H.—103
TAMPLIN, Arthur R.—141
TARAPUR atomic power plant (India)—151
TARRO, Giulio—137
TCE (trichloroethylene)—32, 112, 114
TECHNOLOGY Review (journal)—4
TELLER, Dr. Edward L.—140
TENNESSEE—50, 69, 134, 141-2, 157
TENNESSEE Valley Authority (TVA)—69, 141
TERRY, Luther L.—103-4
TETRA-chloro-dibenzo-dioxin—185-6
TEXACO, Inc.—55
TEXAS—23, 49-50, 125, 136-7, 171-2
THEIS, Judge Frank—158-9
THOMPSON Jr., Judge Gordon—124
THOMPSON, Gov. James R. (Ill.)—171
THOMPSON, Dr. Theos J.—140
THORNBURGH, Gov. Richard (Pa.)—159, 161-6
THREE Mile Island nuclear power plant (Pa.)—6, 159-69, 170-1, 181-2
TOBACCO Industry Research Committee—103
TOBACCO Institute, Inc.—103-4, 107
TORONTO, Canada—21
TORONTO Globe & Mail (newspaper)—96
TOXIC Substances Control Act—3, 18
TRAIN, Russell E.—17, 31, 44, 55-7, 59-61, 99-100, 145-6, 186-9, 193
TRANSPORTATION, Department of—43-4, 72-3
TRICHLOROETHYLENE (TCE)—32, 112, 114
TRINER, Edwin G.—148
TRIS (flame retardant)—35-6
TRUMAN, Harry S.—177
TURKEY Point nuclear power plant (Fla.)—180
2,4,5-T ("agent orange")—185-6

U

UDALL, Rep. Morris K. (D, Ariz.)—164
UDALL, Stewart L.—139-40, 179
UNION of Concerned Scientists—143, 145, 147-50
UNION of Soviet Socialist Republics—10, 120, 138, 170-1, 184-5
UNITED Aircraft Corp.—46
UNITED Automobile Workers—141
UNITED Nations—6, 120-1, 184
U.S. STEEL Corp.—52-3
UNITED Steelworkers of America—33-4, 52, 158
UPJOHN Co.—133-4
UPTON, Dr. Arthur—195-7
URANIUM—140-1, 172-4, 181
UTAH—43, 58, 95, 172, 178
UTILITIES—56-8, 60, 140-2, 147-9, 159-66, 171

V

VAN DUSEN, Judge Francis L.—54
VELSICOL Chemical Co.—36
VERMONT—98, 152, 191
VERNON, Vt.—152
VETERANS Administration—105, 154, 176
VIETNAM—185-6
VINELAND Laboratories, Inc. (Needham, Mass.)—97
VINYL Chloride—31-2
VIRGINIA—30, 37, 49-50, 55, 112, 180, 187-8, 191
VIRGIN Islands—50
VOLPE, John A.—46, 72

W

WALKER, Charles R.—17
WALL Street Journal (newspaper)—97, 118
WALTON League, Izaak (business and civic group)—149
WAMPLER, Rep. William C. (R, Va.)—2-4, 93
WARNER-Jenkinson (St. Louis)—94
WASHINGTON (state)—49, 56, 68, 125, 131, 154, 172, 191
WASHINGTON, D.C.—43, 48, 50-1, 57, 112-3, 152
WASHINGTON, University of (Seattle)—131
WASHINGTON Post (newspaper)—7, 95-6, 107, 129, 131-2, 178
WASHINGTON University Medical Center (George)—137
WATER Hygiene Bureau—98
WATER Pollution—13, 15-8, 26-9, 101-3, 162, 166, 172, 183, 187-8, 191, 195-6. Drinking water quality—98-9. Industrial dumping curbs—99-100. Oil spill cleanup legislation—99
WATER Quality Improvement Act (1979)—99
WAYNE County (Mich.)—130

WEINHOUSE, Sidney—80
WEISBURGER, Elizabeth K.—80
WEISBURGER, John H.—80
WEISS, Dr. Noel S.—131
WEST Germany (Federal Republic of Germany)—64, 170, 173
WHALEN, Robert P.—26
WHELAN, Eugene—96
WILBUR, Dr. J. R.—137
WILDLIFE—17
WILLIAMS, Dr. Michael—14
WILLRICH, Mason—173
WILMINGTON, N.C.—15
WINNEBAGO, Ill.—17
WINNER, Judge Fred M.—54
WISCONSIN—21-2, 83, 180, 184
WISCONSIN, University of—83
WOGAN, Gerald—80
WOLFE, Dr. Sidney M.—109-10
WOMEN—96-7, 106, 122-3, 128-36
WOOLWORTH Co., F. W.—36
WORLD Conference on the Human Environment—175
WORLD Health Organization (WHO)—33, 85, 119-20, 184
WRIGHT, Judge J. Skelly—142
WYDLER, Rep. John W.—181-2
WYNDER, Ernest L.—2
WYOMING—172

X

X-Rays—2, 6, 135-6, 139, 144, 180-2

Y

YALWO, Dr. Rosalyn—126
YELLOWKNIFE, Canada—33

Z

ZAYRE Corp. (Boston)—37
ZICARELLI, Joseph—125
ZIEGLER, Ronald L.—71